ELEMENTS

OF

DENTAL MATERIALS

FOR DENTAL HYGIENISTS AND DENTAL ASSISTANTS

FIFTH EDITION

ELEMENTS

OF

DENTAL MATERIALS

FOR DENTAL HYGIENISTS AND DENTAL ASSISTANTS

RALPH W. PHILLIPS, MS, DSc (deceased)

Emeritus Professor of Dental Materials
Indiana University School of Dentistry
Indianapolis, Indiana

B. KEITH MOORE, PhD

Professor of Dental Materials
Indiana University School of Dentistry
Indianapolis, Indiana

with contributions by
MARJORIE SWARTZ

Emeritus Professor of Dental Materials
Indiana University School of Dentistry
Indianapolis, Indiana

W.B. SAUNDERS COMPANY
A Division of Harcourt Brace & Company
PHILADELPHIA, LONDON, TORONTO, MONTREAL, SYDNEY, TOKYO

W.B. SAUNDERS COMPANY
A Division of
Harcourt Brace & Company

The Curtis Center
Independence Square West
Philadelphia, Pennsylvania 19106

Library of Congress Cataloging-in-Publication Data

Phillips, Ralph W.
Elements of dental materials : for dental hygienists and dental assistants / Ralph W. Phillips, B. Keith Moore;
with contribution by Marjorie L. Swartz. — 5th ed.

   p.   cm.

Rev. ed. of: Elements of dental materials for dental hygienists and assistants. 4th ed., 1984.

Includes bibliographical references and index.

ISBN 0–7216–4298–5

1. Dental materials.   2. Dental hygienists.   3. Dental assistants.   I. Moore, B. Keith.
   II. Swartz, Marjorie L.   III. Phillips, Ralph W. Elements of dental materials for dental hygienists and
   assistants.   IV. Title.

[DNLM: 1. Dental Materials. WU 190 P562e 1994]

RK652.5.P48 1994

617.6'0028—dc20

DNLM/DLC   93-12562

ELEMENTS OF DENTAL MATERIALS:
For Dental Hygienists and Dental Assistants   ISBN 0-7216-4298-5

Printed in the United States of America.

Last digit is the print number: 9   8   7   6   5   4   3

ACKNOWLEDGMENTS

This revision would not have been possible without the assistance of many people. In attempting to give specific acknowledgment, the risk of omission always exists. If I have omitted anyone, I apologize and want to make it very clear that the omission was not intentional. The assistance of all who have helped at every level of this revision has been invaluable and very much appreciated.

I would not have attempted this revision without assurance from Emeritus Professor Marjorie Swartz that she would assist me in any way that she could. Marjorie participated in teaching the dental materials courses for the dental auxiliaries at Indiana University School of Dentistry until her recent retirement. There is no individual in the field who is better qualified to look over my shoulder and ensure that the revision is in keeping with the philosophy and standards established for this text by the late Dr. Ralph Phillips. At the same time, her experience in teaching auxiliaries has helped immensely in efforts to improve the readability and conceptual clarity of the text. I would like to credit her work particularly in the major revision and reorganization of the chapters on dental polymers and dental cements.

The other faculty in the Dental Materials Department, Dr. Yoshiki Oshida and Dr. Mark Winkler, have given generously of their time in reviewing chapters in their areas of expertise and in helping me when I needed ideas about a better way to say something.

I also would like to mention Dr. Nels Ewoldsen, a practicing dentist and a graduate student in the Dental Materials Department. Direct input from a front-line practitioner who is experienced in working with dental auxiliaries and well informed about current dental materials was very important in making decisions about what should be retained, modified, and added in this revision. In particular, Dr. Ewoldsen assisted with the condensation of the chapters related to casting technique and in updating the chapter on dental abrasion and polishing.

Dr. Mark Mallat with the Dental Division of the Indiana State Board of Health graciously took time out of his busy schedule to review the material on dentifrices.

Special thanks are due to Sherry Phillips, our department secretary. This revision was done largely on electronic media, working from computer disc files of the chapters of the Fourth Edition. In theory this was supposed to save labor and reduce the errors that can occur when text is retyped numerous times. However, as with any new technology, there is a learning curve. Sherry was both patient and long suffering through this process. She helped immensely with many of the details, such as keeping track of authorizations to reprint illustrations. Without her efforts, the revision would have taken much longer.

Alana Barra, Mike Holloran, and Mark Dirlam in the Illustrations Department at Indiana University School of Dentistry assisted with new illustrations, made black and white prints from an assortment of unconventional original copy, and helped resurrect usable originals for a number of illustrations that were reprinted from previous editions and other texts.

Selma Ozmat, Editor of Health-Related Professions at W.B. Saunders Company, and her staff have been both helpful and very patient with me. Her expertise helped to make up for my inexperience with the revision of a complete textbook. She has been supportive and very cooperative even when it meant additional work for her group.

My final acknowledgment is to my wife, Diana Moore. A major goal I set when I agreed to be responsible for this revision was to do everything possible to improve the readability of the text without sacrificing the integrity of the information presented. My experience in technical writing for audiences other than materials science professionals is limited. I am very fortunate that my wife, a professional journalist, has had considerable experience editing technical books. After each chapter had been updated and all technical revisions made, it was given to Diana for editing for format, style, and readability. In every case, when I compared my original copy with her suggested changes, the improvement was remarkable. Shortening of complex sentences and paragraphs, making lists of related ideas, setting off important points, and including an outline of each chapter are only a few of the changes that, I think, significantly improve the readability of this text. I hope that both the instructors and students who use this revision will agree. If so, the credit belongs to Diana Moore.

B. KEITH MOORE, PhD

PREFACE

Dr. Ralph Phillips died in May 1991, shortly after beginning the revision for the fifth edition of this textbook. As a consequence, publication of the revision was delayed far beyond the time originally planned.

Although I had helped Dr. Phillips revise specific chapters for previous editions, it was with some reluctance I agreed to be responsible for the completion of the 5th edition of the Elements. My most serious reservation was about my ability to complete the revision in a manner of which Dr. Phillips would have approved. Dr. Phillips had sent the editors at W.B. Saunders an outline of the major changes he planned for this edition. I have tried to follow that outline.

The practice of dentistry has seen some remarkable changes since the publication of the 4th edition in 1984. Major goals of this edition are to include new materials and delivery systems and to show how the changes in dental practice have influenced materials choices and handling.

Before reviewing the changes, I would like to state that the philosophy and objectives as outlined by Dr. Phillips in previous editions have not been changed. The objectives of this text are:

1. To provide the dental auxiliary with a basic understanding of the principles of materials science.

2. To apply those principles to the selection, handling, and better understanding of the various materials currently used in dentistry.

3. To emphasize why materials behave as they do rather than stress specific handling techniques for specific materials.

4. To enable the auxiliary to adapt the knowledge of the basic science and the behavior of existing materials to the new materials and techniques that are rapidly evolving.

5. To create a reference book for the auxiliary to use as needed.

This revision has attempted to bring each chapter up to the current state of accepted dental materials practice. In any rapidly changing field, such an effort requires decisions about the future of new developments. Based on my own opinions about the future of some of the newer materials and techniques, I have made arbitrary decisions about which items are included and excluded. In some cases I have included information about techniques and materials that are not yet in the mainstream of dental practice. The reader is welcome to second-guess my judgment and see how dentistry does evolve over the next four to five years.

Concerns about occupational safety, protection of the environment, disposal of hazardous wastes, and transmission of infectious diseases are vastly changing the practice of dentistry. The impact of these changes on materials selection and handling is specifically addressed in the first four chapters and is followed in discussions of specific materials throughout this textbook.

The safety of dental materials to the patient continues to be a major concern. Dental consumers are becoming increasingly informed about potential health hazards of materials. Dental auxiliary personnel must be knowledgeable about such materials and must play an important role in helping educate patients on making informed decisions about their dental health care.

The demand for esthetic dentistry, which was noted in the 4th edition, has continued to develop. The public is increasingly aware that choices are available for restoration of tooth structure in a "cosmetic" manner. Again, the auxiliary is an important part of the process of dental consumer education.

A quick overview of each chapter in this new edition is probably the best way to illustrate how it differs from the 4th edition. The basic materials science in Chapters 1 through 4 remains unchanged. Specific attention, however, is given to the issues of safety of materials to the patient, dental staff, and the environment.

Chapter 5 has been retitled *Dental Gypsum Products: Dental Plaster and Stone* in keeping with modern dental terminology. This chapter now includes the new ADA classification system for gypsum materials and a discussion of the newer products.

Chapter 6 introduces the concept and requirements of dental impression materials. The inelastic impression materials have been grouped together in the balance of this chapter, and the discussion of these materials has been considerably reduced.

The elastomeric impression materials have been divided into two groups. The water-based materials (hydrocolloids) are discussed in Chapter 7 and the non-aqueous materials (rubber impression materials) in Chapter 8. In both chapters, concerns about safety and infection control are emphasized. Chapter 8 also includes the new automixing cartridge systems, which have become very popular, and visible light-cured impression materials.

Chapter 9, which presents the basic concepts of polymer chemistry and polymeric materials science, has been rewritten in an attempt to make it easier to understand. This chapter also discusses the use of dental polymers in prosthodontic applications, such as complete and removable partial dentures. Other applications discussed include reline materials, tissue conditioners, custom impression trays, and trays for other intraoral applications such as vital bleaching, mouth guards, and extraoral maxillofacial prostheses. The specific discussion of denture fabrication has been reduced.

Chapter 10 is devoted primarily to the direct filling restorative resins. This chapter has been reorganized and extensively revised due to the rapid changes in this area. A classification system is given for the different types of restorative resins currently in use, describing each type in terms of composition and properties in both tables and the text. Clinical applications, including the use of composite resin in posterior occlusal restorations, are discussed. Major attention is given to the visible light–activated composite resins because they have rapidly replaced the older materials. Adhesive resin dentistry, including bonding to both enamel and dentin, is mentioned. The current status of dentin bonding agents, along with the role of the dentinal smear layer, is discussed. The use of composite resins as prosthetic veneering materials and as inlays is described.

Chapters 11 through 13, which cover principles of the science of metals and corrosion, have been edited for improved readability. Chapters 14 and 15, which cover dental amalgam, have been shortened with attention devoted to the high copper content alloys. Chapter 15 relates manipulation of dental amalgam to properties and focuses on current handling practices, which have been considerably changed by the concerns for safety and infection control. The issues of the safety of dental amalgam and the hazards of mercury exposure for both dental staff and the patient are discussed at length.

Chapters 16 through 19 cover the metal alloys and other materials used in dental castings and the casting process. All information related to dental castings has been combined in these chapters. A classification system by clinical application and composition has been provided to help in the understanding of the different alloys. The discussion of the actual casting process and the difficulties encountered has been significantly reduced.

Chapter 20, *Dental Ceramics,* is a new chapter including both new developments and materials previously scattered throughout the text. Recognition of ceramic materials as a distinct group is appropriate in view of their growing applications in esthetic dentistry. New materials and systems include the castable ceramics and computer-aided design and manufacturing (CAD-CAM) of dental restorations.

The two chapters relating to dental cements have been reorganized and extensively edited. Chapter 21 introduces dental cements and discusses their use as restorative materials, liners, and bases. Chapter 22 covers the cements in use as luting agents. The discussion of glass ionomer materials has been expanded to include the latest developments in visible light-cured glass ionomer-resin hybrids. Resin cements also receive greater attention.

Chapter 23, another new chapter, is a general discussion of dental implants, a rapidly growing field of dentistry. It is becoming increasingly likely that the dental auxiliary will assist in implant procedures or help treat patients who have dental implants.

The last two chapters, Chapter 24, *Miscellaneous Materials,* and Chapter 25, *Abrasion, Cutting, and Polishing Materials,* have been updated and edited but cover primarily the same subjects included in the 4th edition.

Many new figures are included in this edition. Color figures have been used for the first time in the discussion of the appearance of dental materials in Chapter 4. Many older figures have been redone; for example, the use of gloves is shown when it is appropriate. Tables also have been revised and new ones added.

Listing objectives at the end of each chapter has been continued and given a new title: *Reviewing the Chapter.* . . . Students have indicated that they find these particularly helpful in reviewing and organizing the material. The objectives have been revised and edited to correspond to the changes in the chapters. The selected reading references at the end of each chapter also have been revised and updated.

As I stated at the beginning of this preface, the philosophy, objectives, and general organization of this textbook have not been changed except as Dr. Phillips indicated the intent to change them for this revision. The text, however, has been extensively edited with the specific goal of improving readability and promoting understanding without sacrificing content. Sentence and paragraph structures have been shortened. Extensive use has been made of lists to clarify and emphasize related ideas or step-by-step procedures. Important points have been set out to draw attention to them. An outline has been provided for each chapter. I assume the responsibility for these changes and hope that Dr. Phillips would have approved.

B. KEITH MOORE, PhD

CONTENTS

CHAPTER 1

INTRODUCTION

HISTORICAL DEVELOPMENTS **AMERICAN DENTAL ASSOCIATION** **SPECIFICATIONS** **FOOD AND DRUG ADMINISTRATION** **REGULATION OF DENTAL MATERIALS**	**OCCUPATIONAL SAFETY IN THE** **DENTAL OFFICE** **THE COURSE IN DENTAL MATERIALS** **Aim of the Course**

The science of dental materials studies the materials used in dentistry to construct dental appliances and tooth restorations. The biological aspects of dentistry are included, but only as they apply to the proper use of materials and their interactions with the oral environment.

HISTORICAL DEVELOPMENTS

The use of dental materials dates before the Christian era. The Phoenicians and Etruscans used gold bands and wires to construct dental appliances. The practice of welding pieces of pure gold foil together in a prepared cavity in a tooth is so old that its origin is not known. Even the use of as complex a material as dental silver amalgam was recorded in an early Chinese dynasty.

In 1728, a dentist named Fauchard de-scribed many types of dental restorations and appliances as well as dental materials. He described a method for the construction of artificial dentures by carving them from ivory. Records document a dentist's obtaining wax impressions of the mouth and constructing a cast with plaster of Paris as early as 1756. Porcelain teeth were introduced late in the 18th century, and other important dental materials were used early in the 19th century. Some materials are used today in essentially the same form.

These early attempts to use dental materials were trial and error—a slow and wasteful method of acquiring knowledge. The patient undoubtedly suffered considerable pain and discomfort as well as poor health while the dentist was learning the best way to practice the craft.

Near the end of the 19th century, the scientific method was used in the study of dental materials. The principles of manipulation finally could be systematically developed. Dr. G. V. Black, the most famous of these early scientists, began his work in 1895. Working diligently for the next 20 years, he developed many of the scientific principles involved in the selection and manipulation of dental materials. Many of those fundamentals are valid for materials used today.

In 1919, a dental research program was organized at the National Bureau of Standards (now called the National Institute for Standards and Technology). This government laboratory actively promotes research on dental materials. It has established principles that have helped place the American dentist at the forefront of the profession worldwide. Other centers of excellence in this discipline have been established at universities and comparable facilities in other countries.

Although the final testing of any dental material occurs in the patient's mouth, the modern method is to develop and test new dental materials in the laboratory first. As the science of dental materials has matured, much has been learned by systematically studying the materials that are known to give adequate performance. As a result, one need not place a gold alloy in a patient's mouth to determine whether it will tarnish or corrode or is sufficiently rigid to withstand the forces involved during mastication. All these properties can be tested outside the mouth, and the success or failure of the material can be predicted largely on the basis of experience.

The properties measured in the laboratory, when properly related and corroborated by clinical evaluation, form the selection criteria that should be part of the professional knowledge of the dentist and dental auxiliary.

AMERICAN DENTAL ASSOCIATION SPECIFICATIONS

In 1928, the American Dental Association (ADA), in cooperation with the U.S. government, sponsored research at the National Bureau of Standards. The ADA Specifications came from these investigations. Today, more than 40 types of dental materials are covered by specifications, with more to follow. Each specification is reviewed and revised continually, considering new research data and clinical experience.

The specifications contain requirements for mechanical, physical, and chemical properties of the materials to ensure their safety, quality, and usefulness. If the dental material meets the specification requirements, the manufacturer can submit it to the ADA for certification. Once such certification is obtained, the manufacturer is permitted to use a Seal of Certification on the product label to signify that it has been certified by the ADA.

One of the first criteria in the purchase of any dental material should be that it meets the requirements of the ADA Specification, if any exists for that material. Although the specific details are omitted in the following pages, the ADA Specifications are referred to frequently. The ADA Council on Dental Materials, Instruments and Equipment periodically publishes a listing of certified dental materials in the *Journal of the American Dental Association.* Current information also can be obtained by calling the ADA headquarters in Chicago.

The development of a specification requires the acquisition of data that relate clinical performance to properties measured in the laboratory. Such data for a new type of dental material may take years to obtain. To guide the use of newer dental materials, the ADA Council conducts the Acceptance Program for evaluating dental products. This activity applies to products for which safety and effectiveness have been established by biological, laboratory, and clinical evaluations but for which physical standards or specifications do not exist. Specific guidelines for acceptance for material—such as composite resins for posterior, occlusal restorations—are formulated by the Council.

Data are submitted by the manufacturer, and if approved, the material is granted a Seal of Acceptance.

Several other countries, particularly Australia, have established counterpart programs. The Fédération Dentaire Internationale, or FDI (International Dental Federation), has been instrumental in the development of international specifications. That activity has been formalized under the auspices of the International Standards Organization (ISO). The ISO is a body of national standards organizations from 51 countries. About 40 specifications for dental materials and devices have now been adopted. Considerable progress thus has been made in achieving a broad range of international specifications for dental materials, instruments, and equipment.

FOOD AND DRUG ADMINISTRATION REGULATION OF DENTAL MATERIALS

The Food and Drug Act of 1906 was amended in May 1976 to give the U.S. Food and Drug Administration (FDA) regulatory jurisdiction over the safety and efficacy of medical and dental materials and devices. This jurisdiction includes virtually all dental materials and devices except those that have specific therapeutic (drug) actions. Even the dental products sold over the counter to the public are included. The activities of the FDA, with the ADA Specification and Acceptance programs, provide a crucial framework for standards development and assurance to the dental profession that the materials used are safe and effective.

The safety of dental materials to the patient has been a primary consideration in dental materials research and development. Recent conditions have brought to the forefront other considerations that significantly impact the use of dental materials.

Federal and state agencies, such as the Centers for Disease Control, are developing recommendations for sterilization, disinfection, and barrier techniques to minimize the possibility of transmitting infectious diseases during the practice of dentistry. This directly impacts handling procedures for dental materials and may even result in new physical requirements. High speed dental handpieces, for example, now must be able to withstand sterilization procedures.

All dental personnel who handle dental materials and instruments must be knowledgeable about proper infection control procedures. Failure to do so may compromise the properties of the materials involved or jeopardize the safety of the patient or members of the dental team.

Another consideration relates to responsible disposal of waste materials from dental practice—solids, liquids, and even gases. Materials that are potential carriers of pathogens must be biologically sterilized before disposal. The alternative is to pay for their disposal by a qualified hazardous waste handler.

The typical dental practice also generates other waste that is an environmental disposal problem. Materials that contain toxic heavy metals, such as mercury, must be treated in a responsible manner. Every person on the dental team should be aware that the originator of any hazardous waste material is legally responsible for its ultimate disposal. Regulations concerning waste disposal are likely to grow much more stringent. Dental professionals must keep current with changes that occur.

OCCUPATIONAL SAFETY IN THE DENTAL OFFICE

A dental office with any staff besides the dentist is subject to the same occupational health and safety regulations as any other business or industry. The federal and state Occupational Safety and Health Agencies (OSHA) are responsible for formulating and enforcing provisions that assure a safe working environment for all employees. These regulations are under development for dentistry, but OSHA already is making unannounced inspection visits to dental offices and levying fines for violations.

Various companies supply information and training aids to help the dentist-employer comply with OSHA regulations. One source is the ADA *Regulatory Compliance Manual*, which is continuously updated as new regulations are developed. Each person who handles dental materials should be knowledgeable about potential hazards and trained to handle materials safely.

THE COURSE IN DENTAL MATERIALS

Dental Materials is a required course for dental students. A similar course is included in the training of the dental hygienist or assistant. The scope of the subject for the hygienist or assistant is somewhat different from that intended for the dental student.

The duty of the assistant or hygienist is to be of aid to the dentist at all times.

The chairside assistant needs to be trained primarily in the materials and techniques that are related to operations outside the mouth only. Although assistants don't actually place the cement in the mouth, they should know how to proportion and mix a dental cement. Most dentists depend on them for this operation.

Many of the results expected and the subsequent behavior of the cement are directly dependent on how the cement is manipulated by the chair assistant before it is placed in the mouth. Knowledge about the properties of the cement is necessary for the proper background of the auxiliary. The auxiliary needs to know about hardening time of the cement, the cement's probable usefulness in the mouth, how it is attacked by the mouth fluids, how strong it is, and similar information.

Dental hygienists may not function as chair assistants. They should, however, be able to recognize the dental materials that are placed in the mouth. They also need to understand the weaknesses and strengths so that they can treat the materials properly during prophylaxis and other procedures hygienists may perform. As a matter of patient education, knowledge of the materials and their properties is essential for the hygienist to instruct the patient intelligently concerning oral hygiene.

In settings where expanded duties for hygienists or assistants are taught or practiced, the required knowledge of dental materials becomes broader. In such situations, the auxiliary actually performs selected restorative procedures, requiring a comprehension of the techniques associated with the placement and finishing of certain materials. The scope of this book does not cover those facets in that depth. It does, however, provide an outline of the steps involved and discusses the relevance of manipulative variables to the properties and performance of the restorative material.

Much of the information presented in this book is based on the belief that an educational background is needed for intelligent service. The dental hygienist or assistant is not expected to be intimately involved in the processing or manipulation of denture materials. Nevertheless, if the general principles involved are known, the hygienist or assistant is better prepared to sympathize with and advise a denture patient as required.

Aim of the Course

Although the techniques and dental materials with which the dental assistant is involved are described at some length, the primary intent of this book is not to explain *how* the dentist, hygienist, or assistant should handle the materials. This book emphasizes *why* the particular materials and techniques are used. It also aims to establish criteria of selection so that the hygienist or assistant is thoroughly familiar with both the techniques and the materials used. All dental materials and techniques should be based on sound scientific principles. The purpose of this book is to present these principles.

Because the oral cavity presents unusual conditions, the testing and use of dental materials embrace various sciences. An understanding of the basic concepts in chemistry, physics, engineering, and metallurgy is necessary for appreciating the relation of the material to the oral environment. In addition to theories and practices in the physical sciences, the dentist and auxiliaries must be versed in the biological requirements of den-

tal materials as they relate to clinical techniques and performance.

Reviewing the Chapter

1. Describe the evolution and development of the science of dental materials.
2. Explain the ADA Specification and Acceptance programs and their importance to the profession and the public.
3. Explain the relation of the FDA to dental materials.
4. List other government regulatory agencies that may influence the use of dental materials.
5. Describe the importance of a knowledge of dental materials to the dental auxiliary.
6. Explain the purpose of the course in dental materials.
7. Describe how dental materials influence responsibilities of a dental hygienist and/or dental assistant.

CHAPTER **2**

DENTAL MATERIALS AND THE ORAL ENVIRONMENT

PHYSICAL CONSIDERATIONS
Biting Forces
Temperature Changes
Acidity

BIOLOGICAL CONSIDERATIONS
Microleakage
Temperature Effects
Galvanism
Toxic Effects of Materials

CLASSIFICATION OF RESTORATIVE MATERIALS
Permanent Restorations
Temporary Restorations
Intermediary Bases
Other Materials

The restoration or replacement of tooth structure seldom involves simple problems. The nature of the oral cavity and the limitations that are imposed on dental treatment present complex situations.

PHYSICAL CONSIDERATIONS

The dentist is restricted in the design of the restoration or appliance that can be placed in a tooth or inserted into the mouth. Only a small amount of tooth structure may be removed safely without injuring a vital tooth. Certain areas of the mouth are difficult

to reach. Because the jaw cannot be opened wide enough, visibility of and access to the posterior teeth are limited.

In these respects, the dentist is less fortunate than the construction engineer. The engineer has considerable freedom in designing a bridge or a building to provide resistance to deformation or failure. The physical and biological conditions in the oral cavity often prevent the dentist from using the ideal design for a restoration or an appliance. For example, it may not be possible to provide the bulk of material needed to ensure optimum resistance to fracture when the restoration or an appliance is subjected

6

to masticatory forces. The external contours of a restoration normally are limited to those of the intact tooth.

Many materials that might have ideal physical properties are not suitable for dental use because they are injurious to the patient's health, do not have a pleasing appearance, cannot be readily manipulated by the dentist, or have other limitations. The materials used so efficiently in the construction of skyscrapers are of little use in the oral cavity. Steel rusts and corrodes in the mouth, and it cannot be readily fabricated into small custom restorations, such as inlays and crowns. Concrete also is useless in dental operations. It is too coarse, takes too long to harden, and has many other obvious disadvantages.

The oral cavity is ideally suited for destruction. Dental restorations and appliances do not really belong in the mouth. They are foreign bodies, inert matter installed in a warm, living, moist system. If certain biophysical requirements are met, however, the mouth will tolerate them. In fact, after analysis of the undesirable conditions to which dental materials are subjected, it is surprising that restorations and appliances serve as satisfactorily as they do.

Because of these restrictions, the dentist and auxiliaries must give particular attention to the physical properties of the materials that can be used.

Biting Forces

The average biting force of a person with natural dentition is about 755 newtons (170 lb)* in the posterior part of the mouth. At first glance, a force of this magnitude does not appear to be particularly great. However, expressed in terms of the force being ap-

---

*Throughout the remainder of the text, the term newton is abbreviated N and the term pound is abbreviated lb. In addition, the term megapascal (meganewton per square meter) is abbreviated MPa, and the unit pounds per square inch is abbreviated psi.

plied on an individual tooth or a portion of a tooth, this represents about 193 megapascals (28,000 lb per square inch) on a single cusp of a molar tooth. This is explained further in Chapter 3.

To relate it to common experience, this force is about equal to that created by pressing down on the point of a medium sharp lead pencil with a force of 1333 N (300 lb). Maximum design loads for the floors in office building construction are only 100 lb per square foot (0.7 psi)! Incidentally, the biting force that can be exerted with dentures is markedly less than that of the normal dentition—another reason for preserving the natural dentition for as long as possible. It is difficult to formulate materials that have the strength necessary to prevent them from fracturing during mastication.

Temperature Changes

The temperature in the mouth fluctuates rapidly. An instantaneous temperature change as great as 65°C (150° F) occurs when one drinks hot coffee immediately after eating ice cream. The sudden shock from such a rapid temperature change may crack or craze the surface of the tooth or the restoration.

All substances tend to expand or contract when they are heated or cooled, including the teeth and the materials used in dental restorations. No restorative material expands or contracts at exactly the same rate as the tooth when it is subjected to heat or cold. These differences in the dimensional changes that occur between the restoration and the adjoining tooth structure may result in the material shrinking away from the tooth. The phenomenon is discussed in detail later.

Acidity

The acidity in the mouth (pH) varies greatly. Some foods and beverages (e.g., citrus fruits) are acidic (low pH). In addition, acid is liberated when microorganisms act on food debris present in the mouth. Other foods and liquids may be rather alkaline (high pH). The normal pH in the mouth is about neutral (pH 7.0).

The surfaces of the teeth and dental restorations thus are constantly in contact with substances that are acidic or alkaline. Most nonmetallic materials used in the oral cavity tend to deteriorate in such environments. Even metallic restorations may discolor and corrode when the pH at their surface is altered.

In fact, the conditions that usually prevail in the mouth are conducive to producing tarnish and corrosion, as discussed in Chapter 13. In addition to possessing an optimal pH for initiating corrosion, the oral cavity is warm and moist. It usually contains a host of fluids, food debris, and enzymes. All of these create a favorable environment for the deposition of surface film such as dental plaque—which usually is present on teeth and restorations. Chemical elements and compounds then collect in the plaque and react in an undesirable manner with the surface of the restorative material.

Although the first objective of restorative dentistry is to restore the mouth to normal function, the appearance of restorative materials has become increasingly important. Patients may request or demand aesthetic dental restorations, even in the posterior regions of the mouth. Considerable research is devoted to the development of restorative materials that closely resemble the missing or damaged tooth structure without compromising the properties already discussed.

These and other characteristics constitute the physical demands on tooth structure and the materials used in its replacement. It is extremely difficult to formulate restorative materials that resist fracture, temperature changes, alterations in pH, and discoloration while matching the appearance of natural tooth structure. The conditions in the oral cavity and the particular limitations of each material must be understood when selecting and using dental materials.

BIOLOGICAL CONSIDERATIONS

In addition to possessing the physical and chemical properties that effectively combat such unfavorable environmental conditions, the material must not cause local or systemic injury to oral or other tissues. Strength and resistance to corrosion are unimportant if the material damages the pulp or soft tissue. It should be remembered, too, that the oral cavity is just the beginning of the gastrointestinal system. The biological characteristics of dental materials cannot be isolated from their physical properties.

Microleakage

One of the greatest deficiencies of the materials used in the restoration of the damaged tooth structure is that they do not seal the cavity preparation. The only exception is those materials based on polyacrylic acid (discussed in Chapters 21 and 22). A microscopic space always exists between the restoration and the tooth. Fluids, microorganisms, and debris from the mouth may penetrate the outer margins of the restoration and progress down the walls of the cavity preparation. As explained in subsequent chapters, the dentist and auxiliary attempt to select and use restorative materials in a manner to minimize the leakage. With the materials that currently are available, it cannot be prevented.

This phenomenon, called *microleakage*, may be envisioned as occurring in a manner such as that diagramed in Figure 2–1. The point at which the restorative material is in contact with the tooth structure is referred to as an *interface*. As shown in this figure, the

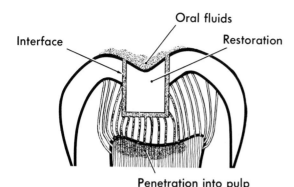

Figure 2–1. Diagram of the microleakage phenomenon. In this case, the leakage of deleterious fluids and debris has extended along the tooth–restoration interface, through the dentin, and into the pulp. (Modified from Massler, M.: *Adhesive Restorative Materials*. Spencer, Ind., Owens Litho Service.)

penetration of injurious agents has occurred along the entire tooth-restoration interface, through the dentin at the floor of the cavity preparation, and into the pulp. Some common observations related to the behavior of restorative materials in the oral cavity can be identified with the effects of microleakage. The seepage of acids and microorganisms could initiate caries around the margins of the restoration. The accumulation of debris in that area certainly enhances the possibility for stain or discoloration to develop.

In some situations, microleakage may cause the tooth to remain sensitive to temperature changes after placement of a restoration. If the leakage is severe, the pulp is continually irritated by the fluids, microorganisms, and debris that penetrate around the restoration, through the dentin, and into the pulp. Such irritation can lead to an inflammatory reaction, resulting in pain and pulp necrosis. The superiority of certain types of materials in reducing postoperative sensitivity has been attributed to their ability to adapt better to tooth structure and thereby minimize microleakage.

The amalgam restoration serves as an example of the relationship between micro-leakage and the clinical behavior of a dental material. The dentist forms the amalgam restoration by condensing the plastic amalgam into the cavity preparation, where it subsequently hardens (see Chapter 15). It is not possible to force or condense the amalgam into perfect contact with all the minute irregularities present in tooth structure. Thus, a microscopic space exists between the amalgam and the tooth. Fluids and debris can penetrate readily into that space.

It is likely that the occasional sensitivity of a tooth that has been restored with amalgam results from the injurious effects on the pulp of the agents that penetrate around the restoration.

This initial pattern of microleakage changes markedly with time. As the amalgam restoration ages in the oral cavity, the leakage decreases significantly, as shown in Figure 2–2. In time, the early leakage becomes minimal or nonexistent. The principal cause of this marked reduction in microleakage is the accumulation of corrosion products, such as tin oxide, in the space between the restoration and the tooth. Such accumulations act as a mechanical block to the passage of fluids down the walls of the cavity preparation.

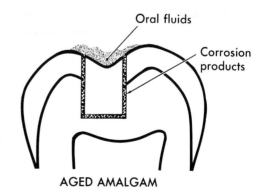

Figure 2–2. Microleakage decreases as the amalgam restoration ages in the oral cavity. Corrosion products accumulate at the tooth–restoration interface, and the mechanical seal is improved. (Phillips, R. W., Swartz, M. L., and Norman, R. D.: *Materials for the Practicing Dentist*. St. Louis, C. V. Mosby Co., 1969.)

When removing an old amalgam restoration, one often can see the corrosion products that have formed along the interface. Such an example is shown in the cross-sectioned restoration in Figure 2–3. The corrosion products have even penetrated the dentin, resulting in some discoloration. The reduction in microleakage with time is an unquestionable advantage of this material, which is rather unique.

Similar examples of the influence of the microleakage phenomenon on the biological and physical behavior of dental materials are cited in the chapters to follow.

Temperature Effects

It has been pointed out that temperature fluctuations in the oral cavity may crack restorative materials or produce undesirable dimensional changes. In addition, temperature changes induced by hot or cold beverages and other fluids may have injurious effects on the pulp.

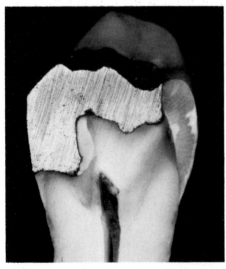

Figure 2–3. Cross section through an amalgam restoration, showing the dark corrosion products that have been deposited beneath the restoration. Discoloration of the dentin is a result of the penetration of metallic ions from corrosion of the amalgam.

Metals conduct heat and cold rapidly. Many popular restorative materials are metallic, thereby posing a problem. If a piece of ice is placed on the outer surface of an amalgam or a gold restoration, within 3 seconds the temperature at the floor of the cavity preparation is the same as that of the surface. The reason many patients complain of sensitivity in a tooth with a metallic restoration when eating hot or cold foods is understandable.

The problem is particularly important in a large restoration. The layer of dentin that remains at the floor of the cavity may be so thin that it does not insulate the pulp against the temperature change that occurs through the amalgam or the gold inlay. The dentist must provide additional thermal protection by placing a layer of a suitable insulating cement under the restoration.

Galvanism

Another potential cause for sensitivity is the small electrical currents created whenever two different metals are present in the oral cavity. For example, assume that an amalgam restoration is placed on the biting surface of a lower tooth and that it opposes a gold inlay in an upper tooth. Because both restorations are wet with saliva, a small battery exists between the two metallic restorations. When the two restorations touch during mastication, the current produced by the battery may irritate the pulp and produce a sharp pain.

Such a situation is diagramed in Figure 2–4. These currents are referred to as *galvanic currents*. A similar effect may occur if a restoration is touched by the edge of a silver fork or aluminum foil from a candy wrapper contacts a metallic restoration. Shock from galvanic currents is a common occurrence in dental practice. The clinical significance of this phenomenon is discussed later.

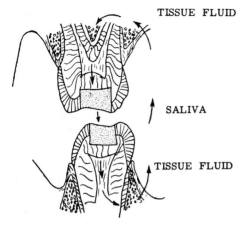

TISSUE FLUID

SALIVA

TISSUE FLUID

Figure 2–4. Schematic drawing of a galvanic cell as it may occur in the mouth. Two opposing restorations, plus saliva, form a battery. Arrows indicate that whenever the restorations touch, the current flows down through the pulp and is carried by the tissue "fluid" up through the saliva and down again through the other tooth.

Toxic Effects of Materials

One other important biological consideration is the effect on living tissue that may be produced by the dental materials. From a physiological standpoint, few, if any, dental materials are totally inert. They may contain a variety of potentially toxic or irritating ingredients. Various types of dental cements, for example, involve the use of a phosphoric acid liquid. The acidity of such materials results in irritation to the pulp unless proper care is exercised to protect it from such injury. Undesirable effects on the pulp also may be produced by the chemical reactions that occur during the setting or hardening of restorative materials after they are inserted into the cavity preparation.

Materials to be used in the oral cavity must be nonirritating to soft tissue. Any material that is used in fabricating an artificial denture, for example, should not produce an allergic or sensitizing effect on the underlying tissue.

To summarize, during and after restoration of a carious tooth, the dental pulp may be subjected to injury from microleakage, thermal shock, galvanism, and chemical irritation. Unless steps are taken to eliminate or minimize these causes of irritation, pulpal reactions and continuing sensitivity result.

Recognizing the importance of the biological characteristics of dental materials, the American Dental Association Specifications contain specific tests that should provide acceptable methods for determining the safety of dental materials. In addition, a principal activity of the Food and Drug Administration is to ensure the patient's safety.

CLASSIFICATION OF RESTORATIVE MATERIALS

The dental hygienist or assistant is concerned primarily with the materials used for restorative dentistry—either assisting the dentist in their manipulation or observing their behavior in the oral cavity. To orient the beginning auxiliary with those materials, a brief resume of the general classification of restorative materials follows. Each type is discussed in detail in the chapters to follow.

One method of classification is based on composition. On that basis, dental restorative materials are composed of metals, ceramics, or polymeric (plastic) substances. A more common classification may be made according to their intended usage in clinical practice. Although each of the materials to be mentioned is discussed in depth in the chapters that follow, this classification provides the reader with a general concept of the scope of materials armamentarium available for restorative dentistry.

Permanent Restorations

No material lasts forever. When one considers the environmental problems associated with the oral cavity, it is virtually impossible to predict the lifetime of any dental treatment. Although the dentist and the auxiliary may appreciate the limitations of the term *permanent,* the patient may not.

Nevertheless, materials used for a permanent restoration are intended to satisfy the objectives of the restoration for periods that may extend 20 years or longer. An ideal restoration is one that lasts as long as the tooth. The metallic restorative materials—amalgam, gold inlays and crowns, and direct filling gold—have the physical properties with greatest potential to date to meet the demands that are placed on the restoration. Therefore, they have traditionally been used when permanency is desired.

In other situations, such as in the anterior portion of the mouth, a restoration that is more like the tooth in appearance than a metallic material is the prime concern. A resin or glass ionomer cement may then be the material of choice, despite the known deficiencies of the current formulations and recognizing that the restoration may require replacement more frequently than certain metallic restorations.

Temporary Restorations

Materials used for a temporary restoration need last only for a short period of time, when compared with the anticipated life of the tooth. In certain cases, such as a treatment material while the pulp heals and until a permanent restoration can be inserted, the required service of the restoration may be only a few weeks. The zinc oxide–eugenol cements are examples of such materials.

Intermediary Bases

Certain materials are placed between the permanent or temporary restoration and the underlying tooth structure. These intermediary bases protect the pulp by affording thermal insulation and blocking the penetration of irritants that may be present in the restorative material. The biological characteristics are more important than the physical properties in such materials. Because of their proximity to the pulp, they must be nonirritating and, preferably, should promote healing of the pulp. Calcium hydroxide and zinc oxide–eugenol cements are the most widely used intermediary base materials.

Other Materials

In addition to these classes, a variety of other substances are used as adjunct materials. These include varnishes for lining the walls of the cavity preparation and cements for retaining gold inlays and crowns.

Many of the restorative materials to be discussed are molded to shape directly in the mouth. These are referred to as direct restorative materials. Others are fabricated outside the mouth by using an accurate model of the oral structures. Such a restoration is an indirect restoration and often is made in a dental laboratory. Because of their importance to the accuracy of the finished restoration, the materials used to construct the necessary models are discussed in this text.

It should now be apparent that the dentist must consider a number of factors when selecting the material best suited for a particular patient. These factors include the following:

- Condition of the pulp
- Esthetics required
- Biting forces that will be placed on the restoration and
- Past experience of the individual dentist and the auxiliaries with a particular type of material

Selected Reading

Autian, J.: General toxicity and screening tests for dental materials. Int. Dent. J. 24:235, 1974.

Council on Dental Materials and Devices: Recommended standard practices for biological evaluation of dental materials. J. Am. Dent. Assoc. 84:382, 1972.

Going, R. E.: Reducing marginal leakage: A review of materials and techniques. J. Am. Dent. Assoc. 99:646, 1979.

Massler, M.: Restorative materials: Biological considerations. In Clark, James W. (Ed.) *Clinical Dentistry.* Vol. 4. Hagerstown, Md., Harper & Row, 1976.

Phillips, R. W.: The new era in restorative dental materials. Oper. Dent. 1:29, 1976.

Reviewing the Chapter

1. Explain the restrictions placed on the dentist in the design and fabrication of a dental restoration and an appliance.
2. List the various factors present in the oral cavity that tend to alter the behavior of dental restoratives.
3. Give the values for (1) biting forces, (2) temperature changes, and (3) acidity fluctuation that occur in the oral cavity.
4. List the various biological considerations involved in the use and performance of dental materials and discuss the role of various regulatory agencies (e.g., the American Dental Association and the Food and Drug Administration) in this regard.
5. Explain the mechanism of the phenomenon of microleakage and its implications for the dental restoration. Also describe the differences between various types of restorative materials in this regard.
6. Explain, by means of a sketch, what is meant by *galvanism* and *galvanic currents*.
7. Classify restorative materials in regard to the usage intended.

CHAPTER 3

STRUCTURE AND PROPERTIES OF DENTAL MATERIALS:
Adhesion and Elasticity

To understand the proper use of a dental material, it is necessary to be familiar with its physical and chemical properties. With such knowledge, one can better predict how the material will react under conditions of actual use.

When the dentist constructs a gold inlay or a bridge for a patient, for example, it is expected that the restoration will not bend out of shape or fracture in use. The success of the gold crown usually can be predicted if the physical and chemical properties of the alloy are known. In determining which alloy to use, the dentist asks the following questions:

- What is its strength?
- How far can it be bent without permanent distortion?
- How hard is it?
- Will it discolor?

Such properties determine how the gold alloy will behave in the oral cavity. The same may be said for all dental materials, although the pertinent properties vary with the type of material and the demands placed on it.

All these properties can be measured accurately. This and subsequent chapters discuss the ways in which these properties are measured as well as the technical names of the properties and how they can be applied.

SOLIDS

The mechanical and physical properties of any material depend on its internal structure. An understanding of the atomic nature of matter, therefore, permits one to better understand the properties and the behavior of the gross structure.

There are three states of matter: solid, liquid, and gas. Most of the materials used in dentistry are solids. Many were liquids at some point in their use or fabrication and then were changed into solids by cooling or chemical reaction.

A *solid* is a state of matter that occupies a definite volume of space and whose shape does not depend on a container. If an object *feels* hard and unyielding, one concludes that it is a solid. A solid is said to be *rigid* or to possess rigidity. If it possesses rigidity, it usually can be described as *crystalline*. Such a solid is characterized by a regular arrangement of its atoms or molecules with respect to one another.

Assume that the balls shown in Figure 3–1 are atoms. Note that they are regularly spaced in the pile. Such an arrangement of atoms is called a *space lattice*. Atoms in a crystal of gold are arranged in this manner. The ultimate structure of gold is composed of a repeated pattern of individual space lat-

tices, each one oriented in a definite three-dimensional relation with the others.

The simplest form of a lattice is diagramed in Figure 3–2. The atoms are as large and as close together as possible, but their relationship is easier to understand as shown in Figure 3–2. The atoms are held in position by interatomic forces, not by wires, as shown in Figure 3–2.

The lattice shown in Figure 3–2 is called *cubic* because the repeat pattern is cubic. There are 14 possible types of space lattices. Others have different geometric forms, such as hexagonal or rhombic. Most crystalline materials used in dentistry form a cubic type of lattice.

The atoms in a space lattice tend to maintain their position relative to one another—their *interatomic distance*. The normal or equilibrium interatomic distance is the distance at which the force of attraction between the atoms is equal to the force that repels them. Therefore, crystalline materials resist forces that either compress or stretch the space lattice.

Some apparently solid materials possess a structure in which the molecules tend to be arranged at random—similar to the molecules in a liquid. Such a material is said to be *amorphous*. (Amorphous literally means without form.) Glass, for example, is amor-

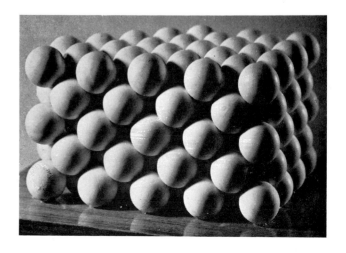

Figure 3–1. A model of a space lattice from a crystal of gold. (From Rogers, B. A. *The Nature of Metals.* Cleveland, Ohio, American Society for Metals, [ASM International, Materials Park, Ohio], 1951, p 21.)

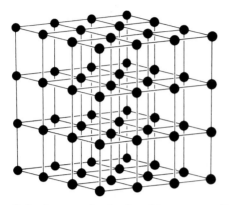

Figure 3–2. Diagram of a simple cubic structure. (From Van Vlack, L. H. *Elements of Materials Science.* 4th ed. Reading, Mass., Addison-Wesley Publishing Co., © 1980. Reprinted with permission of the publisher.)

phous. A long, straight glass tube feels hard and rigid, yet if it is suspended at its two ends, in time it bows or flows under its own weight. Because the property of *flow* is characteristic of a liquid, the glass cannot, strictly speaking, be classified as completely solid.

Amorphous structures, although possessing many characteristics of a solid, may flow under certain conditions. In comparison, crystalline structures are rigid at all temperatures below their melting point.

Another difference is that amorphous substances do not possess a definite melting or freezing temperature or a well-defined range of temperature over which the change of state occurs. Ice, a crystalline substance, is either entirely solid or entirely liquid, depending on its temperature. It becomes water under normal conditions above 0°C (32°F). Amorphous waxes gradually soften over an ill-defined range of temperature and do not exhibit definite melting and freezing points.

The properties of solid materials are intimately related to their atomic structure.

BONDING AND ADHESION

There are essentially two ways of attaching solid structures together. One is through mechanical mechanisms and the other is through the phenomenon of adhesion.

Mechanical Bonding

Strong attachments can be accomplished by *mechanical bonding,* or *retention.* Two pieces of wood, for example, often are held together by a screw, nail, or bolt. Mechanical bonding can occur on a finer level by penetration of a liquid glue into very small surface irregularities, such as crevices and pores in a solid surface. When the glue hardens, the multitude of the projections that are embedded in the surface provide "fingers" for mechanical attachment and retention.

This type of retention is used frequently in dentistry. As described in Chapter 22, the retention of a crown is enhanced by the mechanical attachment of the cementing agent. The liquid cement penetrates into irregularities that exist on the internal surface of the crown and into the porosities that are present in the tooth structure. On setting, the cement projections aid in holding the crown in place.

Another example of mechanical bonding is the use of the resin (plastic) restoration. Before the resin filling material is inserted into the cavity preparation, the tooth enamel is treated with phosphoric acid for a short period. This is referred to as the *acid etch* technique, described in Chapter 10. The acid treatment produces minute pores in the surface of the enamel. When placed into the preparation, the resin flows into these pores. On hardening, these resin projections improve the mechanical retention of the restoration.

Adhesion

It is obvious from the preceding illustrations that mechanical bonding as discussed does not require intimate attraction between the atoms and molecules of the substances involved. In the acid etch technique, for example, there is no real interaction between the molecules of the resin and those of the enamel. A more tenacious bonding is possible if the atoms or molecules of the substances being joined are held together by some type of attractive force. When that occurs, then true *adhesion* has taken place.

The phenomenon of adhesion is involved in many dental situations. Adhesion is a principal concern in attempting to solve the problem of microleakage around dental restorations. The retention of dentures probably depends on adhesion—at the interface between the denture and saliva and between the saliva and soft tissues. Certainly, the attachment of plaque or calculus to tooth structure is partially, if not entirely, an adhesive mechanism.

Adhesion is the force that causes unlike atoms or molecules to attach to each other. The substance to which the adhesive is applied is referred to as the *adherend.* Tooth structure, for example, is the adherend to which plaque attaches. The point at which the adhesive is in contact with the adherend is referred to as the *interface*, as noted in Chapter 2.

If the atoms or molecules are the same kind, the attraction is termed *cohesion.* The strength of a material is governed by the cohesive forces of attraction between its atoms or molecules.

Adhesion may involve attractions that are essentially strong physical forces or the bonding may be chemical. A chemical bond between the atoms or molecules of the adhesive and the adherend is referred to as a *primary* bond. These forces are quite strong and the most desirable for adhesion. An example is the dyeing of cloth, in which the dye is held to the cloth by a primary bond. When primary bonding is involved, the adhesion is termed *chemisorption.*

The most common type of adhesion involves physical forces, or *secondary* bonds.

These are called *van der Waals* forces. This physical attraction does not provide as strong a bond as when a chemical union occurs. The use of a paint or a glue usually involves such bonding.

Wetting

For either chemical or physical adhesion to occur, the adhesive and adherend must be in intimate contact. Unless they are within 0.0007 micrometer* (0.00003 inch) of each other, the attractive force is negligible.

To achieve this intimate contact, the adhesive usually is a liquid. A liquid is more apt to flow easily over the entire surface of the adherend and come in contact with all the small roughnesses that may be present. Such a characteristic is referred to as *wetting.* The better the adhesive flows over and wets the surface of the adherend, the more likely it is that adhesion will occur between the two.

The wetting characteristics of an adhesive usually are determined by measuring the angle formed when a drop of the liquid adhesive is placed on the surface of the adherend. This measurement is called the *contact angle.* If the molecules of the adhesive are not attracted to the surface of the adherend, the adhesive forms a ball, resulting in a large angle.

A familiar example is a drop of water placed on the surface of a frying pan that has an antistick coating. Such a situation is shown in Figure 3–3*A.*

If there is a strong attraction between the molecules of the adhesive and the adherend, the adhesive flows readily over the surface, forming a low contact angle. An example of an adhesive with a low contact angle is shown in Figure 3–3*B.* The ideal adhesive

---

*Micrometer often is also called micron. The symbol for *micrometer* is μm, which is used throughout the text.

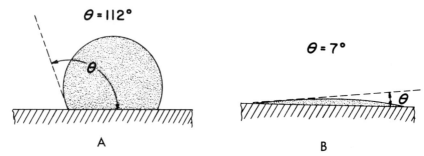

Figure 3–3. *A,* An illustration of a high contact angle formed when a liquid does not wet the surface of a solid. The angle is represented by the angle θ. *B,* An illustration of a low contact angle, which is formed when the liquid flows, freely wetting the surface.

spreads out into such a thin film that the contact angle is zero.

Factors That Influence Wetting

A number of factors influence the ease with which the adhesive spreads over a surface. One of the most important is the reactivity of that surface—the *surface energy.* If the atoms on the surface are eager to attract other atoms to them—in other words, if they have high energy—then it is relatively easy to find adhesives that will bond to that surface. The greater the surface energy of the adherend, the more readily the adhesive reacts with it. The energy is related to the composition of the material, its atomic structure, and other factors.

Most metals have a high surface energy and, therefore, are relatively easy to wet with a suitable adhesive. In contrast, a commercial plastic known as Teflon often is used in situations in which one wants to prevent substances from sticking to the surface—as the antistick coating for frying pans, for example. The principal reason that Teflon is resistant to adhesion is that it has a very low surface energy.

Surface irregularities can prevent an adhesive from completely wetting the adherend. Air pockets may form in small pits or cracks and prevent the adhesive from penetrating into that area.

The cleanliness of the surface is of particular importance. Any debris or surface contamination prevents the adhesive from coming into the intimate contact necessary to produce adhesion. A film of water only one molecule thick on the surface of a solid inhibits contact of the adhesive, as does an oxide film on a metal.

Adhesion and Tooth Structure

Many of the fundamentals of adhesion can be related directly to dental situations. Because the surface energy of metallic restorative materials is higher than that of tooth enamel, debris inherently accumulates more rapidly on the surface of the restoration. This in turn may partially account for the higher incidence of marginal caries around dental restorations.

The wettability of enamel surfaces also is reduced by a topical application of an aqueous fluoride solution. The reduced wettability results in less retention of plaque on the enamel surface over a period of time. Conceivably, one of the reasons for the success of topical fluoride therapy is that fluoride-treated teeth stay cleaner longer.

Throughout this text, reference is made to the problems associated with the microleakage that occurs between nonadhesive restorative materials and tooth structure. Certainly the lack of adhesive systems complicates restorative dental procedures and reduces the lifetime of restorations. Dental materials science has been criticized for its inability to provide adhesive dental materials. If one applies to the dental situation the principles that influence adhesion, the problem is readily understood.

Few of the conditions essential for adhesion are present in the oral cavity. Enamel and dentin are inhomogeneous in composition, being partly organic and partly inorganic. An adhesive that would wet and adhere to the organic component of the tooth would not be as apt to adhere to the inorganic portion. Adhesion thus would occur on isolated sites only and would not be uniform over the entire surface.

The surface of the prepared cavity is marred by surface imperfections, such as tubules, pits, and fissures. This inherent morphologic roughness is increased by scratches produced by the dental burs and cutting tools used in removing tooth structure and preparing the cavity. It is difficult to design an adhesive that will flow into these minute irregularities and wet the entire surface area of the cavity preparation. Furthermore, this surface roughness acts as concentrators for stress whenever the adhesive is subjected to thermal or mechanical stress. The localized high stress concentration eventually could break the adhesive bond at that point.

Microscopically, the tooth surface is covered with a tenacious film of debris that forms when the dentist prepares the cavity. Thorough cleaning or brushing of the surface cannot remove this debris completely. Because even slight surface contamination prevents wetting of an adherend, the prepared tooth is far from ideal from this standpoint.

Of major importance is the presence of water. A microscopic, single-molecule-thick layer of water is always present on the tooth surface. This film prevents the adhesive from coming into intimate contact with the tooth.

Surface moisture is impossible to remove by dehydration without the use of temperatures or agents that could produce serious injury to the pulp. Unless the adhesive forms a low contact angle with water (called *hydrophilic behavior*), it will not even wet the water-covered surface.

Thus, the inhomogeneous, rough, contaminated and wet tooth structure presents conditions that are not favorable for the development of a dental material that would provide true adhesion in the oral environment.

Research in this field is promising, however, and the goals are worthy of the challenges presented. An adhesive that would prevent microleakage could replace many materials now used in restorative dentistry. Also, the technique for placement of the material would be simplified because the mechanical retention of the filling material in the cavity preparation, as is now required, would be unnecessary. This book discusses some of these concepts and the problems associated with bonding, particularly in regard to the use of restorative resins and dental cements.

FORCE, STRESS, AND STRAIN

Force, defined as any push or pull on an object, is measured in units of newtons or pounds. Dental restorations are constantly subjected to forces of various types, such as those of biting and chewing. It is important that the effect of the biting forces on the dental material be known. Otherwise, the wrong material might be selected, and the restoration might be bent or broken during chewing.

As discussed in detail, *stress* is the reaction with which an object resists an external force. Force can be measured in newtons or pounds, but the concept is meaningless unless it is known *where* the force is applied and the *direction* in which it is acting. For example, the force resulting from the weight of a 10-kg object lying on the top of a desk has meaning. The force is directed downward on the desktop. On the other hand, a force of 98 N has no meaning because the statement does not indicate where and how the force acts.

Another point to be considered is the resistance of the desk to the force. With a downward force on the desk of 98 N, the desk also must push upward with a force of 98 N in reaction (one of Newton's famous laws). If it did not do so, it would collapse or move. The magnitude of the desk's "reaction" force is equal to 98 N, but its direction is upward or opposite to the applied force, usually called the *load*. The internal force of the desk in resisting the applied force or load is called the *stress*. A stress is a force, but it is *inside* the structure or body on which the load is acting.

When a force acts on a solid object, its atoms or molecules are slightly displaced from their equilibrium interatomic spacing. As discussed earlier, the interatomic forces act to resist this displacement. This is the fundamental explanation for the stress or reaction force. In other words, the matter is changed in shape by the force. The amount of change in shape (deformation) is called the *strain*. Consequently, it follows that when the load (or external force) produces a stress in the structure, it also produces a strain.

Stress is measured in units of force per unit area. As an example, consider a wire that is being stretched. Assume that the wire is 0.01 square cm² in cross-sectional area. If the load is 98 N, by definition the stress is

$$\frac{98}{0.01} = 98 \text{ MN/m}^2 = 98 \text{ MPa} \qquad 3-1$$

In the metric system, stress usually is expressed as meganewtons per square meter (MN/m²) or megapascals (MPa), whereas in

the English system, it is expressed as pounds per square inch (lb/in², or psi). The relation between these units and others used in this text can be found in the conversion table in the Appendix.

The rationale for considering the behavior of a material in terms of stress rather than simply as the force or load applied is a practical one. Let us say that one has two sticks of a dental plaster, but one is larger in diameter than the other. It will take more force to break the larger stick because of the greater bulk of material. Suppose that the larger stick was 1 cm in diameter (0.8 cm² in cross-sectional area) and that it fractured at a force of 2195 N. The smaller stick, 0.5 cm in diameter (0.2 cm² in cross-sectional area), fractured at a force of 549 N.

Now assume that one was to report the strength of the plaster only on the basis of the load or the force necessary to fracture the plaster sticks without taking into consideration the variation in the specimen size. Two different values would be given for the strength of the plaster, even though the material was the same in each case. Such data would be meaningless because there could be as many values for the strength of that particular plaster as there were for the sizes of the specimens tested.

Calculation of stress solves this problem because it eliminates the variable of specimen size and provides a value that is characteristic of the material independent of its size. This is illustrated below where the stress is calculated for the two sticks of plaster when fractured:

$$\frac{\text{Force}}{\text{Cross-sectional area}} \quad \frac{2197 \text{ N}}{0.8 \text{ cm}^2} = 27.4 \text{ MPa (stress)}$$
$$\frac{\text{Force}}{\text{Cross-sectional area}} \quad \frac{549 \text{ N}}{0.2 \text{ cm}^2} = 27.4 \text{ MPa (stress)} \qquad 3-2$$

Despite the difference in the force required to fracture the large and small sticks, the stress and the true breaking strength of the plaster are identical in the two specimens.

Strain is measured in terms of deformation or change in dimension per unit dimension. Assume that a wire 5 cm in length is stretched 0.0015 cm when the load is applied. By definition the strain is

$$\frac{0.0015 \text{ cm}}{5 \text{ cm}} = 0.0003 \text{ cm/cm} = 0.0003 \text{ (strain)} \qquad 3\text{-}3$$

The rationale for expressing deformation in this manner is the same as that for reporting strength values in terms of stress. If everything else is comparable, the longer the specimen, the greater the change in length. Under a given load, for example, a rubber band 2 cm in length will stretch twice as much as one only 1 cm in length. Thus, if the data were reported simply in terms of change in dimension rather than as strain (change in dimension per unit length), it would be virtually impossible to standardize the reporting of data on the deformation of a material when stressed.

Stress and strain are two entirely different quantities. A stress is a force per unit area with magnitude and direction, but a strain is expressed as a magnitude only. Note that the magnitude of the strain is the same no matter what system of units is used because the same unit appears in both numerator and denominator. Strain is a unitless quantity.

Types of Stress and Strain

There are three types of stress:

1. *Tensile stress* results from a load that tends to elongate a structure, such as the wire discussed previously. A tensile stress always is accompanied by a *tensile strain.*

2. *Compressive stress* is a stress that opposes a load that compresses a structure. The stress in the desk that opposes the downward force exerted, for example, is essentially compressive in character. A compressive stress always is accompanied by a *compressive strain.*

3. *Shear stress* is induced when a structure is rotated, twisted, or deformed by sliding one part parallel to another. Shear stress and strain can be illustrated by a simple experiment. Place this closed book on the table and move the top cover toward the open edge (opposite the spine) of the book. Note that the cover and pages move parallel to each other. A shear stress has thus been induced in the book, with an accompanying *shearing strain.*

It is virtually impossible to induce only one type of stress in a structure. When a wire is stretched, for example, the atoms slide over one another and produce a shearing action. Furthermore, as the wire is stretched, it becomes slightly smaller in diameter. At that point, compressive stresses are being induced. Thus, although one type of stress may predominate, the other two types are invariably present, particularly in the complex pattern of forces exerted on dental structures during mastication.

ELASTICITY

Elasticity is the property of a body that permits it to be deformed by an applied load and then assume its original shape when the load is removed. Sometimes a rubber band is called a "rubber elastic" because it can be stretched and yet return to its original shape when the force or load is removed. In this instance, the strain is completely *elastic.* In contrast, a piece of putty is said to be *inelastic* or *plastic* because when it is deformed, it remains deformed after the load is removed. In other words, the strain is *permanent.*

The rubber band can be permanently deformed as well. If it is stretched too much, it will not return quite to its original length. The maximum stress that a structure can withstand without being permanently deformed is known as the *elastic limit.*

STRESS-STRAIN CURVE

A detailed examination of the relation between stress and strain reveals a number of important properties that are useful in determining the nature and behavior of materials. For example, let us do a tensile stress experiment on a piece of wire used in orthodontics. The cross-sectional area of this wire is 0.01 cm². The wire is placed in a testing apparatus and stretched by gradually applying a tensile load. As this occurs, the stress and strain can be measured.

The results of the experiment are shown in the first two columns of Table 3–1. The wire was stretched by pulling on it with a load of 98 N. The change in length, *deformation*, was measured over a wire length of 5 cm. As shown in the second column of Table 3–1, the change in length was 0.0025 cm. Next, a load of 196 N was applied, and the length of wire was stretched 0.0050 cm, and so on, until the load was 882 N when the wire was stretched a total of 0.0290 cm.

The stress can be calculated for each increment of load. Because the wire was 0.01 cm² in cross-sectional area, the stress under a 98-N load would be

$$\frac{98}{.01} = 98 \text{ MN/m}^2 = 98 \text{ MPa} \qquad 3\text{–}4$$

The stress values at each load are recorded in the third column of Table 3–1.

By definition, the strain is the change in length divided by the length of the wire. Consequently, the result obtained for the change in length (second column) is divided by the length of the wire to determine the strain, as shown in the fourth column.

Suppose that the load is increased to 196 N and that the total increase in length (including that obtained when the 10 kg load was applied) is measured and found to be 0.005 cm. As before, the stress is computed to be

$$\frac{196}{.01} = 196 \text{ MPa} \qquad 3\text{–}5$$

and the strain is

$$\frac{0.005}{5} = 0.001 \text{ cm/cm} = 0.001 \qquad 3\text{–}6$$

As the tensile load on the wire is increased—as shown in the first column of Table 3–1, with resulting increases in total length as in the second column—an important relation between the stress and the strain can be derived. If the third and fourth columns of the table are plotted, with stress values on the vertical axis and the corresponding strain values on the horizontal axis, the graph for wire A shown in Figure 3–4 results.

The curve represents the relation between tensile stress and tensile strain for this wire from stresses of 0 to 882 MPa. A similar relation could be demonstrated between shear stress and shear strain or compressive stress and compressive strain. The stress-strain relationship for metals used in dentistry normally is expressed in terms of tensile stress. An important exception is any brittle material, such as dental amalgam, where it is more convenient to subject the material to a compressive stress in the determination of its stress and strain properties.

TABLE 3–1. Stress-Strain Data for an Orthodontic Wire

Load (N)	Total Change in Length (cm)	Stress (MPa)	Strain (cm/cm)
98	0.0025	98	0.0005
196	0.0050	196	0.0010
294	0.0075	294	0.0015
392	0.0100	392	0.0020
490	0.0125	490	0.0025
588	0.0150	588	0.0030
686	0.0175	686	0.0035
784	0.0215	784	0.0043
882	0.0290	882	0.0058

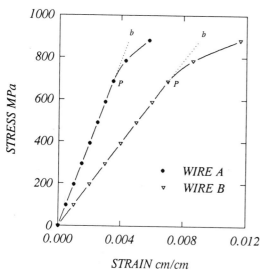

Figure 3–4. Stress-strain curves for two orthodontic wires. The proportional limit *(P)* is the same for the two wires.

PROPORTIONAL LIMIT

By placing a straight-edged ruler on the curve for wire A (see Fig. 3–4), it can be noted that the "curve" is a straight line from 0 to P. If this line is continued upward, the dotted line from P to b results, and it is obvious that the actual stress-strain line begins to curve at P. It is a mathematical fact that when the graph of two quantities results in a straight line, the two quantities are directly proportional to each other. In other words, for all stresses equal to the stress at P or below, each stress is directly proportional to its corresponding strain (Hooke's law). Whenever the stress induced in wire A is increased by 98 MPa, the corresponding increase in strain always is 0.0005 cm/cm. The stress at P is known as the *proportional* limit. At stresses greater than P, the stress is no longer proportional to the strain, as can be noted by studying columns three and four in Table 3–1.

The proportional limit is an important physical property. At stresses that exceed the proportional limit, the structure does not return to its original shape when the external force is removed. In other words, a permanent deformation occurs. The proportional limit occurs at essentially the same stress as the elastic limit, previously discussed. Another term used in the same connection is *yield point*, or yield strength.

Although essentially the same numerically, these three quantities (proportional limit, elastic limit, and yield point) theoretically are measurements of somewhat different properties. For our purposes, the terms can be used interchangeably.

The proportional limit of wire A is 686 MPa (see Fig. 3–4). If the wire is subjected to a tensile stress greater than this, it does not return to its original length. The proportional limit can be determined also for compressive or shear stresses.

When a dental restoration is stressed, the stress should not exceed the proportional limit. Otherwise, the strain or deformation is permanent and the restoration no longer fits. Therefore, a high proportional limit is desired for a material used in a partial denture, a bridge, or any dental restoration or appliance subject to masticatory forces.

MODULUS OF ELASTICITY

If the inlay or bridge is adjacent to another tooth and if the elastic deformation or strain under stress below the proportional limit is considerable, the deformation during function may be sufficient to cause the adjacent teeth to be moved. Likewise, the deformation could be so great that the restoration might be moved away from the adjoining tooth structure, reducing the intimate adaptation originally present. Microleakage would, therefore, increase. Consequently, it is necessary that the restoration be sufficiently stiff or rigid so that its change in shape is negligible when a stress is induced.

The property that defines the rigidity of the material under stresses below the elastic limit is called the *modulus of elasticity*, or *Young's modulus*, and is calculated as

$$\frac{Stress}{Strain} = Modulus\ of\ Elasticity =$$

$$Young's\ Modulus \qquad 3\text{-}7$$

As previously noted, the stress value used in making this calculation must be equal to or less than the proportional limit.

According to this relation, the less the strain for a given stress, the greater the magnitude of the modulus of elasticity. For example, the proportional limit of wire A used for stress-strain curve A shown in Figure 3-4 is 686 MPa. The strain that accompanies the stress is 0.0035 cm/cm, as indicated in Table 3-1. The modulus of elasticity of the wire would be

$$\frac{686}{0.0035} = 196\ GPa^* \qquad 3\text{-}8$$

The modulus of elasticity is expressed in units of force per unit area or stress. This high value indicates that the wire is rigid and stiff.

To better understand the practical significance of this property, it is useful to consider the same property of rubber. When a rubber band is stretched, little stretching force is needed to produce a considerable strain. The rubber band is considered to have high flexibility or low stiffness.

Assume that a rubber band is stretched with a load that results in a stress of 1.37 MPa and a resulting strain of 2 cm/cm. Its modulus of elasticity would be

$$\frac{1.37}{2} = 0.686\ MPa \qquad 3\text{-}9$$

The low modulus indicates a high degree of flexibility with practically no rigidity in contrast to the wire. If the rubber were used for an inlay, every time the rubber inlay con-

---

*1 gigapascal (GPa) = 1000 MPa

tacted food during chewing, it would rebound with little or no breaking up of the food.

Although this illustration is admittedly farfetched, there was an attempt to construct denture teeth that contained a resilient layer of rubber, but they proved to be impractical. This example illustrates the necessity for a high modulus of elasticity for most dental restorative materials. In fact, the higher the modulus of elasticity, the more satisfactory the restoration is likely to be, provided that its proportional limit also is high. In other words, the restoration should not bend, compress, or otherwise be strained perceptibly during mastication.

Consequently, the modulus of elasticity is as important as the proportional limit in judging the proper physical properties for a dental material. To recapitulate, the modulus of elasticity is a measure of the rigidity or stiffness of a material, and the proportional limit is a measure of its ability to be stressed without being permanently deformed. Ideally, both should be high in magnitude for an efficient tooth restorative material. Both are expressed in terms of force per unit area or stress (MPa, psi, etc.).

RELATIONS BETWEEN PROPERTIES

In certain cases, a definite relation exists between certain properties. If one knows the value for one mechanical or physical property of a given material, an accurate prediction often can be made as to the approximate values for other properties of the material.

This is not true when the proportional limit and modulus of elasticity are compared. Examine the curves shown in Figure 3-4. In addition to wire A, which has been used as a basis for discussion so far, a stress-strain curve for another orthodontic wire, B, has been plotted. Note that the proportional limit (P) is the same for both wires. At or below the proportional limit, the strain induced in wire B is twice that of wire A for a given stress. As previously calculated, the modulus of elasticity for wire A is 196 MPa. The modulus of elasticity for wire B is

$$\frac{686}{0.007} = 98 \text{ GPa} \qquad 3\text{--}10$$

Although the stress necessary to permanently deform the two wires is the same, the modulus of elasticity of wire A is higher than that of wire B. Hence, wire A is less flexible and more rigid than wire B.

Selected Reading

Beech, D. R.: Adhesion and adhesives in the oral environment. J. Aust. Coll. Dent. Surg. 5:128, 1977.

Brauer, G. M.: Adhesion and adhesives. In von Fraunhofer, J. (Ed.): *Scientific Aspects of Dental Materials.* London, Butterworths, 1975.

Buonocore, M. G.: *The Use of Adhesives in Dentistry.* Springfield, Ill.: Charles C Thomas, 1975.

Glantz, P.: On wettability and adhesiveness. Odont. Rev. 20(Suppl. 17): 1, 1969.

National Institute of Dental Research: *Adhesive Restorative Dental Materials—II.* Public Health Service Pub. No. 1494. Washington, D.C., U.S. Government Printing Office, 1966.

Van Vlack, L. H.: *Elements of Materials Science.* 4th ed. Reading, Mass., Addison-Wesley, 1980.

Reviewing the Chapter

1. Describe the relation between the internal structure and the properties of a material.

2. List the three states of matter and their characteristics.

3. Describe what is meant by a *space lattice* and its components (e.g., interatomic distance).

4. Explain the difference between *crystalline* and *amorphous* structures. Give examples of each.

5. Name the basic mechanisms of bonding substances together and illustrate dental applications of each.

6. Describe the difference between *adhesion* and *cohesion.*

7. List the various components in an adhesive bond.

8. Describe the two types of adhesion and give examples of each.

9. Explain the wetting phenomenon and describe the factors that influence it.

10. Illustrate the *contact angle test* and discuss its role in predicting adhesion.

11. Discuss all the problems of adhesion as related to tooth structure. Explain the effect of topical fluorides on the surface energy of enamel.

12. Define *stress* and *strain* and list the three types.

13. Construct a stress-strain curve and use it to define proportional limit, elastic limit, yield, and modulus of elasticity. Discuss the dental application of those properties.

14. Discuss the relation between the various mechanical properties of a material.

CHAPTER 4

PROPERTIES OF DENTAL MATERIALS: Permanent Deformation, Rheology, Thermal Properties, and Color

ULTIMATE STRENGTH

DUCTILITY AND MALLEABILITY
Measurement of Ductility

FLOW AND CREEP

TOUGHNESS

HARDNESS

ABRASION RESISTANCE

RELAXATION

RHEOLOGY

THERMAL PROPERTIES
Thermal Conductivity
Coefficient of Thermal Expansion

SELECTION CRITERIA

COLOR
Dimensions of Color

OTHER FACTORS

When fabricating a dental restoration or appliance, the dentist often needs to exceed the proportional limit. The orthodontic steel wire discussed in Chapter 3, for example, must be bent into the shape required for the appliance. A permanent deformation is necessary in this case. Consequently, a study of dental materials must include the part of the stress-strain curve above the point where the material has completely elastic characteristics—that is, where the curve describes the behavior of the wire when it is being permanently deformed.

As noted in Figure 3–4, whenever the stress is greater than the proportional limit, the straight line becomes curved. The relation between stress and strain is no longer in direct proportion.

Because the modulus of elasticity is a property associated with the behavior of a material below the point at which permanent deformation occurs, it cannot be computed at stresses above the elastic limit. When the load is removed at such stress values, the total strain does not disappear, resulting in a permanent deformation of the wire.

If the tensile load is increased progressively beyond the values shown in Table 3–1, the stress finally increases to the extent that the wire is pulled apart or fractured.

A complete stress-strain curve is shown in Figure 4–1. Note that the stress drops slightly before fracture at point BS. Thus, the true strength of this wire is somewhat greater than the stress measurement made at the point of fracture. This discrepancy can be attributed to the fact that the wire continues to stretch during the application of the load. This decreases the cross-sectional area of the wire and thereby lowers the apparent stress required for fracture.

ULTIMATE STRENGTH

The greatest stress a structure can withstand without rupture is known as the *ultimate strength*, or simply, *strength*. (The term *ultimate* often is omitted for the sake of brevity.)

Assuming that the stress and strain are ten-

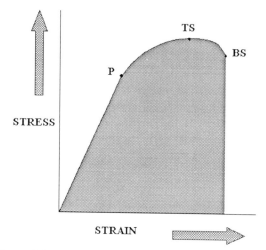

Figure 4–1. Stress-strain curve as determined by application of a tensile stress. The point of permanent deformation, proportional limit, is shown at *P*. The ultimate tensile strength is shown at *TS*. Toughness can be determined by measuring the total shaded area under the curve.

sile, as in Figures 3–4 and 4–1, the maximum stress before fracture is termed the *ultimate tensile strength*—point TS in Figure 4–1. If the stresses are compressive, the maximum stress is called the *ultimate compressive strength* or *crushing strength*. The tensile strength of many materials is lower than the corresponding compressive strength.

DUCTILITY AND MALLEABILITY

Another property of the wire or dental appliance that may determine its usefulness is the extent it can be stretched or bent without fracture. Sometimes the dentist needs to bend or contour a dental appliance to obtain a better fit. The ability of a material to withstand permanent deformation under tensile stress without fracture is known as *ductility*. If the metal is being compressed, its ability to withstand permanent deformation under compressive stress without rupture is known as *malleability*.

If a metal or an alloy can be readily pulled into a wire, for example, it is said to be *ductile*. If the metal can be hammered or rolled into a thin sheet, it is *malleable*. Gold is the most ductile and malleable metal known. Many metals used in dentistry are both malleable and ductile.

Both ductility and malleability are indicative of the ability of a metal to be bent, contoured, or otherwise permanently deformed without fracture. The properties differ somewhat in their general relations to stress. A ductile substance usually is strong, but strength is not a necessary property for malleability. Both strength and ductility are indicative of plasticity. Because ductility is more easily measured, the plasticity of a dental material usually is assessed in terms of its ductility.

Measurement of Ductility

The ductility of a dental material usually is measured by the percentage of change in length after it has been fractured in tension. Using the wire discussed in Chapter 3, two marks are placed on the wire a specified distance apart. The wire then is pulled apart under tension. The broken pieces are removed from the testing machine, and the two ends of the wire are carefully placed back together. The increase in distance between the two marks is measured, and the percentage of elongation is computed as follows:

$$\text{Percentage of Elongation} = \frac{\text{increase in length}}{\text{original length}} \times 100 \qquad 4\text{-}1$$

The percentage of elongation is the percentage of increase in length after the wire has been fractured. It follows, therefore, that the greater the percentage of elongation, the greater the ductility.

Other methods for measuring ductility include determining the reduction in the cross-sectional area of the wire at the fractured ends. The percentage of elongation is the test most commonly used in dentistry.

Low ductility indicates the *brittleness* of a material. A brittle material is not necessarily lacking in strength. A thin fiber of glass may have a small percentage of elongation yet possess great tensile strength.

FLOW AND CREEP

Some materials continue to deform permanently under a load even though the load is held constant. For amorphous or noncrystalline solids, this continuing deformation is referred to as *flow*. The slow bending of a glass rod under its own weight when it is supported at its two ends is an example of flow. Other examples of this type are given in subsequent chapters. As described in Chapter 3, this deformation is related to the fact that amorphous materials are not true solids.

In dental materials, flow is measured under compressive stress. A cylinder of material is placed under a certain compressive stress for a certain time. After the stress is removed, the flow is measured by the percentage of shortening in length of the cylinder at the end of the test. Flow has been used to evaluate the tendency of dental waxes and certain impression materials to deform under a constant load.

Creep, a somewhat synonymous term, is used in reference to crystalline materials. A creep test evaluates the tendency of dental amalgam to deform under a constant applied load. The amalgam specimen is tested after it has completely hardened—which could be 1 day or even 1 week after the amalgam is prepared.

The chapters on amalgam point out that the creep of a commercial alloy may be an important factor in the potential for marginal deterioration of the clinical restoration. In general, creep is significant only for crystalline materials used at temperatures near their melting points.

TOUGHNESS

Another property associated with a material's ability to resist fracture is *toughness*. Very simply, the tougher a material, the more difficult it is to break. Technically, toughness can be defined as the total energy required to cause fracture.

Toughness is measured by calculating the total area under the stress-strain curve. This is demonstrated by the shaded portion in Figure 4–1. Most tough materials are strong and have high ductility.

Certain restorative materials are improved by increasing their toughness. In Chapter 21, the longevity of one type of zinc oxide—eugenol cement—is extended by making it tougher.

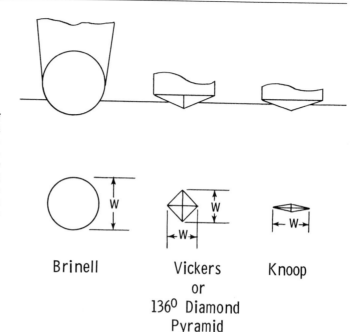

Figure 4–2. Diagrammatic representation of various hardness indenter points impressed into a surface. The dimensions of the indentation that are measured and used to determine the hardness number are arbitrarily designated by *W*. In the Brinell test, a steel ball is used and the diameter of the indentation is measured. The Vickers test makes use of a diamond pyramid point, as does the Knoop.

Brinell

Vickers
or
136° Diamond
Pyramid

Knoop

HARDNESS

Hardness is defined as the resistance of a solid to penetration. Such penetration may range from touching the object with the finger or fingernail to scratching it with a knife blade or similar object.

Hardness is a difficult property to define because it can be measured in many ways. For dental purposes, the surface hardness of a material is measured generally in terms of its resistance to indentation.

A number of instruments are available for determining hardness. Basically, most consist of a small indenter point applied to the surface of the material under a specified load. Then the imprint of the point—the size of the indentation produced—is measured with a microscope. Alternatively, the depth to which the point penetrates into the solid can be measured. The harder the material, the smaller the indentation; the softer the material, the longer the indentation. Three types of indenters commonly used for determining the hardness of dental materials are

diagramed in Figure 4–2. Certain tests are more applicable for one type of material than for another.

The oldest test is the Brinell. A hardened steel ball is pressed into the surface of the material under a specified load. A spherical impression is formed, diagramed in Figure 4–2. The diameter of the impression is measured, and the Brinell Hardness Number (BHN) is obtained by dividing the load placed on the indenter point by the area of the indentation. The harder the material, the smaller the indentation and the higher the hardness number.

Computation of the surface area of a spheroidal indentation is somewhat complex. As a matter of convenience, tables that list the hardness numbers for all diameters of indentations within the range of the instrument have been prepared.

The Brinell test is useful for measuring the hardness of ductile materials, such as metals. Materials that are very brittle or exhibit a great deal of elastic recovery cannot be measured accurately by this test. Glass fractures when indented, as does tooth enamel or dental porcelain.

A different problem arises with materials that have a high degree of elastic recovery. When the point is removed, the material recovers elastically. The depression left by the steel ball is smaller than that which was present before the indenter was removed. Therefore, the size of the impression measured does not accurately depict the actual penetration that occurred or the true hardness of the material. This is readily illustrated by forcing a nail into a piece of rubber. When the nail is removed, the hole left in the rubber is much smaller than the nail.

The Vickers test uses a square-based diamond point instead of a steel ball (see Fig. 4–2). Vickers also is called the diamond pyramid hardness (DPH) test. The diagonals of the indentation are measured and used to calculate its area. As with the Brinell test, the Vickers Hardness Number (VHN) is given by the load divided by the area. Although the sharp cutting edge of this indenter penetrates brittle materials without fracturing, a highly elastic material presents the same problem as with the Brinell test.

The Knoop test (see Fig. 4–2) is widely used in dentistry. As with the Vickers, a diamond indenter is used. The Knoop Hardness Number (KHN) is computed on the basis of the measured long axis of the indentation. The shape of the diamond makes it possible to imprint brittle substances without fracturing the surface. This is shown in Figure 4–3, which shows Knoop indentations on enamel.

The Knoop test is equally versatile for elastic materials. The configuration of the indenter is such that all the elastic recovery occurs across the short axis of indentations. This is somewhat like making a knife cut in a piece of rubber. The rubber spreads the width or thickness of the knife. When the knife is removed, this space disappears but the length of the cut remains. The Knoop

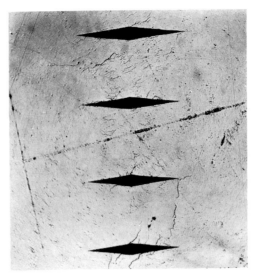

Figure 4–3. Knoop impressions in tooth enamel (× 100).

test can be used with any type of material—whether brittle, such as tooth enamel, or ductile and very elastic, such as dental plastics.

As discussed in subsequent chapters, a hardness test is valuable in assessing the properties of a dental material. The BHN (or KHN) is directly proportional to the tensile strength and proportional limit of dental gold alloys. Consequently, the strength of the alloy can be estimated by measuring hardness without destroying or fracturing the object tested.

ABRASION RESISTANCE

Sometimes hardness is used as a measure of the ability of a material to withstand abrasion and attrition. In general, the harder the material, the less likely it is to wear. This rule has many exceptions, however. A rubber tire is quite soft, but it resists wear better than a wooden tire.

Any laboratory wear test reflects only the wear that occurs under the particular test conditions to which the specimen is subjected. Thus, a dental material that would satisfactorily resist a simulated toothbrush abrasion test might abrade rapidly under the attrition produced during chewing.

Abrasion resistance is a function of many properties. In general, though, relatively hard materials are used whenever possible in the replacement of lost tooth structure because they are less apt to be abraded during mastication and toothbrushing. They are also less likely to deform, as previously noted.

RELAXATION

Whenever a substance is permanently deformed, the internal stresses and strains present are permanent. The atoms in a space lattice are permanently displaced from their regular positions and, therefore, the lattice is disarranged. In amorphous substances, some molecules are too close together and others are too far apart after the substance has been permanently deformed.

Such a situation is not stable. Over time, the displaced atoms slowly but surely move back to their proper relation. The higher the temperature, the faster this diffusion or rearrangement occurs. After the normal regularity is restored, the stresses and strains disappear and the substance is said to have relaxed. This phenomenon is known as *relaxation.*

If a sufficient number of atoms change their positions during relaxation, the shape or contour of the structure changes. It was stated in Chapter 3, for example, that putty is not elastic. If the putty is molded into a certain shape, however, the molecules may be sufficiently displaced that there might be a change in the molded shape when they relax—warpage or *distortion* occurs as a result.

Many examples of relaxation are given in the pages that follow. A wax impression may be taken of a tooth by softening the wax and forcing it over the tooth. When the wax is removed from the tooth, the molecules disarranged by the molding process may relax. The entire impression may be distorted to the extent that it is useless. In the precision work required in dentistry, the distortion causes unacceptable inaccuracy. Considerable space is devoted in subsequent chapters to the importance of technique and steps in manipulation that can minimize such distortions.

RHEOLOGY

Up to this point, our discussion of the physical properties of dental materials has been restricted to the behavior of solids subjected to different types of stress. As mentioned in Chapter 3, many, if not most, of these solid materials were liquids at some point in their dental application.

- A large number of materials, such as direct filling resins, cements, and impression materials, are placed into the mouth in a liquid condition and then undergo a transformation to a solid.
- Other materials, like gypsum products and casting alloys, are shaped as liquids into structures that solidify outside the mouth.
- As previously noted, amorphous solid materials, like waxes and resins, more closely resemble liquids than they do solids and flow under relatively small applied stresses.
- Certain dental materials are used entirely as liquids—prophy pastes, toothpastes, fluoride treatment gels, and acid etching solutions.

The success or failure of these materials may depend as much on their behavior as liquids as it does on their properties as solids. Thus, the manner in which liquids deform or flow when subjected to stress is important in dental applications.

The study of the flow of liquids is the science of *rheology*. A liquid at rest cannot support a shear stress. Once it begins to flow, however, a liquid tends to resist the force causing the motion. This is quite noticeable when trying to stir a thick liquid like molasses. This resistance is called *viscosity*. Different materials have different viscosities. Water, which is easy to stir, has a low viscosity compared with molasses.

The viscosity of most liquids decreases rapidly as the temperature is raised. If the material exhibits *thixotropic* behavior, viscosity also can depend on the previous mechanical treatment of that material. If a thixotropic material is stirred rapidly and its viscosity is measured, a lower value is found than if the same material is allowed to rest for several hours before measurement. In other words, thixotropic materials become thin when stirred but are thick on standing.

Prophy pastes often are advertised as "thixotropic." Such a paste does not tend to drip or fall from the brush or cup but spreads easily over the tooth once the handpiece is activated.

THERMAL PROPERTIES

Thermal Conductivity

One important thermal property of a dental material is its *thermal conductivity*, or ability to transmit heat. Thermal conductivity is measured by determining the rate at which heat can be transmitted through a given cross-sectional area of a specimen of the material during a given time interval. The higher the value, the greater the thermal conductivity.

When used for constructing an artificial denture, a poor thermal conductor prevents heat exchange between the soft tissues and the mouth itself. With such a material, the patient does not have a normal sense of hot and cold while eating or drinking. From this standpoint, a denture base made of metal, which conducts heat readily, is more natural and pleasant than one made from a plastic.

For a metallic tooth restorative material, the situation is reversed. Here the thermal conductivity should be as low as possible. The temperature in the mouth may vary from close to 0° C (32° F) when a person is eating ice cream to as high as 60° C (140° F) when drinking hot coffee. These extremes in temperature can produce sensitivity or pain and even permanent injury to the tooth pulp. Enamel and dentin, natural tooth substances, have relatively low thermal conductivities and thus insulate the pulp from temperature changes in the mouth. Ideally, a restorative material should be an effective insulator and provide protection from such thermal shocks. Most metals have relatively high thermal conductivities.

In many situations, the cavity preparation is quite deep, with little dentin separating a metallic restoration from the pulp. Because the diffusion of heat or cold through a substance is governed not only by the material's inherent thermal conductivity but also by its thickness, a thin layer of dentin is not adequate to provide insulation from the metal conductor. The effect of thickness is easily appreciated by thinking of the use of pot holders for handling hot cooking utensils. Although the holders are composed of materials that are good insulators, frequently two instead of one are needed to avoid being burned.

The dentist often adds an additional layer of insulating material on top of the dentin to provide adequate protection to the pulp. The thickness of this insulating layer and of the remaining dentin is as important as the thermal conductivity of the substances themselves. This point is discussed at length in Chapter 21.

Coefficient of Thermal Expansion

Another important thermal property is the amount of dimensional change that takes place in the restorative material and the tooth during temperature fluctuations in the mouth.

Almost all materials expand when they are heated and contract when they are cooled. The extent of thermal expansion and contraction is a characteristic of each particular material. The thermal expansion (or contraction) of a material is measured by the *linear coefficient of thermal expansion*, which is the change in length of a material per unit length when the temperature is increased 1° C. A few substances have a negative coefficient of thermal expansion—they actually contract slightly when heated.

The linear coefficients of thermal expansion for tooth structure and a number of dental materials are shown in Table 4–1. As can be noted, the amount of expansion for 1 mm of material with a 1° C change is small. Nevertheless, such a change can be important under certain circumstances.

If the tooth and the restorative material expand the same amount when their temperatures change, the dentist would have little reason to consider dimensional change. As noted from Table 4–1, however, the linear coefficients of thermal expansion for teeth and restorative materials are not equal. Not one of the materials expands or contracts exactly the same amount as the tooth,

although the change in temperature of tooth and restoration is the same.

Amalgam's linear coefficient of expansion is 2.2 times greater than that of the tooth (see Table 4–1). This means that when hot food is taken into the mouth, the amalgam expands more than twice as much as the tooth. In the last column in this table, the coefficient of thermal expansion of the dental material is divided by that of the tooth crown. Dental amalgam also contracts 2.2 times as much as the tooth when both are in contact with cold foods. In the latter instance, the space between the restoration and the tooth might be increased to the extent that mouth fluids or bacteria could seep into the space, with caries eventually resulting.

Similar ratios between the thermal changes of other restorative materials and the tooth are given in Table 4–1. Note that only the glass ionomer cement expands and contracts about the same amount as tooth structure. In contrast, restorations with acrylic resin (PMMA) may expand and contract 7.1 times as much as tooth structure. These materials can be used by the dentist because other factors, to be discussed later, aid in the reduction of the discrepancies. As discussed in Chapter 10, acrylic resin has been replaced by newer formulations (composites). One advantage of these newer materials is that they have a lower coefficient of thermal expansion, as seen in Table 4–1.

The ideal situation of equal thermal expansion and contraction of tooth and restoration is not as yet realized in practice, and this is of concern to the dentist. This factor is discussed further in other chapters.

SELECTION CRITERIA

The practical importance of some of the discussion presented in these last two chapters might well be questioned. The proportional limit, modulus of elasticity, and tensile

TABLE 4–1. Linear Coefficients of Thermal Expansion (α) for Various Types of Dental Materials

Material	α (°K^{-1} × 10^{-6})	α Relative to Tooth
Tooth	11.4	1.0
Dental amalgam	25.0	2.2
Acrylic resin (PMMA)	81.0	7.1
Pit and fissure sealant	85.0	7.5
Composite resin	35.0	3.0
Direct filling gold	14.0	1.2
Gold casting alloy	15.0	1.3
Aluminous porcelain	6.6	0.7
Silicone impression material	210.0	19.0
Glass ionomer cement	10.2	0.9

strength of the gold alloy to be used in dentistry, for example, are tested in the form of a rod under tensile stress. The question may be: How is such a test related to the performance of the same alloy in the form of an inlay cemented in the mouth?

The tests that have been described can be related to the dentist's experience. A certain dental material has been found to be satisfactory over a long period. This material then can be subjected to the tests described, and its proportional limit, modulus of elasticity, and similar properties determined.

When a new material becomes available, its properties can be determined and compared with the properties of the material whose past clinical performance has been satisfactory. If the properties of the new material are equal or superior to those of the old one, the dentist can use the new material with reasonable assurance that it is at least as good.

It is not necessary, therefore, to subject a particular material to the same type of stresses as those found in the mouth. Nor is it necessary to test it in the shape of a crown or a bridge. Tensile testing of the material in the form of a rod or compression testing of a cylinder on a comparative basis usually is sufficient to ensure that the material will serve adequately as a bridge, denture, or other dental appliance.

The American Dental Association (ADA) Specifications have been formulated on the basis of such judgments. As discussed in Chapter 1, these specifications provide the most valuable criteria of selection when choosing materials. If an ADA Specification or comparable specification exists for a certain material, materials certified to meet that specification should be chosen.

COLOR

The preceding discussion has been concerned with those properties required to permit a material to properly restore the function of damaged or missing tissues. An increasingly important goal of modern dentistry is to give restorations and prosthetic appliances the color and appearance of the natural teeth and soft tissues. Aesthetic or cosmetic dentistry is assuming an ever-growing priority. The search for an ideal general purpose, direct-filling, tooth-colored restorative material is one of the challenges of current research. This section briefly discusses the underlying scientific principles involved in aesthetic dentistry.

Light is a form of radiant energy that can be detected by the human eye. The eye is sensitive to certain wavelengths only, referred to as visible light, as seen in Figure 4–4. The combinations of wavelengths present in a beam of light determine the property called *color.*

The human eye cannot detect other wavelengths of light, such as ultraviolet light and infrared. For an object to be visible, it must either give off light or reflect light shown on it from an external source. Dental interest concerns reflected light.

The phenomenon of vision—and certain terminology—can be illustrated by considering the response of the human eye to light coming from an object. The light is focused on the retina of the eye and converted into nerve impulses that are transmitted to the brain.

The eye is most sensitive to light in the green-yellow range and least sensitive at either extreme—red or blue—as shown in Figure 4–5. (For this reason, fire trucks now are commonly painted yellow-green instead of the traditional red.) These signals are processed by the brain to produce the perception of color. In a scientific sense, one might compare the human eye to an exceptionally sensitive instrument for analyzing and differentiating color.

Although this type of knowledge explains the nature of the light coming from an object

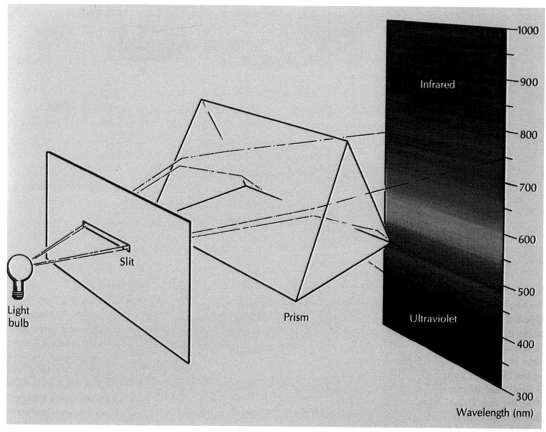

Figure 4–4. Spectrum of visible light ranging in wavelength from 400 nm (violet) to 700 nm (red). One nanometer (nm) is 10^{-9} m. (From Phillips, R. W.: *Skinner's Science of Dental Materials,* 9th ed. Philadelphia, W. B. Saunders Co., 1991.)

and the response of the eye, it does not relate to the usual concept of color and is not useful in specifying the color of an object. The following section describes the terms used in communicating color information. The color of a tooth as seen by the dentist, for example, must be related to the laboratory technician to duplicate that appearance in a crown or bridge.

Dimensions of Color

Color can be described in terms of its three components: *hue, chroma,* and *value.*

Hue refers to the characteristic associated with the color of an object, whether it is blue, green, red, or some other color. Hue relates to the predominant wavelengths present and the names associated with those wavelengths, as seen in Figure 4–6.

Chroma indicates the strength for a particular hue. The higher the chroma, the more vivid the color (see Figure 4–6).

Value is associated with the luminance of an object—how bright or dark it is. On a color television set, for example, value would be the adjustment knob to control brightness. In the same manner, one can recognize the control knobs that regulate hue and chroma of the television picture.

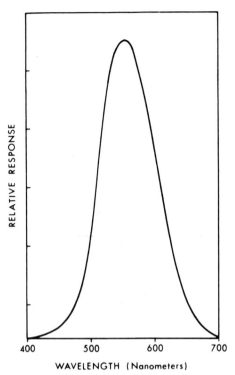

Figure 4–5. Relative response of the human eye at different wavelengths. (With permission from O'Brien, W. J., and Ryge, G.: *An Outline of Dental Materials.* Philadelphia, W. B. Saunders Co., 1978 [Adapted from Billmeyer, F. W., Jr., and Saltzman, M.: *Principles of Color Technology.* New York, Interscience, 1966].)

Color matching in the dental operatory or laboratory usually is done by the use of a *shade guide*, like the example seen in Figure 4–7. This guide is used in much the same way as paint chips are used to select the color for a house paint. The dentist uses the guide to specify the color to the dental technician, who can then mix the correct shade. The guide shown in this figure, originally developed for Vita porcelain, has been adopted for use with composite restorative resins and glass ionomer cements.

Objects of dental interest are visible because they reflect light from an external source. The color of these objects depends on the nature of the incident light. Most people have made that observation when attempting to match the color of articles of clothing. A color match that was good under the fluorescent light in a store looked very different when viewed outside under natural light. This effect, called *metamerism*, is common in dentistry. Color matching to a shade guide should be checked under at least two different light sources, one of which is natural daylight, if at all possible.

In addition to the considerations mentioned, natural teeth absorb light of wavelengths too short to be visible—in the ultraviolet region in Figure 4–4. This energy is released at wavelengths in the visible part of the spectrum between 400 and 450 nm. This blue-white *fluorescence* contributes to the vital appearance of natural teeth. A restorative material that does not duplicate this ability appears dull or even dark when compared with adjacent tooth structure. This poses additional color-matching problems because incandescent lamps, such as operatory lights, contain little, if any, ultraviolet energy.

OTHER FACTORS

The previous discussion was limited to the criteria used in the selection of a dental material on the basis of its mechanical and physical properties. Still other factors must be considered before the dentist and auxiliary choose a material.

Figure 4–6. Color wheel showing the panorama of hues (colors) and how they blend into one another. If the wheel is sectioned along the A-B diameter, the lower figure results. This shows variation in chroma horizontally and value vertically. (Courtesy of Minolta Camera Co., Ltd., Osaka, Japan.) (From Phillips, R. W.: *Skinner's Science of Dental Materials*, 9th ed. Philadelphia, W. B. Saunders Co., 1991.)

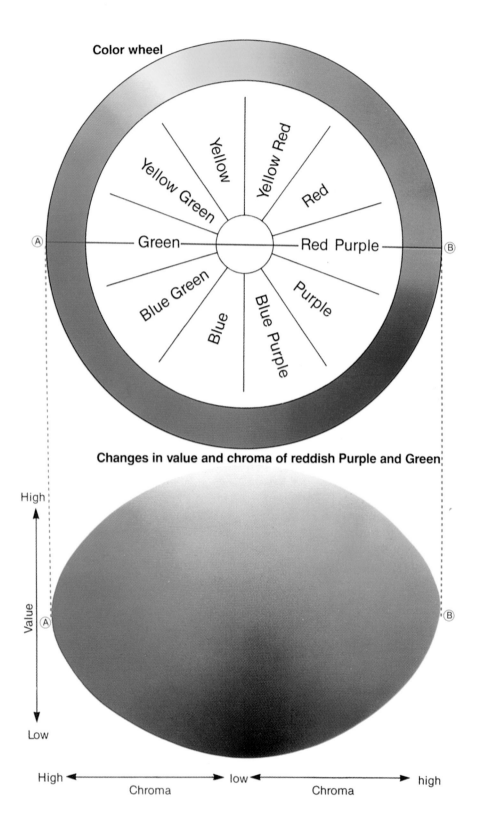

Color wheel

Yellow
Yellow Red
Yellow Green
Red
Green
Red Purple
Blue Green
Purple
Blue
Blue Purple

Ⓐ

Ⓑ

Changes in value and chroma of reddish Purple and Green

High

Value

Ⓐ

Ⓑ

Low

High ← → low ← → high

Chroma

Chroma

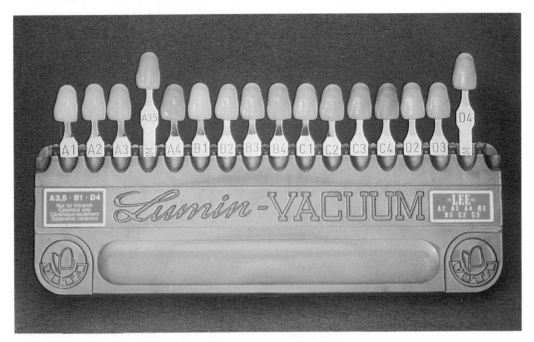

Figure 4–7. Shade guide used for selecting color of a dental restorative material. (Courtesy of Dr. Lloyd L. Miller.) (From Phillips, R. W.: *Skinner's Science of Dental Materials*, 9th ed. Philadelphia, W. B. Saunders Co., 1991.)

Note that the auxiliary is included as an important factor in this process. Sales representatives often spend most of their time in the office talking to the auxiliary personnel about the merits of a material. The auxiliary is nearly always involved in the manipulation of the material, which plays a key role in its properties. Also, an appreciation of the relation between properties and clinical performance provides a useful background for communication with the patient and the dentist, as discussed in Chapter 1.

In addition to the physical properties, one must have assurance as to the safety of the material—its toxicity and compatibility with oral tissues. Biological testing is an integral part of ADA Specifications and a requirement for approval by the federal Food and Drug Administration.

The material selected must be one that can be readily handled by the dentist or the auxiliary. People differ in their preferences about handling characteristics, such as how fast the material hardens and the desired fluidity or ease of trimming or carving. A research study on the flow of dental cements had clinicians mix different materials with varying amounts of powder and liquid. The operator then rated the mix as too thick, too thin, or just right. Opinion about which materials fell into each group varied considerably. These factors are important considerations in the selection of a material.

Assuming that the new product under consideration has the necessary physical and biological properties and can be handled easily, one other question remains to be answered: the clinical documentation. Although properties provide excellent screening tests for predicting behavior in the oral cavity, the final test is to evaluate the performance by placing the material in the mouth in carefully controlled studies. This is particularly essential when the composition of the material varies from previously established formulations.

In the following chapters, attention is given to the importance and proper weighing of the physical and biological properties of dental materials, their manipulative characteristics, and the clinical evaluations of their effectiveness.

Selected Reading

Harper, R. H., R. J. Schnell, M. L. Swartz, and R. W. Phillips.: In vivo measurements of thermal diffusion through restorations of various materials. J. Prosthet. Dent. 43:180, 1980.

McLean, J. W.: *The Science and Art of Dental Ceramics.* Vol. 1. *The Nature of Dental Ceramics and Their Clinical Use.* Chicago, Quintessence Publishing Co., 1979.

Reviewing the Chapter

1. Illustrate how *toughness* is measured and explain its dental significance.
2. Illustrate how *ultimate strength* is measured and explain its dental significance.
3. Define *ductility* and *malleability* and explain how they are measured. How are these properties used in formulating and selecting dental materials?
4. Explain *flow* and *creep.* Give examples of the importance of these properties.
5. Explain the general method used in measuring hardness and list the various types of tests.
6. Discuss the relation between *hardness* and *abrasion resistance* of a material. What are the limitations in measuring abrasion resistance of a dental restorative material?
7. Explain the *relaxation phenomenon* and the resulting distortion.
8. Identify the two important thermal properties of dental materials and explain the dental significance of each.
9. Describe all the various considerations involved in the selection of restorative materials.
10. Define the term *rheology* and explain why the mechanical behavior of liquids is important in dentistry.
11. Explain what the property called *viscosity* measures. Is the viscosity of a particular material always the same? What might cause the viscosity to change?
12. Explain why the *color* of a dental material is an important consideration in restorative dentistry.
13. List the factors that affect the perceived color of a particular object.
14. Define *hue, value,* and *chroma.*
15. How does a dentist specify color to the technician or dental laboratory?
16. Define *metamerism* and give an example. What precaution should be observed when attempting to match color in the dental operatory?

CHAPTER 5

DENTAL GYPSUM PRODUCTS:
Dental Plaster and Stone

DENTAL PLASTER
Manufacture of Plaster
Setting of Hemihydrate
Water-Powder Ratio

SETTING TIME
Control of Setting Time

SETTING EXPANSION
Control of Setting Expansion

STRENGTH

HARDNESS AND ABRASION
RESISTANCE

MANIPULATION
Proportioning
Mixing

CLASSIFICATION OF GYPSUM
PRODUCTS
Impression Plasters (Type I)
Model Plaster (Type II)
Dental Stone (Types III and IV)
Dental Stone (Type V)

CONSTRUCTION OF THE CAST OR
MODEL

CARE OF GYPSUM PRODUCTS, DIES,
AND CASTS

INFECTION CONTROL CONCERNS

Gypsum, the dihydrate of calcium sulfate ($CaSO_4 \cdot 2H_2O$), is the most common sulfate mineral. It occurs widely in a massive form known as rock-gypsum, a dull-colored rock. Less common is the fine-grained variety, *alabaster*.

If gypsum is ground and heated *(calcined)*, some water is removed to form plaster or plaster of Paris. The powder then can be mixed with water to re-form gypsum or set plaster. Plaster is widely used in industry for building interiors, forming molds to shape pottery, and so forth. In its pure form, it is compounded into dental plaster for the construction of dental appliances and restorations.

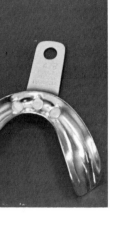

Figure 5-1. Impression trays for obtaining impressions of the upper arch *(left)* and the lower arch *(right)* of an edentulous mouth.

DENTAL PLASTER

Dental plaster never is used for mouth restoration. As a laboratory material, it plays a vital role in a number of dental procedures. In many situations, the dentist needs an accurate three-dimensional model of the patient's dentition. In orthodontics, for example, these models are part of the patient's clinical record along with the dental chart and radiographs. The orthodontist uses these models to plan treatment, design and construct appliances, and follow the changes in tooth alignment through the course of treatment. When a prosthodontist constructs an artificial denture, the patient cannot be kept in the dental office during the considerable time needed for denture construction. The dentist also cannot construct the denture directly in the patient's mouth. A model of the endentulous mouth is required.

Dental gypsum products, plaster and stone, are used to construct these models. The student is probably familiar with a similar use for plaster of Paris. This material is sold in hobby shops, along with rubber molds, for various small craft objects. The plaster is mixed and poured into the mold and hardens into a three-dimensional object.

The dental procedure is similar. The dentist first constructs the mold of the patient's mouth, called an *impression.* At one time, plaster commonly was used as the material for making the mold. Today, more convenient materials are used (see chapters on impression materials). To use plaster as an impression material, the dentist follows this procedure:

1. An *impression tray,* shown in Figure 5-1, is selected. The tray on the left resembles the contour of the upper arch in reverse, and the other tray, the contour of the lower arch in reverse.

2. The dentist mixes the plaster and water to form a paste-like mass, which is placed in the impression tray.

3. The filled tray is then carefully placed in the patient's mouth and the soft mix is impressed against the mouth tissues.

4. When plaster is mixed with water, it is said to *set* or harden by chemical reaction. When the plaster sets, the *impression* of the mouth is withdrawn and used in subsequent operations.

A typical impression of an upper arch made with plaster is shown in Figure 5–2. Note that it is a *negative* reproduction of the mouth structures.

To obtain a *positive*—a three-dimensional

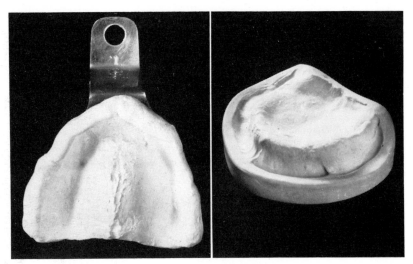

Figure 5-2. Plaster impression of an edentulous upper arch.
Figure 5-3. Stone cast obtained from the impression.

model of the patient's mouth—a mix of plaster and water could be poured into the impression and allowed to set. Generally, however, a similar but harder material known as *dental stone* is used.

When the impression and the material added are separated, an exact model or *cast* of the patient's mouth is obtained (Fig. 5–3). With a cast or model of both the upper and the lower arches, the dentist can construct the denture in the patient's absence.

A similar technique was used to obtain models of mouths that have natural dentition, but many problems were caused by the use of plaster or other brittle materials. The plaster impression had to be broken into pieces to remove it from the mouth! Modern dentistry has *elastomeric* (rubbery) impression materials available. Today, the use of plaster is limited to pouring the impressions, made from these elastomeric materials.

Manufacture of Plaster

Knowing how plaster is made is essential in understanding why plaster sets when mixed with water.

Gypsum is mined. It is then ground into small pieces, placed in huge kettles, and heated. When the temperature reaches 100° to 120° C (230° to 250° F), steam (water vapor) is driven off. The reaction is as follows:

$$2CaSO_4 \cdot 2H_2O + heat \rightarrow (CaSO_4)_2 \cdot H_2O + 3H_2O$$

gypsum   + heat → plaster   + steam 5-1
  (calcium sulfate   (calcium sulfate
    dihydrate)   hemihydrate)*

Note that the chemical change is simply a matter of heating the gypsum so that it loses three molecules of water to form calcium sulfate hemihydrate. The water suddenly leaves the particles as steam, producing pressure that breaks up the particles into finer crystals. These are then dried and ground further to obtain the variety of particle sizes necessary to provide a plastic mass when the powder is mixed with water (Fig. 5–4).

Two basic types of calcium sulfate hemihydrate are manufactured. Plaster, as just described, is made by heating the gypsum at

*Calcium sulfate hemihydrate also is written $CaSO_4 \cdot \frac{1}{2} H_2O$.

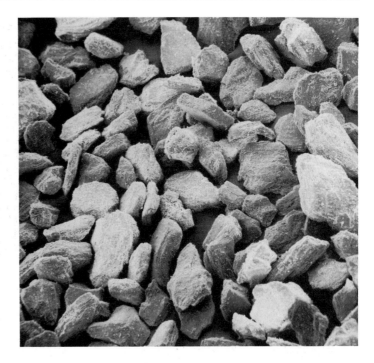

Figure 5–4. Powder particles of plaster of Paris. Crystals are irregular in shape and have a porous, spongy surface (× 400). The fine particles normally present have been removed. (Courtesy of B. Giammara and R. Neiman.)

atmospheric pressure. Sometimes it is referred to as the *beta-hemihydrate (β)* form. Another method involves heating gypsum under steam pressure. The end product is designated *alpha-hemihydrate (α)*, which is the essential constituent of *dental stone.* If the gypsum is dehydrated in a solution of calcium chloride, a somewhat smoother crystal type is created—also called the α-hemihydrate form (Fig. 5–5). This product is principally used in stones that serve as dies used in the fabrication of cast metal restorations.

Remember that plaster and dental stones are identical chemically. As shown in Figures 5–4 and 5–5, however, the shapes of the powder particles are different. The powder particles of plaster are rough, randomly shaped, and porous. Similar particles of stone are smooth, well crystallized, and less porous.

Setting of Hemihydrate

If either dental stone or plaster is mixed with water, a hard substance is formed. According to the reaction just described, when the gypsum is heated, either α-hemihydrate (dental stone) or β-hemihydrate (plaster) is formed and water is driven off. It follows that if water is added to either type of hemihydrate, the reaction can be reversed, again forming gypsum:

$$(CaSO_4)_2 \cdot H_2O + 3H_2O \rightarrow 2CaSO_4 \cdot 2H_2O + heat$$

plaster/stone + water → gypsum + heat
(calcium sulfate   (calcium sulfate   5–2
hemihydrate)   dihydrate)

The gypsum is the hard, rigid material that forms the impression or cast as previously described.

Heat also is a product of this reaction. This heat is known as the *exothermic heat* of reaction. The amount of heat given off during the reaction is exactly equal to the amount of heat required to form the hemihydrate from the dihydrate (gypsum).

The setting reaction is quite interesting. Plaster is slightly soluble in water; 0.8 gram of plaster will dissolve in 100 milliliters of

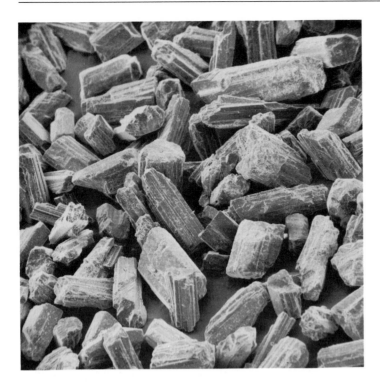

Figure 5–5. Powder particles of dental stone. Crystals are more regular in shape and have a smoother surface than those of plaster. Fine particles have been removed, as in Figure 5–4 (× 400). (Courtesy of B. Giammara and R. Neiman.)

water,* forming a saturated solution. This dissolved plaster immediately reacts with water by the setting reaction shown above to form a solution of gypsum in water. That solution is supersaturated with respect to gypsum, however, because the solubility of gypsum is only 0.2 g/100 ml of water. Thus, gypsum precipitates from the solution. Plaster continues to dissolve, accompanied by the precipitation of more gypsum, usually on crystals that have already formed. These crystals continue to grow until all the plaster has turned to gypsum.

Under the microscope, the crystals of gypsum form in clusters, branching from a common center, as shown in Figure 5–6. The centers of the crystal growth are *nuclei of crystallization*. In this case, the nuclei may be small gypsum crystals, which were not changed to the hemihydrate during the orig-

inal heating or calcination. These gypsum nuclei act as seeds from which the gypsum crystals grow.

Water-Powder Ratio

The situation depicted in Figure 5–6 is unrealistic because the centers of nuclei of crystallization are far apart. In practice, every milliliter of hemihydrate-water mixture contains a large number of nuclei close together. The nuclei are so close together that the gypsum crystals intermesh as they grow and become entangled with one another during growth. This intermeshing gives the final gypsum product its strength and rigidity. Figure 5–7 does not represent a usable mix of plaster. Excess water was used so that the individual crystals could be seen.

The amount of water used when mixing a gypsum material affects the strength and hardness of the gypsum—the more water used, the fewer gypsum crystals per unit vol-

*In the remainder of the text, the term gram is abbreviated g, and the term milliliter is abbreviated ml.

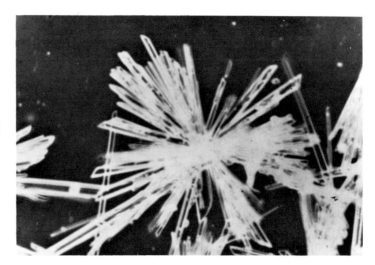

Figure 5–6. Gypsum crystals forming during the reaction between plaster and water in a dilute solution of hemihydrate. (Courtesy of D. C. Smith.)

ume. Conversely, the less water used, within certain limits, the more gypsum crystals created and the greater the intermeshing. The greater intermeshing increases the strength, rigidity, and hardness.

For best results, therefore, the water and powder should be properly proportioned to control the physical properties of the plaster or stone. A typical proportion for dental stone is 30 ml of water per 100 g of dental stone powder. Because 1 ml of water weighs 1 g, the proportion of water to powder (dental stone)—known as the *W/P ratio*—is 30/100 or 0.30. If 28 ml of water were mixed with 100 g of powder, the W/P ratio would be 0.28.

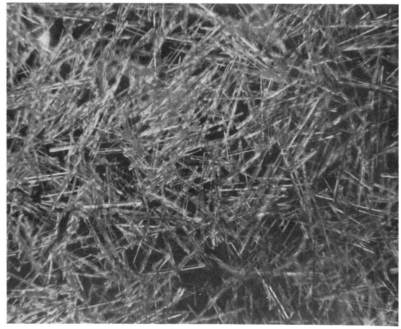

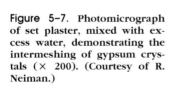

Figure 5–7. Photomicrograph of set plaster, mixed with excess water, demonstrating the intermeshing of gypsum crystals ($\times$ 200). (Courtesy of R. Neiman.)

The optimum W/P ratios for dental stone and plaster differ markedly. As noted earlier in this chapter, the β-hemihydrate powder particles are irregular in shape and porous, whereas the α-hemihydrate powder particles are regular in shape and not porous (see Figs. 5–4 and 5–5). There is a minimum W/P ratio that can be used—sufficient water must be provided for the setting reaction to take place. For that reaction to occur, the minimum water required is 18.62 ml for 100 g of hemihydrate. Additional water usually is needed to wet the powder particles so that they can be mixed into the water and the mix will pour into the impression or impression tray. This excess water, similar to a lubricant, is known as *excess water* or *free water*.

Imagine two vessels of the same volume and shape. Suppose that one of the vessels is filled with small spherical sponges and the other vessel is filled with Ping-Pong balls of the same size. Now suppose that water is poured into both of the containers in sufficient amount to float the sponges and the balls so that they can be stirred and poured from the container. Which vessel requires more water?

In a similar manner, dental plaster requires more water than does an identical weight of dental stone because of the rough surface and porosity of the β-hemihydrate particles in contrast to the smooth, dense α-hemihydrate particles.

Consequently, the lowest possible W/P ratio for most dental plasters is about 0.50, whereas that of some dental die stones may be as low as 0.19.

SETTING TIME

The setting time for a gypsum material can be defined as the elapsed time between the start of mixing and the time when the set material hardens sufficiently to use. The dentist needs adequate working time to mix the plaster, to fill the tray, and to carry the material into the mouth before the plaster has hardened unduly. An impression plaster should set in 3 to 4 minutes from the time mixing begins. If the plaster impression previously discussed required 20 to 30 minutes to set in the patient's mouth, the discomfort to the patient would make its use impractical.

The term "hard enough to use" is subjective and depends on the type of gypsum product and its application. For quantitative purposes, the hardening rate usually is measured with some type of penetration test similar to the concept of measuring hardness described in Chapter 4.

Because the setting reaction begins as soon as the water and gypsum product are mixed, the crystallization of dihydrate is a continuous process until all the hemihydrate has reacted. The working time can be defined as the time elapsed from the start of mixing until the mix has begun to thicken appreciably. This is a subjective term, which also depends on the application. In general, the working time and setting time change in a similar manner. The following discussion about the relation of hardening rate and handling variables is related to the setting time.

Control of Setting Time

As might be expected from the general theory, the greater the number of nuclei of crystallization per unit volume, the faster the gypsum crystals intermesh and the sooner the plaster or stone reaches a consistency that resists penetration. In other words, the setting time is shortened. With this principle in mind, one could predict the factors that influence the setting time.

MANUFACTURING PROCESS. If more gypsum (dihydrate) crystals are left in the plaster after manufacture, there will be a greater number of nuclei of crystallization resulting in a shorter setting time.

W/P RATIO. As previously described, the addition of more water reduces the number of nuclei per unit volume and, consequently, the setting time is prolonged. Therefore, the greater the W/P ratio, the longer the setting time, and vice versa.

MIXING. Within practical limits, the longer and the more rapidly the gypsum product is mixed, the shorter the setting time. Nuclei and gypsum crystals that start to form are broken up by the mixing and so the number or concentration of the nuclei increases.

TEMPERATURE. The effect of the temperature of the water used for mixing on setting time is erratic and varies with the particular product. Little change usually is seen between 0° and 50° C. Above 50° C, the setting time usually increases.

ACCELERATORS AND RETARDERS. The best method for regulating the setting time is to add chemicals to the plaster or dental stone. This is done during the manufacturing of the material. If the chemical shortens the setting time, it is called an *accelerator.* If it lengthens the setting time, it is known as a *retarder.*

- Potassium sulfate is the best accelerator. Ordinary table salt accelerates the setting if it is used in small amounts. If too much is used, it increases the setting time.
- Borax is an excellent retarder, although sodium citrate is used principally in dental stones. As discussed in Chapter 7, certain colloids or gels also retard the setting of dental stones.

SETTING EXPANSION

All gypsum products expand during setting. This setting expansion normally is 0.1 to 0.3 per cent when measured between two points. If the hemihydrate is allowed to set under water, however, the expansion may be two or more times greater than in air. This latter expansion is called *hygroscopic setting expansion* to distinguish it from the normal type.

Control of Setting Expansion

As previously described, plaster may be used to obtain an impression of the mouth, with the use of an impression tray. If the impression expands during setting, an error is introduced because its final form is larger than the mouth parts involved. More than likely, the impression also will be warped because the setting mass is restricted from expanding in certain directions by the impression tray.

If a cast is constructed in this impression with a dental stone that has considerable setting expansion, the cast also will warp for the same reason, as shown in Figure 5–8. If a denture is constructed on this cast, its palate will be too high, and the denture will rock on the hard palate in the mouth. Under these circumstances, the setting expansion is harmful and should be reduced or eliminated.

A similar argument can be followed for dental stone used to construct a die on which a metal cast restoration is fabricated. In this case, the errors that can be tolerated are even smaller because a rigid metal casting is being made to fit accurately on a rigid tooth. Although setting expansion cannot be eliminated, the manufacturer can reduce it

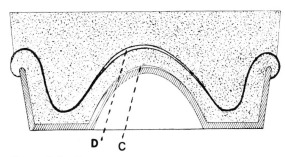

Figure 5–8. If a stone cast is constructed in a warped impression *(C)*, further warpage occurs at *D*.

considerably with the use of accelerators and retarders. Potassium sulfate, for example, not only accelerates the set but also reduces setting expansion. The manufacturer adds potassium sulfate to the stone, but then the setting becomes too fast. This effect can be counteracted by adding a retarder, such as borax or a citrate, both of which also reduce setting expansion. In this manner, setting expansion of some stones can be reduced to as low as 0.08%.

STRENGTH

With the exception of impression plaster, great strength often is desired in a dental plaster or stone. Inadequate strength may result in fracture or distortion of the cast or mold during fabrication of the dental appliance.

Because set gypsum is a brittle material, the strength of a gypsum product usually is determined under compressive stress. The compressive strength of a set gypsum product is directly related to the amount of water used in mixing. The greater the W/P ratio, the weaker the product.

Such a relation might have been predicted on the basis of the previous discussions. The more water used, the farther apart the gypsum crystals and, consequently, the less the intermeshing of the crystals. Because crystalline intermeshing provides strength and rigidity, the strength is reduced in such a case.

As previously noted, dental plaster requires more water for mixing than does dental stone. It follows, therefore, that the dental stone cast is stronger than a cast made with dental plaster. The maximum compressive strength of a set dental plaster is about 27.5 MPa (3980 psi), whereas the maximum compressive strength of a set dental die stone may be 127.5 MPa (18,000 psi). For this reason, dental stone rather than plaster is used to construct casts and dies.

The strength of a gypsum product is decreased if any water is present in excess of that needed for the chemical reaction with the hemihydrate. Because excess water is always needed so that the material can be mixed and poured, such water is present in varying amounts according to the W/P ratio used. This excess water is referred to as *free water*, as previously noted, because it is not used in the setting reaction.

Immediately after a gypsum material has hardened, this excess water is present between the crystals of dihydrate. The strength of the material when free water is present is known as its *wet strength*. After about 24 hours, the free water has evaporated, and the cast is completely dried. The strength measured then is known as the *dry strength*. The dry strength of a gypsum product is approximately twice its wet strength. A gypsum cast or die should never be subjected to high stresses until the material is completely dry.

HARDNESS AND ABRASION RESISTANCE

Hardness of gypsum materials usually is measured in the conventional manner described in Chapter 4. A hardness test suitable for a brittle material should be used. Decreasing the W/P ratio used to mix plaster or stone increases its hardness as well as its strength.

The hardness and strength of gypsum products are directly related. The factors that increase or decrease strength do the same to hardness.

The abrasion resistance of stone is an important property in certain dental procedures. If a wax pattern is to be carved and finished on a stone die, the metal instrument used to carve the wax may abrade and destroy adjacent areas of the stone die. In such situations, the need for the stone to have a high resistance to abrasion may be more important than its strength or hardness. For this reason, proper manipulation is essential to assure maximum abrasion resistance. Special treatments can be used to increase the wear resistance of the stone surface, but they usually have only a modest effect on that property and may adversely affect other desirable properties, such as dimensional accuracy and surface detail.

MANIPULATION

Application of the basic principles presented to proper manipulation technique is discussed in the following paragraphs.

Proportioning

The effect of the W/P ratio on the properties of the set gypsum product has been discussed repeatedly. If the strength, setting time, and setting expansion of the plaster or stone cast are to be properly controlled, *the powder and water must be proportioned by weighing on a balance.*

Because 1 ml of water weighs 1 g, water can be measured accurately by volume, but powder can be measured by weight only. A cupful of flour may vary considerably in amount according to whether the flour is placed in the cup lightly or packed tightly. Similarly, the plaster or stone powder must be weighed to obtain an exact amount.

Nor can one mix the powder and water by eye and obtain the best possible results. If the mix is too thin and more powder added after the stirring begins, one gets two different mixes, each crystallizing at a different time. If the mix is too thick, more water might be added, moving the gypsum crystals already formed further apart. In addition, the crystallization is abnormal and the strength is decreased. Only in instances in which strength and setting expansion are unimportant can such careless procedures be used.

Dental gypsum products can be weighed accurately on a simple, inexpensive spring scale of the type sold for kitchen use. Preweighed packages of dental stones are available from most manufacturers.

Mixing

The water and powder commonly are mixed in a rubber plaster bowl with a stiff metal or plastic stirrer or spatula. A typical plaster bowl and spatula are shown in Figure 5–9.

One precaution to observe is to avoid incorporation of air during mixing. Air bubbles reduce the strength of the set material, cause surface inaccuracies, and produce an unsightly cast or impression, as shown in Figure 5–10. For this reason, water should be placed into the mixing bowl *first* and the powder should be sifted into the water. Air is almost certain to be trapped in the mix if the powder is dumped in or if the water is poured into the powder.

If a dental vibrator is available, the bowl with the water and powder can be placed on the vibrator for a few seconds to free any air bubbles that are present. Otherwise, the bowl can be rapped sharply on the bench to remove air.

The mix should then be stirred rapidly with a stiff-bladed spatula. At the same time, the blade should be wiped against the sides and bottom of the bowl to ensure that all the powder is mixed. Mixing can be done with the bowl resting on the vibrator to remove air bubbles, or the bowl can be bounced lightly on the bench occasionally during mixing.

Probably the best way to mix plaster or stone is under vacuum, using a mechanical mixer. A mixer of this type is shown in Figure 5–11.

When the mixture appears to be smooth and uniform, after about 60 seconds of hand mixing or 20 to 30 seconds of mechanical

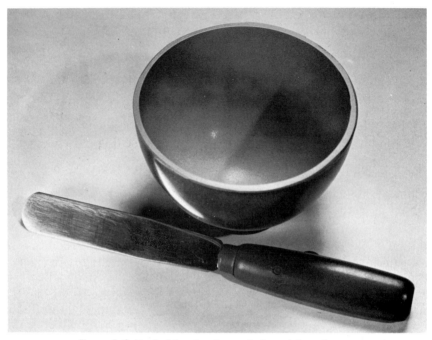

Figure 5-9. Typical bowl and spatula for mixing plaster.

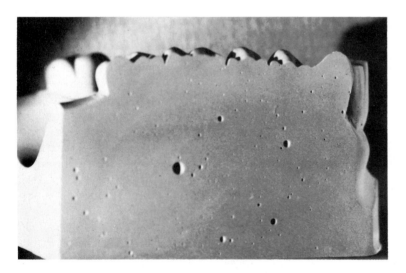

Figure 5-10. Section through a cast in which the stone was not mixed correctly. Note the gross porosity.

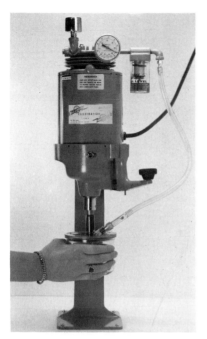

Figure 5-11. Mechanically mixing a gypsum product under vacuum. (Courtesy of Whip-Mix Corp.)

mixing, the material can be poured into the tray or impression. When properly manipulated, a plaster or stone cast should be smooth and dense, such as that shown in Figure 5–12.

CLASSIFICATION OF GYPSUM PRODUCTS

The classification system used in the ADA Specification for Dental Gypsum Products is based on their clinical application and is widely used. Table 5–1 lists this system along with traditional terms used to describe the different products.

The requirements for physical properties differ for the various types. For example, the allowable setting expansion decreases from 0.30 per cent for a Type II plaster to 0.10 per cent for a Type IV stone. Naturally, the minimum compressive strength permissible increases from a Type I to a Type IV product. Table 5–2 lists some of the more pertinent properties for the five types of gypsum material.

Impression Plasters (Type I)

As previously discussed, an impression plaster should have a low setting expansion and a relatively short setting time to ensure accuracy and comfort to the patient. The properties are regulated by the addition of modifiers—accelerators and retarders—to the powder by the manufacturer.

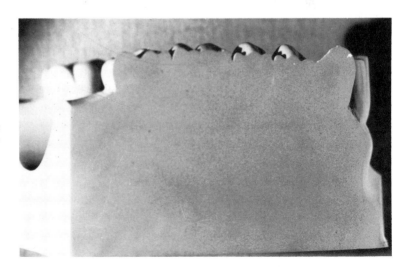

Figure 5-12. Section through a cast made from a correctly mixed dental stone.

TABLE 5-1. Classification of Dental Gypsum Products

	ADA Classification	Traditional Terminology
Type I	Impression plaster	Impression plaster
Type II	Model plaster	Lab or model plaster
Type III	Dental stone	Class I stone, cast stone, or hydrocal
Type IV	Die stone or high-strength dental stone	Class II stone, densite or improved stone
Type V	High-strength, high-expansion die stone	

ADA, American Dental Association.

Great strength is neither required nor desired in impression plasters. Even when taking impressions of edentulous patients, undercut regions will be present. This usually does not create a problem when removing the impression from the mouth; the tissue is soft and resilient.

When the impression is poured with a hard brittle stone, however, a problem arises in separating the cast from the impression. It may be necessary to break the impression material to do so. For this reason, a higher W/P ratio is used for mixing impression plaster than usually is used with other gypsum products. Not only does the thinner mix reduce the strength, but also there is less increase in temperature because of the exothermic heat. The chief requirement for the mixture is that it be sufficiently thick or viscous that it will not run out of the impression tray when the tray is inserted into the mouth.

Model Plaster (Type II)

Model plaster is supplied commercially for general use in the dental laboratory. The bet-

ter grades contain modifiers to regulate the setting time and expansion. They are used for work in which precise setting time, strength, and setting expansion are not important, such as the construction of a model or cast for demonstration, study, or display purposes. Formerly, model plaster was used for the construction of dental casts, but dental stone is now used for this purpose.

Dental Stone (Types III and IV)

Dental stone usually is composed of α-hemihydrate. It also contains modifiers (about 2 per cent), which are added to regulate the setting time and setting expansion of the stone. More time should be allowed for the setting of a dental stone than for the setting of impression plaster.

Dental stone originally is white. To distinguish its appearance from ordinary plaster, it usually is colored buff, although some manufacturers supply it in many pastel shades. The color is not a factor as far as the properties of the stone are concerned.

At least two types of dental stone are available. The stone described previously often is referred to as a *Class I stone* or *cast stone* (see Table 5-1) and would be a *Type III gypsum* according to the ADA Specification. It is used extensively for the construction of casts. The dry compressive strength of such stone ranges from 49.0 to 68.62 MPa (7100 to 9900 psi).

When constructing a cast on which a gold

TABLE 5-2. Properties of Gypsum Products

Type	Setting Time (min)	Setting Expansion (%)	Strength at 1 hr (MPa)	W/P Ratio
I	4	0.15	3.9	0.50-0.75
II	12	0.30	8.8	0.45-0.50
III	12	0.20	20.6	0.28-0.30
IV	12	0.10	34.3	0.22-0.24
V	12	0.30	48.0	0.18-0.22

casting is to be fabricated, a strong and hard stone model is required. Such a cast, which is a reproduction of a tooth containing a prepared cavity, is called a stone *die*. Part of the technique for constructing the inlay or crown is to mold a wax replica of the gold restoration on the die. This procedure requires that the wax be carved flush with the die, using a sharp-edged instrument. The die material must be strong and hard so as not to be damaged by the carving instrument.

As noted earlier, the abrasion resistance of the die is of particular importance under these circumstances. A *Class II* stone or *die stone* (Type IV gypsum) is used in such cases. This type is characterized by a powder with somewhat larger particles, although the particles are nonporous and smooth, as indicated in Figure 5–13. A comparison of these particles with those in Figure 5–4 for Class I stone indicates this difference.

Class II stones can be mixed with less water than Class I stones, as shown in Table 5–2. The dry compressive strength of Class II stone may be 78.4 MPa (11,400 psi) or greater. The surface hardness of a Class II stone also is greater. In fact, the difference in hardness is greater than the difference in strength. The setting expansion of Class II stone is lower than for Class I stone. A lower setting expansion is needed in situations in which high accuracy is required—a stone die.

For die stone to attain these properties, the powder and water must be carefully proportioned. The chief reason for using a die stone is to obtain strength. An improperly proportioned and mixed stone–water mixture may result in a weaker product than a properly mixed model plaster.

Dental Stone (Type V)

Type V gypsum products (high-strength, high-expansion die stone) are the most re-

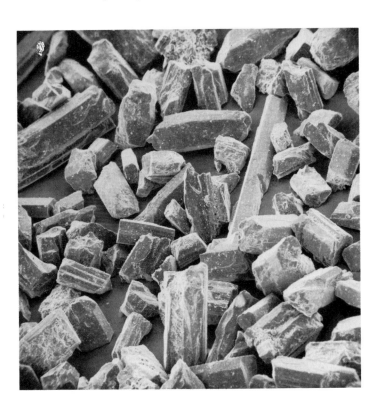

Figure 5–13. Powder particles of die stone (Type IV gypsum; × 400). (Courtesy of B. Giammara and R. Neiman.)

cent additions to dentistry. These may have dry compressive strengths as high as 138 MPa (20,000 psi). Their hardness also usually is higher than the typical Type IV stone. Careful control in the manufacturing process allows the Type V stones to be mixed at W/P ratios as low as 0.186. This in turn increases strength and hardness.

The setting expansion increases as well, and most of the very high strength die stones exceed the 0.10% expansion limit for Type IV gypsum. Whether this additional expansion will cause problems can be determined only by trial. In some cases where a pattern constructed on a die will be cast in an alloy with high shrinkage, the additional expansion can be beneficial.

The α-hemihydrate also is an essential ingredient in making dental *investments*. These materials, discussed in Chapters 18 and 19, provide the mold into which gold alloys are cast in the construction of metal restorations. The gypsum binder is necessary to provide the strength required in the investment to withstand the force of the alloy as it is forced into the mold.

CONSTRUCTION OF THE CAST OR MODEL

Details for construction of the cast vary according to the impression material used. These are described as each type of impression material is discussed.

Some general principles can be given, however. The impression is first rinsed with water to clean it of dried saliva, blood, and similar debris. Then it usually is subjected to some type of infection control procedure. An impression removed from the patient's mouth must be considered biologically contaminated and a potential vector for transmission of pathogens. Details of the disinfection procedure depend on the type of impression material used. After disinfection,

the interior of the impression should be dried to eliminate drops of water.

The objective when pouring the mixed gypsum material into the impression is to fill the impression without trapping air bubbles between the impression and the gypsum or within the cast itself. This is most easily done by following these steps:

1. Add a small amount of mix at one end of the impression, and allow this material to flow down the length of the interior, wetting all the impression interior surface. Gentle vibration on the dental vibrator assists in this process.

2. Carefully pour the balance of the mix into the impression, again using the dental vibrator. Although the mix may appear stiff and viscous in the mixing bowl, it flows readily when gentle vibration is applied.

3. Once the impression has been filled with gypsum material, place it on the bench and allow it to set undisturbed until the gypsum product has reached an initial set.

4. Allow the gypsum product to harden for the length of time recommended by the manufacturer before attempting to separate the cast or model from the impression.

The wet strength of gypsum products, as noted, is low compared with their dry strength, and the values reported are measured after 1 hour. Premature attempts to separate the cast from the impression will probably result in a broken cast, especially if one of the high elastic modulus (very stiff) impression materials is used.

CARE OF GYPSUM PRODUCTS, DIES, AND CASTS

Unmixed gypsum products (hemihydrate) are sensitive to changes in the relative humidity of the atmosphere. Both plaster and stone powders should be stored in air-tight containers when not in use. The container should not be left opened any longer than necessary. Under no circumstances should moisture be allowed to come into contact with the contents. Special care should be taken that the scoop or spoon with which the powder is removed is dry and clean.

Exposure to moisture through direct contact or exposure to high-humidity air may cause the setting reaction to start. The result will be a marked change in setting time and a reduction in strength and hardness of the set material. Long exposure to moisture may prevent the setting entirely. A film of gypsum, caused by the moisture, appears on the surface of the hemihydrate particles, as shown in Figure 5–14. This gypsum layer inhibits or even prevents the water from contacting the powder particle.

Gypsum models, casts, and dies are dimensionally stable after the gypsum product has set. Care must be exercised, however, if the set gypsum is brought in contact with water. As noted, gypsum is soluble in water

to the extent of 0.2 g/100 ml. Fine detail and dimension are quickly lost from a stone cast exposed to running water. When a technique requires the surface of the cast to be wet, it should be soaked in water saturated with pieces of set gypsum (dihydrate).

INFECTION CONTROL CONCERNS

Because of the difficulty of disinfecting some types of impression materials, dental gypsum products that contain disinfecting agents are available commercially. The properties of some of these materials compare favorably with conventional products that do not contain these agents. As always, the best assurance of adequate performance is to choose a product that meets the ADA Specification for Gypsum Products.

Selected Readings

Dilts, W. E., Duncanson, M. G. Jr., and Collard, E. W.: Comparative stability of cast mounting materials. J. Okla. Dent. Assoc. 68:11, 1978.

Fairhurst, C. W.: Compressive properties of dental gypsum. J. Dent. Res. 39:812, 1960.

Mahler, D. B.: Hardness and flow properties of gypsum materials. J. Prosthet. Dent. 1:188, 1951.

Toreskog, S., Phillips, R. W. and Schnell, R. J.: Properties of die materials: A comparative study. J. Prosthet. Dent. 16:119, 1966.

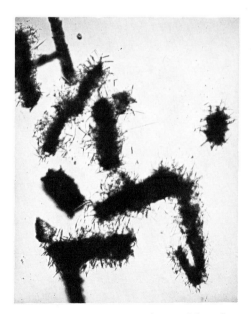

Figure 5–14. Hemihydrate powder particles after exposure to moisture in the air. Crystals of gypsum can be seen growing from the surface of the particles. (Courtesy of H. K. Worner.)

Reviewing the Chapter

1. List the various dental materials made from gypsum. Explain the differences in their structure and properties, including the ADA Specification classification.
2. Define *impression, cast, stone die,* and *investment.*
3. Show the setting reaction that takes place when plaster is mixed with water. Include a description of the crystal formation.
4. Defend the importance of the correct

W/P ratio in the handling of gypsum products.

5. Define *setting time* and explain how it is measured.

6. List the factors that influence the setting time of plaster or stone.

7. Discuss the variables that influence the setting expansion of a gypsum product. What is meant by *hygroscopic setting expansion?*

8. List the factors that influence the strength of plaster or stone. What is the difference between the dry and wet strength?

9. Describe step by step the manipulation of stone and the construction of a cast.

10. Explain the importance of correct care of the plaster or stone powder, especially as related to moisture contamination.

CHAPTER 6

DENTAL IMPRESSION MATERIALS:
Inelastic Materials

INTRODUCTION TO IMPRESSION MATERIALS

The function of a dental impression material is to make a negative copy (replica) of an oral structure. This structure may be an entire arch or a single tooth. It may be an edentulous arch (one without teeth), as discussed in Chapter 5. This replica must be accurate because it is used as a mold into which a material (probably a gypsum product) is poured and hardens to become a cast or die or model (a positive replica) of the oral structure.

The fundamental requirement for an impression material is that it can be placed into the mouth as a semiliquid material, which will flow and adapt itself around the structures of interest. The material must then set (*harden*) into a solid that is rigid enough to be removed from the mouth without becoming permanently deformed. Two different sets of physical properties are important in dental use. One is the rheological behavior of the impression material in liquid state (its flow). The other is concerned with the mechanical (elastic) properties of the material after it sets.

Several other characteristics of dental impression materials also are of interest.

- *Accuracy* within the limits of the clinical application is a primary consideration. This includes the ability to reproduce the size and shape of the oral structure and to copy fine details—in some cases as small as 0.025 mm.
- The *dimensional stability* of the impression after it has been removed from the mouth is another practical consideration that may affect the accuracy.
- For materials that harden (set) by a chemical reaction, the *working time* available between the start of mix and placement in the mouth is important.
- The amount of time required to *harden* in the mouth is significant for all types of materials.
- Because relatively large amounts of an impression material are placed into the mouth for a short period of time, the *biocompatibility* and *aesthetics* (odor and taste) must be considered.
- The impression material must be *chemically compatible* with whatever material will be used to pour the cast or die. Although this usually is a gypsum product, various resins and electroplated metals sometimes are used.

The use of plaster of Paris as an impression material is described in Chapter 5. Plaster, however, is only one of several materials that can be used to obtain a dental impression.

CLASSIFICATION OF IMPRESSION MATERIALS

Impression materials can be classified in several ways. One is according to the manner in which they harden. Plaster of Paris, for example, hardens by a chemical reaction

within the material, as do the zinc oxide and eugenol impression pastes, the irreversible hydrocolloids, and the rubber impression materials, all of which are discussed in the following chapters.

Impression compound softens when heated and then solidifies when it cools to mouth temperature with no chemical change taking place. Such materials are classified as *thermoplastic* substances. Although the reversible hydrocolloid materials, described in Chapter 7, may not be classified strictly as thermoplastic materials, they are liquefied by heat, and they do solidify—or gel—when they are cooled.

In Table 6–1, the classification of the various impression materials is based on their mechanism of hardening and their respective thermal behaviors. Another way to sort out these materials is according to their use in dentistry.

As previously noted, an impression made

TABLE 6–1. Classification of Dental Impression Materials

Material	Setting (Hardening) Mechanism
A. Inelastic Materials	
1. Impression plaster (Type I gypsum)	Chemical reaction
2. Impression and tray compound	Cooling to mouth temperature
3. Zinc oxide–eugenol impression paste	Chemical reaction
B. Aqueous Elastomeric Materials (Hydrocolloids)	
1. Irreversible hydrocolloid (alginate)	Chemical reaction
2. Reversible hydrocolloid (agar)	Cooling to 15°–20° C
C. Nonaqueous Elastomeric Materials (Rubber)	
1. Polysulfide rubber	Polymerization reaction
2. Polyether rubber	Polymerization reaction
3. Addition silicone rubber	Polymerization reaction
4. Addition silicone rubber (polyvinyl siloxane)	Polymerization reaction

with plaster of Paris is not elastic and cannot be removed over undercuts without the impression being fractured. Compound also is inelastic. If an impression of teeth is made with impression compound, the compound either flows or fractures when the impression is withdrawn over the undercuts, and the tooth form is not preserved.

Although plaster and compound have been used for all types of dental impressions, they are best suited for obtaining impressions of edentulous mouths, and thus are classified as impression materials for use in complete denture prostheses.

On the other hand, the hydrocolloid and rubber base impression materials, discussed in subsequent chapters, are elastic, and thus can be used in taking impressions of teeth when it is necessary to reproduce the crown or an undercut. These materials have mechanical properties that permit considerable elastic deformation, but they return to their original form on removal of the stress, much as a rubber band does. An appropriate term for such a material behavior is *elastomeric*.

IMPRESSION COMPOUND

When impression compound is used to make an impression of an edentulous mouth, it is softened by heat, inserted in an impression tray, and pressed against the tissue before it hardens. The compound is permitted to cool, and after hardening, the impression is withdrawn from the mouth. This impression is referred to as the *primary* impression.

The rigid primary compound impression may then be used as a tray on which other types of impression materials may be carried to be placed against the tissues. A mix of impression plaster may be placed in such a tray, and a final impression then obtained by spreading the plaster over the compound. The thin layer of plaster reproduces the fine detail of the denture area and, when used in this manner, is referred to as a *corrective* impression material. This impression is known as the *secondary* impression. Secondary impressions may also be taken with the zinc oxide and eugenol pastes and the elastomeric impression materials.

Composition

In general, compounds are a mixture of waxes, thermoplastic resins, a filler, and a coloring agent.

One of the first substances used as an impression material was beeswax—still an ingredient in some modern products. Because such waxes are brittle, compounds such as shellac, stearic acid, and gutta-percha may be added to improve the plasticity and workability. When used in this manner, these substances are referred to as *plasticizers*.

A *filler*, such as French chalk, usually is added to increase strength and plasticity. Fillers are small particles of inert materials that are chemically different from the principal substance to which they are added. The influences of the addition of fillers to a matrix material is discussed in greater detail in Chapter 10. At this time, it is sufficient to mention that if factors such as particle size and concentration are controlled, then the filler can improve substantially many properties of the matrix material.

Thermal Conductivity

The thermal conductivity of impression compound is very low; it conducts heat poorly. This property should be taken into consideration during the heating and cooling of the material. When the compound is heated, the outside portion softens before the inside. Because it is important that the compound be uniformly soft when it is placed in the tray, adequate time must be allowed for the material to be heated uniformly throughout its mass.

Flow

The flow of impression compound can be beneficial, but it can also be a source of error. After the compound has softened and while it is being pressed against the tissues, a continuous flow is desirable. The material should flow easily so that every detail of the soft tissue will be accurately reproduced. The high degree of flow should occur at a temperature that is safe and comfortable for the patient. Once the compound has solidified on cooling, however, flow should be at a minimum so that distortion will not occur when the compound is removed from the mouth. Typical flow behavior for impression compound is shown in Figure 6–1.

Distortion

Stress is induced while the impression is being obtained, and although it can be min-imized by proper handling, some stress is always present in the final impression. Because impression compound has essentially a noncrystalline structure, a stressed condition is more apt to occur in it than in a crystalline material. This stress may be released once the impression has been removed from the mouth. The safest procedure is to construct the cast or die within the first hour after the impression has been obtained—before any release of stress can occur.

OTHER USES

Although impression compound seldom is used today as an impression material, it does find applications in most dental offices. It is popular for use as a *border molding material* for application to the impression trays used with rubber impression materials. In this application, the compound defines the margins of the impression and helps to retain the rubber impression material within those limits.

Another application is as an adhesive to assemble or align models or appliances in the laboratory.

ZINC OXIDE–EUGENOL MATERIALS

The reaction that occurs when powdered zinc oxide is mixed with eugenol makes it possible to compound a number of materials useful in dental procedures. Zinc oxide and eugenol formulations, often abbreviated as *ZOE*, are used as luting cements, temporary and root canal filling materials, surgical dressings, bite registration pastes, and impression materials for edentulous mouths.

The basic composition of all these materials is the same: zinc oxide and eugenol (or suitable substitutes for eugenol) and rosin.

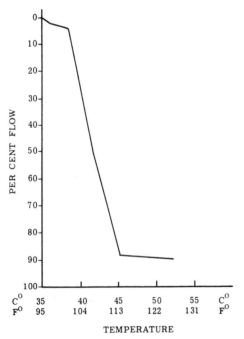

Figure 6–1. Flow of a typical impression compound at different temperatures. This material meets ADA Specification no. 3 for dental impression compound.

Plasticizers, fillers, and other additives are incorporated as necessary to provide the desired properties for the particular use of the product.

ZOE IMPRESSION PASTES

Impression pastes are used as secondary impression materials within the primary impression or within a custom impression tray, using the following procedure:

1. A primary impression may be taken with compound.
2. A zinc oxide and eugenol paste is then spread over the compound impression and the corrective impression taken to record the fine details of the soft tissues.
3. The impression is withdrawn after the paste has hardened.
4. The hardening occurs by a chemical reaction.

Although ZOE is used infrequently as an impression material today, the chemistry of the setting reaction is identical with that of the other types of ZOE materials listed above. The use of these materials is discussed in Chapters 21 and 22.

Composition and Chemistry

The zinc oxide and the eugenol usually are formulated into pastes and dispensed in separate tubes, as shown in Table 6–2.

The type of zinc oxide is critical, particularly the fineness of the powder. A small amount of water also must be present because a completely dehydrated zinc oxide will not react with eugenol. Unfortunately, the water may reduce the *shelf life* (ability to be stored without deteriorating) of the commercial product. Therefore, these materials should not be purchased in large quantities.

The addition of rosin produces a smoother mix and influences the speed of the reaction.

TABLE 6–2. Composition of a Zinc Oxide– Eugenol Impression Paste

Components	Composition (%)
Paste A	
Zinc oxide	87
Vegetable or mineral oil	13
Paste B	
Oil of cloves or eugenol	12
Rosin or gum	50
Filler	20
Lanolin	3
Balsam	10
Accelerator and coloring	5

Courtesy of E. J. Molnar.

Other soluble chemicals, such as calcium chloride, zinc acetate, and glacial acetic acid, also can be incorporated in either paste to serve as accelerators. Although the addition of water decreases the setting time of a zinc oxide–eugenol product, water should not be classified strictly as an accelerator. Too much water may retard the rate of reaction.

Because oil of cloves contains 70 to 85 per cent eugenol, sometimes it is preferred to eugenol because it reduces the burning sensation in the soft tissues when the impression is first placed in the mouth. The vegetable or mineral oil in paste A acts as a plasticizer and provides a smoother and more fluid mix. Olive oil also acts as a plasticizer and aids in reducing the irritating effect of eugenol. If the mixed paste is too thin before setting, a filler such as talc may be added to either paste.

The reaction between zinc oxide and eugenol is complex and not completely understood. Apparently, not all the zinc oxide reacts with the eugenol, and some free eugenol remains as well. The principal compound resulting from this reaction is long, thin crystals of zinc eugenolate. The hardened mass may be visualized as particles of zinc oxide bound together with a matrix of zinc eugenolate. This structure is shown in Figure 6–2.

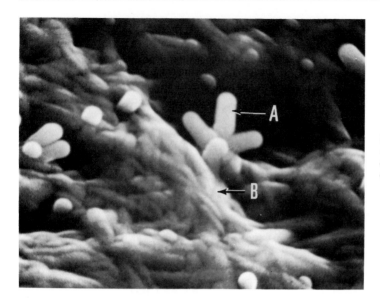

Figure 6-2. Structure of zinc oxide–eugenol cement. *A*, Particles of zinc oxide powder embedded in *B*, a matrix of zinc eugenolate.

Setting Time

As with all impression materials, control of the setting time of the zinc oxide–eugenol mixture is of prime importance to the dentist. Sufficient time must be allotted for mixing, filling the tray, and seating the impression in the mouth. Once in the mouth, the material should set rapidly to prevent any inaccuracy caused by unavoidable movement of the tray, which may occur while the paste is still soft.

As described earlier, the composition of the individual pastes influences the setting time. The type and amount of accelerator are, unquestionably, the most important factors in the control of the setting time. Small changes in the amount of accelerator incorporated in the paste can affect the setting time markedly.

The ratio of zinc oxide and eugenol also influences the rate of setting. Consequently, it is important that the proportions of the two pastes be measured before mixing. The setting time for most brands of ZOE impression pastes is decreased as temperature and humidity increase. Thus, these materials usually set more rapidly in the mouth than on the mixing pad. On a hot day and with high humidity, the setting time may be so short that the material sets on the mixing pad or in the tray before the impressions can be made.

Control of Setting Time

There are several methods by which the setting time can be altered, within certain limits:

1. If the paste sets too slowly, the reaction rate can be increased by adding an accelerator, such as a small amount of zinc acetate. Water is not a reliable accelerator.

2. When the setting time is too short, the cause usually is high humidity or temperature. Cooling the spatula and mixing slab may help to lengthen the setting time, provided the temperature is not so low that moisture condenses on the slab. The addition of certain inert oils or waxes, such as mineral oil or petrolatum, also may retard the setting. The rigidity of the hardened material may be reduced; however, unless such agents are used with care, an unhomogeneous mix results.

3. The setting time can be controlled to a certain extent by altering the ratio of the zinc oxide paste to the eugenol paste. Whether the setting will be accelerated or retarded depends on which paste contains the accelerator.

4. The mixing time affects the setting time to a limited extent. Usually, the longer the mixing time, the faster the paste hardens.

Fluidity and Consistency

Pastes that flow readily when carried into the mouth are preferred because they prevent compression and movement of the soft tissues. The zinc oxide and eugenol pastes are superior to compound in this respect because their consistency can be regulated by the composition of the paste. Thus, the dentist can select a paste that is very fluid or one that is more viscous and, with proper control of the manipulation, can be certain of the desired flow at the time the impression is obtained. One of the prime requirements of any impression material is its ability to accurately reproduce the details of the oral tissue.

Dimensional Stability

Shrinkage during hardening (less than 0.1 per cent) is negligible. Likewise, no significant distortion occurs if the impression is stored after removal from the mouth, provided that the tray material used to form the original impression was stable.

Mixing Technique

Although a glass mixing slab can be used, mixing of the two pastes usually is accomplished on an oil-impervious paper. The following procedure is recommended:

1. The correct proportion of the two pastes is obtained by squeezing out two lengths of paste of the same length onto the mixing slab. The diameters of the strips of pastes should be equal to the openings in the tubes.

2. In mixing, both sides of a flexible stainless steel spatula are wiped in the yellow-brown paste.

3. The yellow-brown paste then is smoothed into the lighter-colored paste.

4. Mixing is continued for about 1 minute, until a uniform color is obtained.

OTHER TYPES OF PASTES

Zinc oxide–eugenol pastes often are placed over oral tissues after extractions or periodontal surgery to aid in retaining a medicament and to promote healing. The ingredients of such pastes are essentially the same as those of impression pastes, although they may contain more eugenol. The amount and particle size of the filler are different also. The use of ZOE as a cementing media is discussed in Chapters 21 and 22.

Bite Registration Pastes

The materials used for recording the occlusal relationships between natural and/or artificial teeth include impression plaster, compound, wax, resin, elastomeric impression materials, and metallic oxide pastes. Zinc oxide–eugenol pastes often are used as such recording materials in the construction of complete dentures and fixed or removable partial dentures. One such product is a noneugenol type. Plasticizers, such as petrolatum, and silicone often are added to reduce the tendency of the paste to stick to the mouth tissues. Bite registration pastes follow conventional zinc oxide–eugenol–resin formulations.

Noneugenol Pastes

The use of eugenol has certain disadvantages, the principal one being that some patients find the odor and taste disagreeable. A number of chemicals produce a reaction with zinc oxide in a manner comparable to eugenol. The one most commonly used is a carboxylic acid. Several noneugenol impression pastes are available.

One form of this acid that is especially valuable is ortho-ethoxy-benzoic acid, commonly abbreviated *EBA*. It can be used as either a liquid or a powder. EBA is also used in zinc oxide–eugenol cements and is discussed in Chapters 21 and 22.

Selected Reading

Asgar, K., and Peyton, F. A.: Physical properties of corrective impression pastes. J. Prosthet. Dent. 4:555, 1954.

Hempton, J. B., and Vevan, E. M.: Proportioning zinc oxide–eugenol impression pastes. Aust. Dent. J. 9:186, 1964.

Vieira, D. F.: Factors affecting the setting of zinc oxide–eugenol impression pastes. J. Prosthet. Dent. 9:70, 1959.

Reviewing the Chapter

1. Establish a classification system for impression materials based on (1) method of hardening, (2) elastic characteristics, and (3) use in dentistry.
2. Define *thermoplastic* and give a dental materials example.
3. Explain the differences between *primary impression, corrective impression,* and *secondary impression.* Describe how each is used.
4. Discuss the composition of dental compound. What is meant by *plasticizer, core,* and *matrix* in this regard?
5. Explain the difference between *impression compound* and *tray compound.*
6. Explain why an impression compound needs to have different flow characteristics at oral temperatures and at the temperature at which it is inserted into the mouth. Draw a graph to show the flow of a certified material plotted against temperature.
7. Describe the procedures in softening compound and constructing the cast. What things may distort the impression?
8. Give the fundamental requirement for a material to be used as a dental impression material, and explain why two sets of physical properties must be considered.
9. Define the following characteristics of a dental impression material:

   Accuracy
   Stability after setting
   Working time
   Setting time
   Biocompatibility and aesthetics
   Compatibility with cast and die materials

10. List the various dental uses of zinc oxide–eugenol impression pastes.
11. Describe how such pastes are used in taking a secondary impression within a compound tray.
12. List the chemicals involved in the setting reaction and give the structure of the set material. What factors and chemicals affect the setting time of ZOE?
13. What other chemical often is used to replace eugenol? Why is it substituted?
14. Describe the correct proportioning and mixing of such a paste. Is the final impression dimensionally stable?
15. Give some additional dental applications for the ZOE chemistry besides its use as an impression paste.

CHAPTER 7

AQUEOUS ELASTOMERIC IMPRESSION MATERIALS: Dental Hydrocolloids

In a broad sense, impression materials may be classified as either inelastic or elastomeric, as shown in Table 6–1. Inelastic materials, such as plaster, were the first impression materials used in dentistry and are acceptable for certain uses, such as impressions for complete dentures. Because the plaster is inelastic, the impression cannot be removed from around the crown of the tooth or from undercuts without fracture or distortion.

Various types of elastomeric impression materials have replaced the inelastic ones for most dental purposes. These materials stretch elastically when removed over a tooth and then spring back to their original shape. The impression is a faithful negative reproduction of the mouth structures, regardless of the presence of tooth contours or undercuts around which the material is removed.

These flexible materials can be regarded as general purpose impression materials. They can be used for making impressions in the construction of partial dentures, crowns, or bridges with greater accuracy and ease than was possible with inelastic materials. They also have largely replaced the inelastic materials for complete denture impressions.

An explanation of the indirect technique for constructing a cast metal restoration is appropriate at this point. First, an impression of the tooth and the prepared cavity is obtained, as diagrammed in Figure 7–1A. The impression then is poured with stone to produce a model, or *cast,* of the tooth or teeth and the prepared cavities (Fig. 7–1B). The stone model is removed from the impression (Fig. 7–1C). This model is referred to as the die. The wax pattern, which is an exact replica of the structure to be cast, is now formed on the die, and the gold casting is fabricated from the pattern (Fig. 7–1D). Before the development of highly accurate elastomeric impression materials, wax patterns for cast metal restorations were constructed directly in the patient's mouth—an inconvenient and time-consuming process. The indirect technique allows dies to be sent to a dental laboratory for the construction of the cast restoration.

There are two general categories of elastomeric impression materials, as shown in Table 6–1. The first to be discussed is water-based materials, hence the name *aqueous elastomers.* The second category is synthetic rubber–type materials called *nonaqueous elastomers.*

HYDROCOLLOIDS

A more common name for the water-based impression materials is *hydrocolloid.* Colloids are suspensions of molecules—or groups of molecules—in some type of dispersing medium. Colloidal systems involve particles of a size between the small particles

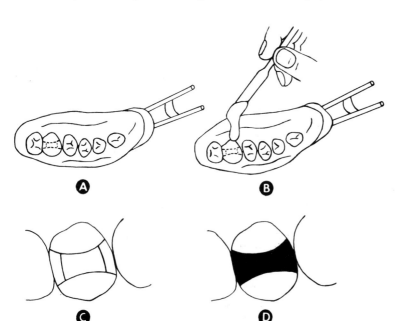

Figure 7–1. Schematic drawings of steps involved in the indirect technique. A, The elastic impression is taken. B, The impression is filled with a suitable gypsum die material. C, An enlarged drawing of a section through the stone cast shows the die of the prepared cavity. D, A wax pattern is fabricated on the die, and a gold casting is made from the pattern.

of a true *solution* and the large ones present in a *suspension*. A liquid colloid may be referred to as a colloidal *sol*.

A colloid has two phases: the dispersed particles and the dispersion medium that contains the particles. The term *hydrocolloid* indicates that the dispersion medium is water. Jell-O powder after hot water has been added to it is an example of a hydrocolloid in the sol condition. Hydrocolloid sols possess the capacity to change into a jelly or *gel* under certain conditions. When the liquid Jell-O is placed in a refrigerator, a gel eventually results as the sol is cooled.

The temperature at which this change from the sol state to a rubbery semisolid material takes place is known as the *gelation temperature*. This gelation process is *reversible* because the gel can be *reliquefied* (returned to the sol condition) by allowing the Jell-O to sit at room temperature for a period of time. Thus, the change from the sol to the gel, and vice versa, is essentially a physical effect induced by a change in temperature. The reaction may be summarized as:

$$Sol \rightleftarrows Gel \qquad 7\text{--}1$$

Because the change from sol to gel is reversible, these materials are called *reversible hydrocolloids.*

As the temperature of a reversible hydrocolloid sol is lowered, secondary forces of attraction cause the particles of the dispersed phase to agglomerate into *fibrils* that intermesh and become tangled. The final gel is composed of a brush-heap arrangement of these fibrils with water trapped between the branches and is not chemically different from the original fluid sol. When in the sol condition, the solid phase is suspended in water. In the gel condition, the water is suspended in the tangled branches of gel fibrils.

A gel also can be formed from a sol by a chemical reaction. The structure of such a gel is similar to that of one formed by cooling. The fibrils are held together by primary chemical bonds, however, and cannot be reliquefied by heating. Such a material is referred to as an *irreversible hydrocolloid*, and the gelation reaction can be described as:

$$Sol \rightarrow Gel \qquad 7\text{--}2$$

Gel Strength

Hydrocolloid gels are relatively weak elastic solids that are subject to *tensile fracture* (tearing) and flow. Such a gel can exhibit sufficient strength and elastic strain to be used as a dental impression material if the stress is applied rapidly and not maintained for a prolonged time—in other words, if the impression is removed from the mouth with a quick jerk.

Dimensional Stability

Because a large fraction of the volume of a hydrocolloid gel is occupied by water, the water content of such a gel has a considerable influence on the dimensional stability of the impression material. Loss of water results in shrinkage; uptake of water produces swelling.

A hydrocolloid gel exposed to air rapidly loses water by evaporation and by exuding fluid in a process called *syneresis*. If a hydrocolloid gel is stored in contact with water, it sorbs additional water by the process of *imbibition*. Either one leads to unacceptable dimensional changes (distortion of the impression).

Dental Hydrocolloids

Having described the nature of the two types of hydrocolloids, the remainder of this chapter focuses on their use as dental impression materials. Both types are referred to simply as *hydrocolloid impression materials.*

IRREVERSIBLE HYDROCOLLOID— ALGINATE

The transformation from sol to gel (gelation) of irreversible hydrocolloid, more commonly called *alginate*, occurs by means of a chemical reaction. Once the gel has formed, it cannot be changed back into the sol condition by physical means. In dental use, a powder is mixed with water to form a viscous sol, which is carried into the mouth in a perforated or solid impression tray. The sol then forms an elastic gel through a series of chemical reactions. After the gel has formed, the impression is removed from the mouth.

Alginate impression materials are used for making impressions in areas in which partial dentures are to be fabricated. They are also used in the fabrication of study models for orthodontic treatment, for making primary impressions in edentulous mouths, and as corrective materials in secondary impressions of all types.

They generally are not used in the indirect techniques. Alginate does not reproduce fine detail as reliably as do the other elastomeric impression materials. Careful examination of a stone die poured in an alginate impression usually reveals a slight rounding of any sharp angles or margins that are present in the original cavity preparation. The density of the surface of the stone die is also inferior. These defects may be due either to the somewhat more porous surface of the impression material or to a reaction between the stone and the irreversible hydrocolloid.

Alginates are widely used because of their low cost, convenience and ease of manipulation, need for minimal equipment, and acceptable accuracy for many dental procedures.

Composition and Chemistry

The following is a typical formula for an alginate impression material powder:

Potassium alginate	15%
Calcium sulfate	16%
Zinc oxide	4%
Potassium titanium fluoride	3%
Diatomaceous earth	60%
Trisodium phosphate	2%

The chief ingredient, from the standpoint of the chemical reaction, is the soluble potassium alginate, from which the material gets its common name. Obtained from sea kelp, alginate dissolves reasonably well in water to form a viscous sol. Alginates are common ingredients in various food products, such as ice creams, in which they are used as thickening agents. Once this sol—contained in an impression tray—is placed against the mouth tissues, it must be changed into an elastic gel that can be removed without distortion. A number of methods bring about this change, but the simplest is to react the soluble alginate with calcium sulfate, producing the gel structure of insoluble calcium alginate.

Because the reaction must take place in the mouth, it must be delayed until the impression material powder can be mixed with water, placed in the tray, and carried to the mouth. To delay this reaction and provide adequate working time, a third soluble salt, such as trisodium phosphate, is added to this solution. The added salt is known as a *retarder*. The calcium sulfate reacts first with the trisodium phosphate before reacting with the soluble alginate. As long as any trisodium phosphate is present, the gelation reaction between the alginate and calcium sulfate is prevented.

If suitable amounts of calcium sulfate, potassium alginate, and trisodium phosphate are mixed together in proper proportions with water, the following reaction takes place:

$$2\ Na_3PO_4 + 3\ CaSO_4 \rightarrow$$
$$Ca_3(PO_4)_2 \downarrow + 3\ Na_2SO_4 \qquad 7\text{--}3$$

Trisodium phosphate + calcium sulfate →
calcium phosphate + sodium sulfate

When the supply of trisodium phosphate is exhausted, the calcium ions begin to react with the potassium alginate as follows:

$$K_nAlg + \frac{n}{2} CaSO_4 \rightarrow \frac{n}{2} K_2SO_4 + Ca_{\frac{n}{2}}Alg$$

7–4

Potassium alginate + calcium sulfate →
   potassium sulfate + calcium alginate

Other soluble alginate salts, such as sodium alginate, also can be used. There are also many retarders that can be used as effectively as trisodium phosphate.

The final structure of the gel is a brush-heap network of calcium alginate fibrils holding the excess water and particles of the filler. Diatomaceous earth is the usual filler. When added in proper amounts, a filler increases the strength and stiffness of the alginate gel and ensures a firm surface that is not tacky. Zinc oxide also is used as a filler.

Because the stone surface can be softened appreciably by the alginate impression, other ingredients are added to improve the surface of the gypsum die. Alginates are the most likely of all the impression materials to interfere with the setting reaction of gypsum products. For this reason, complex fluorides, such as potassium titanium fluoride, are added to serve as accelerators for the setting of gypsum.

The presence of soluble fluoride in alginate should not result in any undesirable systemic effect for the patient. Because absorption of the fluoride ion into the oral cavity can result in a temporary elevation of the body fluoride levels, however, it is prudent to make sure that no remnants of the impression material are left in the mouth. The patient also should be cautioned not to swallow any remnants inadvertently. This is particularly true for the pediatric patient, who may be receiving other fluoride therapy, such as topical fluorides, which also increase the amount of fluoride present in the oral cavity. Alginate impression materials

usually are scented and flavored to make them more acceptable to the patient, possibly tempting a child to "sample" them.

Because the exact proportion of each chemical varies with the type of raw material used by the manufacturer, the amount of retarder is carefully adjusted to provide proper gelation time. If about 15 g of powder of the composition listed are mixed with 50 ml of water, gelation occurs in 2 to 4 minutes at normal room temperature.

Shelf Life

Alginate impression materials deteriorate rapidly at elevated temperatures, in the presence of moisture, or under both conditions. When this happens, the material usually becomes thin during mixing, resulting in reduced strength and higher permanent deformation when removed from the mouth. Thus, alginate impression materials should never be stored in an area where the temperature may be high (such as a cabinet over a radiator or near a heating pipe). Only as much material as will be used in 1 year should be purchased at a time. The material should be dated on receipt so that the oldest material can be used first.

The alginate impression material is dispensed either in individually sealed, preweighed packets of powder or in a can in bulk form. The individual packets reduce the chance of moisture contamination of the alginate and make it easier to obtain a correct water-powder ratio. If the bulk package is used, the lid should be replaced firmly on the can immediately after the powder has been dispensed. Moisture contamination from the air may produce erratic setting times with the powder that remains in the can. Even with proper care, repeated opening of the can increases the amount of moisture contamination. If it is anticipated that the entire can of powder will not be completely used within a few months, it is prudent to buy the material in the form of packets.

Before use, the can of bulk material should be tumbled to fluff up the powder and mix the various ingredients. The dispensing cup should be slightly overfilled without packing. The blade of the spatula is then used to scrape off the excess from the top of the cup.

Care should be exercised to avoid inhaling dust from alginate powder during handling. The diatomaceous earth filler contains particles of finely divided silica; this material has been identified as an occupational health hazard if inhaled. The can of alginate should be allowed to set momentarily after fluffing and then held away from the face when opened. "Dust-free" alginates are being marketed and have become quite popular.

Manipulation

Gelation Time

The gelation time, measured from the beginning of mixing until the gelation occurs, is important because sufficient time must be allowed for the dentist to mix the material, load the tray, and place it in the patient's mouth. A prolonged gelation time is tedious for both the patient and the dentist. On the

other hand, premature gelation, which begins before the filled impression tray is placed in position in the mouth, results in a distorted and useless impression. Once the gelation starts, the material must not be disturbed because any fracturing of the fibrils is permanent. The optimal gelation time is between 3 and 4 minutes at a room temperature of 20° C (68° F).

Several methods can be used to measure gelation time, but probably the best method is to observe the time from the start of mixing until the material is no longer tacky or adhesive when touched with a clean, dry finger. At this point, the material also loses its glossy appearance and becomes rubbery when depressed.

Two types of alginates are designated in the American Dental Association Specification no. 18. Type I (fast-setting) must gel in not less than 60 seconds or more than 120 seconds. Type II (normal-setting) must gel between 2 and 4.5 minutes.

The best method for controlling the gelation time is to alter the temperature of the water used for mixing the alginate material. As shown in Figure 7–2, the effect of the temperature of the water on the gelation time of an alginate impression material is quite dramatic: the higher the temperature,

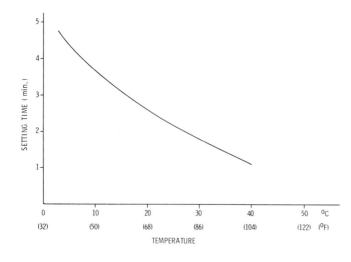

Figure 7–2. The effect of water temperature on the setting time of an alginate impression material. (Courtesy of J. Cresson.)

the shorter the gelation time. In many areas in the United States, tap water temperature can vary from below 40° F in the winter to above 85° F in the summer. The importance of having the mixing water at room temperature is evident. In hot weather, special precautions should be taken to provide cool water for mixing so that a premature gelation will not be obtained. Under most circumstances, it is better to err by having the mix too cool rather than too warm because alginate has a short working time. If the desired setting time cannot be achieved by varying the water temperature within reasonable limits, it is better to select another product that has the desired setting time instead of resorting to other modifications in the manipulative technique.

Increasing the water-powder ratio used to mix alginate is not recommended. Although it increases the setting time, it also adversely influences the strength and dimensional accuracy of the impression material.

Mixing

Maximum gel strength is required to prevent fracture and to ensure elastic recovery of the impression on its removal from the mouth. All the manipulative factors affect the gel strength. Because too little or too much water used in mixing weakens the final gel, the correct W/P ratio specified by the manufacturer should be used. Using preweighed packets of powder is the most accurate method for proportioning the powder. Bulk alginate can be measured by volume if a careful, consistent measuring technique, as previously described, is used. The necessity for implementing infection control procedures makes the use of predispensed unit dose dental materials much more attractive.

The mixing time is particularly important. The strength of the gel can be reduced as much as 50 per cent if the mixture is not complete. Insufficient spatulation results in

failure of the ingredients to dissolve adequately so that the chemical reactions can proceed uniformly throughout the mass. On the other hand, if the mixing time is unduly prolonged, the gel is broken up as it forms, decreasing the strength. The directions supplied with the product should be adhered to in all respects.

As with gypsum products, the water should be measured and placed into the clean, dry mixing bowl first. All suppliers of alginate impression materials provide graduated plastic cups for measuring the water by volume. The weighed powder is placed into the water and incorporated by careful spatulation.

Improper mixing of alginate impression materials is all too common. Proper technique is necessary to rapidly dissolve the powder particles without incorporating air. A vigorous figure-eight motion is used, with the mix being swiped or smashed against the sides of the rubber mixing bowl, as shown in Figure 7–3.

A mixing time of 1 minute is sufficient. The result should be a smooth, creamy mixture that does not drip off the spatula when it is raised from the bowl.

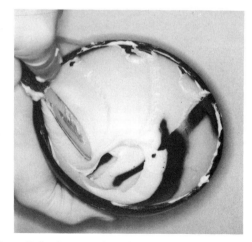

Figure 7–3. The mix of an alginate impression material is made by a vigorous *swiping* of the mix against the sides of the rubber mixing bowl.

The alginate mixture is placed in a suitable tray, which is carried into place in the mouth by the dentist. Plastic, disposable impression trays, shown in Figure 7–4, are most commonly used. Provision for retention of the impression material within the tray is essential in any impression-taking process. Perforated trays retain the material by mechanical penetration of the alginate into the tray perforations. With nonperforated trays, the use of a tray adhesive designed for alginate is imperative.

The strength of the alginate gel increases for several minutes after initial gelation—in some commercial products, it doubles during the first 4 minutes. For that reason, the dentist should not remove the alginate impression from the mouth for at least 2 to 3 minutes after gelation has occurred. This is about the time at which the material loses its tackiness in the mixing bowl. The impression is removed with a quick snap action because the strength and elasticity of the gel increase under an increasing rate of strain, as noted earlier.

Dimensional Stability

The phenomena of syneresis and imbibition are applicable to the alginate materials. Fluctuations in water content—and thus dimensional changes—occur on storage in any medium. These materials are most stable when stored in a humidor at 100 per cent humidity. For accurate results, the die should be constructed immediately after the impression is obtained. There is no adequate method for storing any of the hydrocolloid impression materials.

Construction of the Die

Immediately after removal from the mouth, the impression is thoroughly rinsed under running water and excess water shaken from the impression. The impression should not be dried with an air syringe.

Most infection control protocols prescribe treating the alginate impression with a spray disinfecting agent. Because of problems with dimensional stability, prolonged immersion in such an agent is not recommended. The manufacturer's instructions should be followed for the most appropriate disinfection procedure. Some brands of alginate contain disinfecting agents.

Although pouring gypsum into an alginate impression is not difficult because of the *hydrophilic* nature of the material, care still

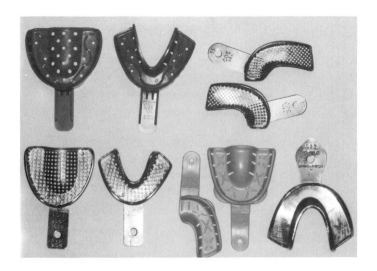

Figure 7–4. Stock metal and disposable plastic impression trays used with alginate impression materials. If nonperforated trays are used, a tray adhesive must be applied.

must be taken to avoid trapping air between the impression and the gypsum. Models that harden in 100 per cent relative humidity have somewhat superior stone surfaces. A humidor can be used or the filled impression wrapped in a damp towel. The use of a humidor is shown in Figure 7–5. The stone cast should not be separated for 30, or preferably 60, minutes. For the irreversible hydrocolloids, remove the cast from the impression at about 1 hour for maximum density of the stone surface.

Common Difficulties

Many of the common difficulties experienced with the irreversible hydrocolloids are summarized here.

Difficulty	Cause
1. Grainy material	a. Improper mixing b. Incorrect water-powder ratio c. Incorrect mixing water temperature
2. Tearing	a. Inadequate thickness of material b. Premature removal from mouth c. Incorrect removal technique d. Material partially gelled when tray was seated in the mouth e. Incorrect mixing or water-powder ratio
3. Irregularly shaped voids on surface of impression	a. Moisture or debris on tissue b. Grainy impression material
4. Rough or chalky stone surface	a. Inadequate cleaning and drying of impression b. Incorrect handling of gypsum c. Premature separation of cast or failure to separate cast after 1 hour d. Incompatibility of brands of alginate and Type IV gypsum
5. Distorted, inaccurate model	a. Delayed pouring of impression

b. Inadequate retention of impression material in the tray
c. Incorrect technique used to remove impression from the mouth
d. Premature removal from mouth
e. Movement of tray during gelation
f. Failure to seat tray in mouth before gelation starts

Summary

Alginate, the most commonly used dental impression material, reproduces detail sufficiently for most dental applications. It is not generally considered adequate for constructing dies for the indirect technique. Incompatibility is experienced between specific brands of alginate and Type IV gypsum products. Some manufacturers of Type IV materials do not recommend their use with alginate. If a Type IV gypsum is to be used, try different products to find a compatible combination of alginate and die stone.

REVERSIBLE HYDROCOLLOID

Historically, reversible hydrocolloid was the first elastomeric impression material introduced into dentistry. It was a major advance over the inelastic materials like impression plaster. The availability of reversible hydrocolloid made the indirect technique practical.

Agar-agar, a substance extracted from a certain type of seaweed, provides a suitable colloid as a base for dental impression materials. When suspended in water, agar-agar forms a liquid sol at temperatures that can be safely used in the oral cavity. It converts to a gel at a temperature slightly above that of the mouth.

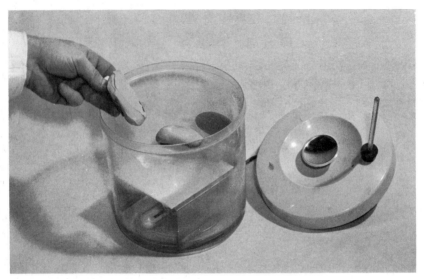

Figure 7–5. A hydrocolloid impression that has been filled with stone being placed in a humidor until the stone hardens. Water is in the bottom of the receptacle. The impression tray is placed on a platform above the water level. A tightly sealed lid provides an environment of about 100 per cent humidity.

The reversible hydrocolloid impression material is placed into the cavity preparation in the sol condition. Water-cooled impression trays rapidly convert the sol into a gel that is firm yet elastic.

Composition

The basic constituent of reversible hydrocolloid impression materials is agar-agar, present in a concentration of 8 to 15 per cent. (The principal ingredient by weight [about 80 to 85 per cent] is water.) Most dental products are blends of several species of agar-agar.

The manufacturer adds small amounts of borax to increase the strength of the gel. As discussed in Chapter 5, borax retards the setting of gypsum products. Thus, the presence of borax is detrimental to the impression material, in that it retards the set of the gypsum die material poured into the impression. If the surface becomes contaminated with the borax during setting—or with the gel itself (colloids also are retarders)—a soft, powdery surface may be formed on the final gypsum cast or die. The problem can be overcome in two ways:

1. Before the impression is filled with stone, it may be immersed in a solution that contains an accelerator.

2. The manufacturer can incorporate a plaster hardener or accelerator in the material itself. Potassium sulfate (approximately 2 per cent) usually is added to commercial dental hydrocolloid impression materials for that purpose.

Preparation of Material

Proper equipment for preparing and storing the hydrocolloid is essential, and the dental office must be organized for this work. Various types of conditioners are available, such as the one shown in Figure 7–6. Syringes inject the fluid material in and around the prepared cavity, and water-cooled trays carry the hydrocolloid into the mouth to form the remainder of the impression.

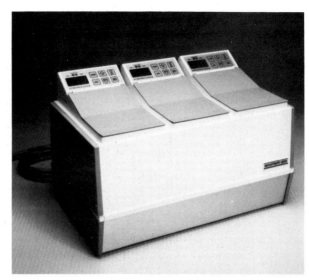

Figure 7–6. Conditioner for the hydrocolloid technique. The various compartments are for liquefying the material, for storage after boiling, and for tempering the tray hydrocolloid. (Courtesy of Van R. Dental Products.) (From Phillips, R. W.: *Skinner's Science of Dental Materials.* Philadelphia, W. B. Saunders Co., 1991.)

Typical syringes and impression trays used with reversible hydrocolloid are shown in Figure 7–7. Water is circulated through the cooling tubes attached to the outside surface of the tray. Some trays are perforated to aid in mechanically holding the impression material to the tray so the impression can be withdrawn over the undercuts around the teeth without distortion.

Unlike most other types of impression materials, reversible hydrocolloid is supplied with all the ingredients combined into a homogeneous gel. Glass cartridges—resembling local anesthetic cartridges—of a low viscosity (very fluid) hydrocolloid are supplied for use in the syringes. A more viscous (heavy body) hydrocolloid used to fill the tray is supplied in plastic tubes that resemble toothpaste tubes. These cartridges and tubes are placed directly into the conditioner for liquefication (Fig. 7–6).

The first step is to produce a fluid sol. The cartridges and tubes are placed in boiling water—a convenient means of liquefying the hydrocolloid. In locations at high altitudes above sea level, the boiling temperature of water is too low, and other liquids may be used. A minimum of 10 minutes of boiling is essential—there is no evidence that longer periods of boiling are harmful. Insufficient boiling leads to a granular, stiff mass of material that will not reproduce the necessary fine detail required in the cavity preparation.

If the material is to be reliquefied after a previous gelling, a minimum of 3 minutes should be added to the boiling time. Each time the agar-agar gel forms, it is more difficult to reliquefy. It is advisable for the auxiliary to mark with a piece of waterproof tape the materials not used after liquefying. This will assist in determining the amount of boiling time required when the material is reliquefied the next day.

After it has been liquefied, the material may be stored in the sol condition until it is needed for injection into the cavity preparation or for filling the tray. One advantage of the reversible hydrocolloid technique is that in the morning, the dental auxiliary can prepare a sufficient number of tubes and cartridges for use throughout the day. The material then is ready for quick use as needed—a time saver in the operatory.

Here again, suitable equipment permits storage of the prepared sol until it is needed.

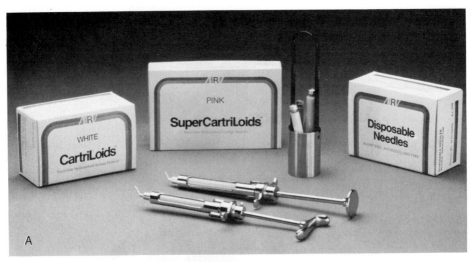

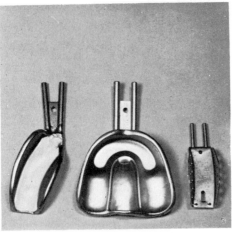

Figure 7–7. *A,* Cartridges of reversible hydrocolloid syringe material and the syringes used to inject the hydrocolloid over the teeth. *B,* Water-cooled trays used to carry the tray hydrocolloid into the mouth. (From Phillips, R. W.: *Skinner's Science of Dental Materials.* Philadelphia, W. B. Saunders Co., 1991.)

A storage temperature of 66° to 69° C (150° to 155° F) is ideal. Lower temperatures may result in some gelation and inaccurate reproduction of fine detail. Because temperatures required in the various steps of preparing the hydrocolloid are critical, those in the different compartments of the conditioner should be checked periodically.

Conditioning

The material that is used to fill the tray must be cooled or *tempered.* This *condition-ing* increases the viscosity of the hydrocolloid so that it will not flow out of the tray and reduces the temperature so that the material will not be uncomfortable to the patient.

Because the rate of gelation is influenced by the temperature at which the hydrocolloid is held, various combinations of temperatures and times may be used. A satisfactory one is to partially gel the material for about 10 minutes at a temperature of 46° C (115° F). The time may be varied for the particular brand of hydrocolloid and for the fluidity preferred by the dentist—the lower the temperature, the shorter the storage time in the conditioning compartment. In any case, the loaded tray should never be stored in this bath for more than 15 minutes because gelation may have proceeded too far, resulting in inadequate flow.

The Impression

To secure maximum detail, the dentist injects the low-viscosity syringe material into the prepared cavity. This material is used directly from the storage bath. While this step is being carried out, the water-soaked outer layer of hydrocolloid is scraped from the tray material that has been stored in the tempering bath. Failure to remove that layer may prevent a firm bonding between the tray material and the hydrocolloid that has been previously injected into the cavity preparation. The tray is then immediately brought into position in the mouth and held under passive pressure.

Gelation of the hydrocolloid is induced by circulating cool water in the tray at about 16° to 21° C (60° to 70° F) for not less than 5 minutes. Circulation of colder water induces rapid gelation and a concentration of stress in the hydrocolloid that is near the tray, resulting in a distortion of the impression. Patient discomfort caused by thermal shock may also result. A minimum 5-minute gelation time is required for gelation to proceed until the gel is strong enough to resist distortion or fracture during removal.

It is never wise for the dentist to hold the impression for a short period and then have the assistant hold it. When this is done, a distortion of the gelling material invariably occurs.

As previously stated, the structure of the gel is such that it resists a sudden application of force without distortion or fracture more successfully than force that is applied slowly. Thus, the dentist removes the impression

with a sudden snapping movement rather than slowly teasing it out.

Wet Field Technique

A technique for taking hydrocolloid impressions in a wet field has recently become popular. It differs from that used with other impression materials in that the tooth surfaces and tissue are purposely left wet. The areas are flooded with warm water. Then the syringe material is introduced quickly and liberally to cover the occlusal and/or incisal areas only. While the syringe material is still liquid, the tray material is seated. The hydraulic pressure of the viscous tray material forces the fluid syringe hydrocolloid down into the areas to be restored, displacing the water on the surface.

Laminate or Combined Reversible-Irreversible Technique

A formulation of syringe hydrocolloid is made that bonds chemically to alginate. Alginate is then used in place of the tray hydrocolloid material in a conventional stock alginate tray. When the cool alginate in the tray contacts the syringe hydrocolloid, the hydrocolloid adheres to the alginate and gels. This technique combines the simplicity of alginate with the detail reproduction of hydrocolloid. Water-cooled trays are not required, and the hydrocolloid conditioner is much smaller because only syringe cartridges are used and they require only two different water baths.

Dimensional Stability

The hydrocolloid gel is composed of fibrils of agar-agar suspended in water. The water content is critical to the dimensional stability of the impression. If water is lost, the gel shrinks. Likewise, if the gel takes up water, the hydrocolloid swells and expands.

Such changes are of great importance to the accuracy of the dental impression.

Various storage media—such as 2 per cent potassium sulfate or 100 per cent relative humidity—have been suggested to prevent dimensional change. Results obtained for one dental hydrocolloid by storing impressions in these and two other media may be seen in Figure 7–8. These results are typical, and they indicate that a relative humidity of 100 per cent best preserves the normal water content. The water content and contraction still are changed, even when the impression is stored in this environment. Even if the water equilibrium could be preserved, distortion probably would occur during storage because of the relaxation of the internal stress always present in the impression.

Because no satisfactory method exists for storing a hydrocolloid impression, the im-

portance of immediately constructing the cast cannot be overemphasized. A vivid example of the dangers involved in not doing so can be seen in Figure 7–9. A gold casting was constructed on a model of a dental cavity preparation. A hydrocolloid impression was taken of that preparation, and the master casting was placed back on a stone die constructed from the impression. If the die is an accurate reproduction of the original model, the casting should fit the stone die. When stored in water, the impression was grossly distorted. On critical dental preparations, inaccuracy can be detected in as little as 15 minutes after the impression is taken from the mouth.

Surface Hardness of the Die

Some form of gypsum ordinarily is used as the cast or die material in a hydrocolloid impression. Every precaution must be taken to ensure maximum surface hardness. The slightest porosity or chalkiness on the die results in inaccuracy and lack of sharp detail. One factor involved is the compatibility of the impression material and the gypsum die material.

A correctly formulated reversible hydrocolloid, as it is now available, has little deleterious effect on the hardness of a Type II or III gypsum cast. The hardness of a Type IV gypsum, however, may be reduced by about one third from contact with a reversible hydrocolloid. In general, the surface character, including hardness, of any type of gypsum correctly proportioned and mixed should be satisfactory after setting in contact with the present commercial reversible hydrocolloids.

At one time, immersing the impression in a 2 per cent solution of potassium sulfate before filling with the mix of dental stone was a recommended practice. A denser stone surface was thus obtained. However, the impression may distort during this storage period. For most modern materials, this

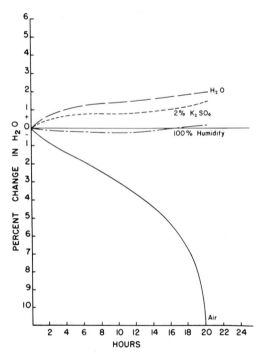

Figure 7–8. Percentage of change in the water content, by weight, of a reversible hydrocolloid impression material when stored in various media. For this brand, 100 per cent humidity produced the least change.

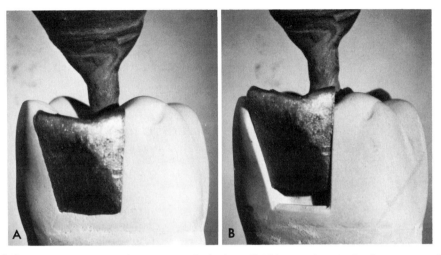

Figure 7-9. Effect of storage on the accuracy of a hydrocolloid impression. *A,* Fit of a master casting on a stone die constructed immediately after the impression was removed from the original die. The fit of the casting on this stone die is comparable to the fit of the casting on the original. *B,* Fit of same casting when the die was constructed after the impression was stored for 1 hour in air. Gross inaccuracy has resulted.

step is no longer required and should not be done unless the user is certain that a detectable improvement in the stone surface will result. The manufacturer's directions can probably be relied on.

Rough stone surfaces result if excess water has collected on the surface of the impression at the time the stone mixture is poured. The excess droplets of water should be gently blotted from the impression. The surface should be shiny and moist but with no visible water film or droplets. The impression should not be dried with an air syringe.

As pointed out in Chapter 5, the manufacturer's directions should be carefully followed in regard to the water-powder ratio when the stone is being mixed. Mechanical spatulation, preferably under vacuum, is a valuable aid in obtaining a denser die surface. The stone is added slowly in small amounts and is mechanically vibrated into the mold under *mild* vibration.

Somewhat superior stone surfaces usually are obtained if the stone hardens in an at-

mosphere of about 100 per cent relative humidity. The filled impression should never be immersed in water while the stone sets. As with alginate, the use of a humidor is the best choice.

Similarly to alginate impressions, the stone die should not be separated from the reversible hydrocolloid impression for at least 30 minutes or, preferably, 60 minutes. Sufficient time must be allowed for the stone to set, and premature removal results in an inferior die surface.

The recommendations for infection control given for alginate should be followed for reversible hydrocolloid. Prolonged immersion in an aqueous disinfectant should be avoided.

Causes of Common Difficulties

Some common difficulties encountered with reversible hydrocolloid impressions are summarized here.

Type	Cause
1. Grainy material	a. Inadequate boiling b. Conditioning or storage temperature too low c. Conditioning time unduly long
2. Separation of tray and syringe material	a. Water-soaked layer of tray material not removed b. Undue gelation of either syringe or tray material
3. Tearing	a. Inadequate bulk b. Moisture contamination at gingiva c. Premature removal from mouth d. Syringe material partially gelled when tray seated e. Incorrect removal from the mouth
4. External bubbles	a. Undue gelation, preventing flow
5. Irregularly shaped voids	a. Moisture or debris on tissue b. Material too cool or grainy
6. Rough or chalky stone cast	a. Inadequate cleansing of impression b. Excess water or potassium sulfate solution left in impression c. Premature removal of die d. Incorrect manipulation of stone
7. Distortion, inaccuracy	a. Impression not poured immediately b. Movement of tray during gelation c. Premature removal from mouth d. Incorrect removal from mouth e. Use of ice water during initial stages of gelation

Summary

The reversible hydrocolloid materials were the first of the elastic impression materials to be developed. Although their use has largely been supplanted by the rubber base materials, these hydrocolloids are capable of producing extremely accurate dies with ex-

cellent reproduction of detail well suited for the construction of wax patterns for cast restorations. They are relatively inexpensive materials and convenient to use. The technique affords a clean and highly controlled procedure.

Selected Reading

Appleby, D. C., Cohen, S. R., Racowsky, L. P., and Mingledorff, E. B.: The combined reversible hydrocolloid/irreversible hydrocolloid impression system: Clinical application. J. Prosthet. Dent. 46:48, 1981.

Ayres, H. D., Phillips, R. W., Dell, A., and Henry, R. W.: Dental duplication test used to evaluate elastic impression materials. J. Prosthet. Dent. 1:374, 1960.

Baum, L., Phillips, R. W., and Lund, M. R.: Textbook of Operative Dentistry. Philadelphia, W. B. Saunders Co., 1981, chap. 16.

Baum, L., and Sponzo, M. T.: Alginate impressions and study models. J. Conn. State Dent. Assoc. 53:35, 1979.

Carlyle, L. W., III: Compatibility of irreversible hydrocolloid impression materials with dental stones. J. Prosthet. Dent. 49:434, 1983.

Civjan, S., Huget, E. F., and de Simon, L. B.: Surface characteristics of alginate impressions. J. Prosthet. Dent. 28:373, 1972.

Eames, W. B., Rogers, L. B., Wallace, S. W., and Suway, N. B.: Compatibility of gypsum products with hydrocolloid impression materials. Oper. Dent. 3:108, 1978.

Setcos, J. C., Vrijhoef, M. M. A., Blumershine, R., and Phillips, R. W: Airborne particles from alginate powders. J. Am. Dent. Assoc. 106:355, 1983.

Skinner, E. W., and Pomes, C. E.: Alginate impression materials: Technic for manipulation and criteria for selection. J. Am. Dent. Assoc. 35:245, 1947.

Stauffer, J. P., Meyer, J. M., and Nally, J. N.: Accuracy of six elastic impression materials used for complete arch fixed partial dentures. J. Prosthet. Dent. 35:407, 1976.

Toreskog, S., Phillips, R. W., and Schnell, R. J.: Properties of die materials: A comparative study. J. Prosthet. Dent. 16:119, 1966.

Wilson, H. J., and Smith, D. C.: Alginate impression materials. Br. Dent. J. 114:20, 1963.

Reviewing the Chapter

1. Describe the difference between the direct and the indirect techniques for fabricating a crown.

2. Understand what is meant by *colloid, sol, gel,* and *fibril.* Relate these terms to a dental hydrocolloid impression material.

3. What is another name for an irreversible hydrocolloid impression material?

4. How is the sol gel transformation produced during the setting of such a material?

5. From a standpoint of the setting reaction, the most important ingredients in a typical alginate impression material powder are a soluble alginate, calcium sulfate dihydrate, and trisodium phosphate. Explain the role of each ingredient and describe the chemistry by which this material gels.

6. What other components usually are present in an alginate powder?

7. What is the shelf life of unused alginate powder? How should it be stored?

8. Discuss the handling and manipulation of an alginate material. Include proportioning, mixing, removal of tray from mouth, pouring, and separation of the cast.

9. How can the gelation time be measured conveniently?

10. How long should the tray remain in the mouth?

11. How can gelation time be adjusted safely?

12. Discuss dimensional stability and gypsum compatibility of the alginates.

13. List common difficulties and the handling errors most likely related to these problems.

14. Describe the components in a reversible hydrocolloid impression material and the structure of the gelled material. How are reversible hydrocolloid impression materials used?

15. Discuss the manipulation of reversible hydrocolloid in regard to the following: (1) required equipment, (2) liquefaction of the material, (3) preparation of the tray material, (4) gelation in the oral cavity, and (5) removal from the mouth.

16. Describe the conditioning unit for hydrocolloid, including the purpose and use of each compartment.

17. Explain the *wet field* technique for use of hydrocolloid.

18. Define *syneresis* and *imbibition.* Explain the significance of these phenomena in terms of the dental impression.

19. What methods can be used for storage of the impression? Are any of these satisfactory?

20. Explain the purpose of treating the impression with a 2 per cent potassium sulfate solution before pouring the cast. Should this be done with all brands of hydrocolloid?

21. List common difficulties encountered with reversible hydrocolloids and the most likely causes for these defects.

22. What is the combined reversible-irreversible hydrocolloid system? What are its advantages?

CHAPTER 8

NONAQUEOUS ELASTOMERS: Rubber Impression Materials

In addition to the hydrocolloid gels, other elastic impression materials are soft and rubber-like. Known technically as *elastomers*, these materials are synthetic rubbers, not gels. These are listed in Table 6–1, which classifies the various impression materials. To distinguish elastomers from the hydrocolloids, American Dental Association Specification no. 19 refers to them as *nonaqueous elastomeric impression materials.*

The elastomeric solid impression is formed by chemical reactions between the various components. The chemical reaction that changes the elastomeric base—called a *liquid polymer*—into the final rubber-like material generally is referred to as curing or *polymerization.* The polymerization process is discussed in detail in Chapter 9. For present purposes, a polymer can be thought of as a chemical compound built up from a very large number of elementary units linked together during the reaction.

Two basic types of polymerization reaction occur. *Addition polymerization* results in the formation of a polymer without the formation of any other chemical compounds. The second type, *condensation polymerization*, produces other chemical compounds called by-products that are not part of the polymer.

Chemically, four types of elastomeric polymers are used for dental impression materials: *polysulfide, condensation polymerizing silicone, addition polymerizing silicone,* and *polyether.* Commercial products representative of the four types are seen in Figure 8–1. Figure 8–2 shows a visible light-cured polyether urethane dimethacrylate, a fifth type developed recently.

Because any or all of these are referred to as *rubber impression materials,* that terminology is used in the following discussion. The composition, chemistry, and properties of each type are presented separately, followed by the manipulative techniques. If handled correctly, all are comparable in accuracy to reversible hydrocolloid in the ability to reproduce oral tissues faithfully.

In addition to the different chemical types, many commercial products are available in different consistencies or viscosities, identified as follows:

- Very high viscosity, which is of modeling clay consistency
- High viscosity, which is referred to as *heavy body* or tray material
- Medium viscosity, often called *regular*
- Low viscosity, referred to as *light body* or *syringe*

The need for these four consistencies is apparent when the clinical techniques used with the rubber impression materials are discussed.

POLYSULFIDE RUBBER— COMPOSITION AND CHEMISTRY

Polysulfide rubber impression materials are supplied in two tubes (see Fig. 8–1): one

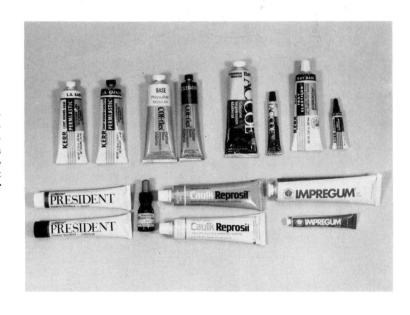

Figure 8–1. Four types of nonaqueous elastomeric impression materials. Two polysulfides are at upper left, and two condensation silicones are at upper right. Two additional silicone products are at lower left and center. A polyether is at lower right.

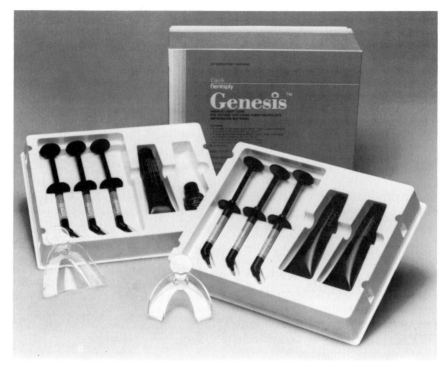

Figure 8–2. Visible light–activated elastomeric impression material. It is a single component system in two viscosities: low and heavy. The light used for curing light-activated composite resins (see Chapter 10) is used to cure the material after it has been placed in the mouth. Notice the transparent impression trays that must be used with this material. (From Phillips, R. W.: *Skinner's Science of Dental Materials*, 9th ed. Philadelphia, W. B. Saunders Co., 1991.)

for the polysulfide rubber base and one for the oxidizing agent.

The polysulfide rubber base is a liquid polymer made into a paste by the addition of certain powdered fillers. Accelerators and retarders also may be added as needed. The basic molecule of the polymer has a sulfhydryl group (SH) attached to a terminal carbon atom.

When this liquid polymer reacts with an oxidizing agent—usually lead dioxide (PbO_2)—the polymer grows or lengthens by polymerization and changes to an elastomeric solid. Sulfur also is added to facilitate the reaction and to provide better properties. The polymer paste usually is white and labeled as the *base*.

The second tube contains sulfur and lead dioxide. Because both these substances are powders, a liquid plasticizer is added to form a paste. The paste often is labeled by the manufacturer as the *accelerator* or *catalyst*. It would more correctly be termed the *reactor* because it contains the ingredient (PbO_2) that produces the reaction that forms the solid rubber. It typically is brown because of the lead dioxide. If an organic peroxide is used as a reactor, the paste may be another color.

The manipulation of these materials is discussed in detail later in this chapter. Basically, the two pastes are proportioned on a mixing pad—usually by squeezing out equal lengths—and then mixed thoroughly with a spatula. The curing reaction begins when the mixing is started and continues in a progressive manner. The mix gains elasticity until it forms a rubbery material that can be withdrawn over the teeth and undercut areas with a minimum amount of permanent deformation.

The polysulfides are not sufficiently dimensionally stable to permit storage of the impression before pouring the cast. The curing reaction for the polysulfides is a condensation reaction (water is the by-product). This leads to a moderate amount of curing shrinkage, which continues after the impression is removed from the mouth.

CONDENSATION SILICONE RUBBER (POLYSILOXANE)—COMPOSITION AND CHEMISTRY

The condensation silicone rubber base material usually is supplied as a paste in a metal tube (see Fig. 8–1). The reactor is in the form of a liquid and may be packaged in a bottle or smaller metal tube. A putty viscosity–class material is available with the condensation silicone rubber materials. It typically is supplied in a jar along with a small bottle or tube that contains the appropriate reactor liquid.

The base material is a silicone polymer called *polysiloxane.* This liquid polymer is mixed with a powdered silica (SiO_2) to form a paste. Polymerization occurs by a condensation reaction between the silicone base and an alkyl silicate, a second silicone compound. The alkyl silicate and tin octoate, a catalyst, are combined to form the liquid component, which may be labeled *accelerator* or *catalyst.* The by-product of the reaction, ethyl alcohol, is rapidly lost by evaporation. This leads to a relatively high curing shrinkage and poor dimensional stability after polymerization.

ADDITION POLYMERIZING SILICONE RUBBER (POLYVINYL SILOXANE)—COMPOSITION AND CHEMISTRY

The addition polymerizing silicone impression materials were developed to overcome the shrinkage problems encountered with the condensation silicone materials. Although these materials are based on silicone polymers, their chemistry and properties are quite different from those of the condensation silicones. They are packaged either as a two-paste system in metal tubes (see Fig. 8–1), or in two plastic jars of putty material. They commonly are available in all four viscosity classes for a given product. A recent innovation in packaging of the addition silicones is a dual-cartridge system for use in a gun that proportions and mixes the two materials automatically, shown in Figure 8–3.

Curing occurs by the addition reaction of two different liquid silicone polymers (in the presence of a platinum salt catalyst) to form an elastic solid. No by-product is formed. Hence, the curing shrinkage is small and the dimensional stability is excellent. One of the two liquid silicone polymers is a polysiloxane terminated by a vinyl group, which is essential to an addition reaction (as seen in Chapter 9). Manufacturers frequently refer to the addition silicones as *poly(vinyl) siloxane* impression materials to distinguish them from the condensation silicones. As usual, powdered solids (*silica*) are added to the liquid polymers to form the two pastes or putties.

POLYETHER RUBBER—COMPOSITION AND CHEMISTRY

The base is a polyether that contains end aziridine rings. Activation occurs by a reactor that consists of an aromatic sulfonate ester.

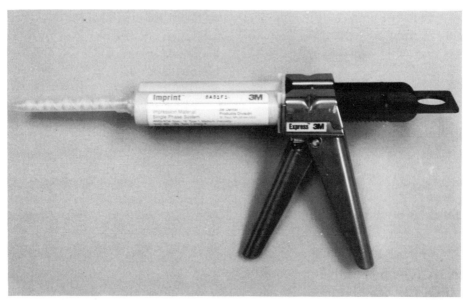

Figure 8-3. Auto dispenser and mixer for addition silicone impression materials. The two components of the impression material are in the dual cartridge. When the trigger is pulled, they are forced into the mixing nozzle and blended as they pass through the spiral *(far left)*. The mixed material emerges from the nozzle tip ready to use. (From Phillips, R. W.: *Skinner's Science of Dental Materials,* 9th ed. Philadelphia, W. B. Saunders Co., 1991.)

Both the base and the reactor are supplied as pastes in collapsible tubes. The base and reactor tubes are not the same size: a smaller nozzle opening on the reactor tube delivers the correct amount of material when equal lengths of both are dispensed. Because the set material is quite stiff, a third component—called a *body modifier* or *thinner*—also is available to reduce the stiffness. The body modifier also reduces the viscosity of the unset material. This may be advantageous because the polyethers usually are marketed in a regular viscosity only (see Fig. 8-1).

Before comparing the properties of the rubber base impression materials, the following section reviews the properties that are desirable from a clinical point of view.

Because the rubber impression materials are used to take impressions for casts and models for the construction of cast appliances, a primary consideration is accuracy.

Casts and models must both duplicate fine detail and accurately preserve the dimensions of the oral structure. This requires that they exhibit a limited amount of dimensional change while they harden into an elastomeric solid. The elastomeric solid also must have sufficient strength and elasticity to be withdrawn from the mouth without distortion or tearing.

A chemical reaction called *polymerization* causes the rubber materials to set. As soon as the two components are mixed, the viscosity begins to increase and the material starts to develop elastic properties. From the start of mixing, the dentist or auxiliary must have adequate time to handle the material and place it securely in the mouth before significant elasticity develops. During the working time, the impression material must possess sufficient flow to cover the oral tissues. Once the impression material is seated in the mouth, it should rapidly attain its elastic properties. Holding a tray of impression material steady in the patient's mouth for an extended period is tedious for both dentist and patient.

Although impression materials normally are in the mouth for only a short period, the usual concerns about biocompatibility are important. The impression material should not result in allergic or toxic reactions. Care should be exercised not to leave torn fragments of impression material in the mouth after removing the impression. Such fragments trapped in the gingival sulcus can result in irritation and inflammatory response of the gingival tissues.

Because most impressions are poured with a gypsum product, the material should be compatible with the setting reaction of gypsum. It should result in a hard surface with fine detail reproduction on the cast or die. And finally, the impression material should be able to be disinfected with an appropriate infection control agent without a loss in detail or accuracy.

PROPERTIES

The properties of the four rubber base materials are summarized in Table 8–1.

Polysulfides

Polysulfides have a strong odor (due to the SH groups) and stain clothing. Careful mixing is required to produce a homogeneous mix that is free of streaks. Both the working and the setting times are relatively long. The curing reaction is accelerated by increased temperature or the presence of moisture. Varying the proportions of the base and catalyst to adjust the curing rate should not be done.

The use of a chilled mixing slab increases the working time if the slab is not cooled so much that moisture forms on it. Adding a drop of water to the mix decreases working and setting times.

Although the permanent deformation after removal from undercut areas is relatively high, this property continues to improve after the material has reached an initial set. Thus, premature removal of a polysulfide impression from the mouth should be avoided.

The stiffness is relatively low; these materials are reasonably flexible. This facilitates removal of the impression from the mouth and separation of the cast from the impres-

TABLE 8–1. Comparative Properties of Rubber Impression Materials

	Polysulfide	Polyether	Condensation Silicone	Addition Silicone
Ease of mix	Fair	Easy	Fair to easy	Easy
Mixing time (sec)	60	30–45	30–60	30–45
Working time (min) at 20°–23° C	3–6	2–3	2–4	2–4
Setting time in mouth (min)	10–20	6–7	6–10	6–8
Cleanup	Difficult	Easy	Easy	Easy
Odor and taste	Unpleasant	Acceptable	Acceptable	Acceptable
Stiffness	Low	Very high	Medium high	High
Dimensional stability after removal from mouth	Moderate	Excellent*	Poor	Excellent
Permanent deformation after removal from mouth	High	Very low	Low	Very low
Wettability by gypsum	Poor	Good	Very poor	Very poor†
Tear resistance	Good‡	Poor	Fair	Poor

*Must be kept dry.
†Material does not fracture easily, but severe distortion occurs.
‡Hydrophilic silicones that contain wetting agents are available.

sion. In comparison with hydrocolloids, however, polysulfides are quite stiff.

The *tear resistance* of an impression material is important. If the tear resistance is high, then the impression is not likely to fracture and leave impression material trapped in the interproximal or subgingival areas. The polysulfide rubbers are good in this respect. Considerable permanent deformation may occur during removal from the mouth, however, if impression material is caught in these spaces.

Polysulfides are hydrophobic and have a high contact angle with a water-based material like gypsum. Care must be exercised when pouring them to avoid trapping air bubbles.

Condensation Silicone Rubber Impression Materials

Condensation silicone rubber impression materials are odor free, clean to handle, and relatively easy to mix. Proportioning is done by squeezing out a measured length of base material and adding the specified number of drops of liquid reactor. Varying the amount of reactor is the recommended way to adjust the working and setting times, although increased temperature also accelerates curing. Working times tend to be rather short.

The permanent deformation of condensation silicones is superior to that of polysulfides (see Table 8–1). The dimensional stability is inferior, however, and a condensation silicone impression should be poured as soon as possible after removal from the mouth. The contact angle of unset gypsum on a condensation silicone is even higher than on a polysulfide. Care must be taken to avoid trapped air when pouring the impression.

Addition Silicones

Addition silicones are odor free, clean to handle, and easy to mix. The working and

setting times are quite short. The curing reaction can be retarded by lowering the temperature of the materials and the mixing pad. Refrigeration of the materials is highly recommended; it increases working time by as much as 1 minute without appreciably changing the setting time in the mouth. Alternatively, a liquid retarder (supplied by some manufacturers) can be added to the mix.

Base-catalyst ratios should *not* be altered from those recommended. The polymerization reaction for addition silicones is very sensitive to contamination by other chemicals. Polysulfide rubber, in particular, severely retards the setting of addition silicone. Mixing spatulas, pads, and syringes used with addition silicone should not be used with other type materials. Rubber gloves, rubber dam, and even some vinyl gloves have been reported to inhibit the setting of this material.

Addition silicones have excellent dimensional stability; most manufacturers claim that pouring can be delayed for up to 7 days. The set material is stiff, and difficulty may be encountered in removing a full arch impression from the mouth. When separating the cast from the impression, care should be exercised to avoid fracturing the gypsum. The tear resistance of the silicones is poor, but the material does not suffer appreciable plastic deformation before fracture.

The contact angle of the gypsum mix on the impression material is similar to that discussed for condensation silicone. *Hydrophilic* addition silicones that contain wetting agents are available and considerably easier to pour than the hydrophobic materials. Wetting agents also can be applied to the impression surface before pouring.

Polyether

The permanent deformation of polyether is comparable to that of addition silicones.

Because the polyether curing reaction produces no by-product, the curing shrinkage and dimensional stability also are quite good. Polyethers sorb water and swell, however. Thus, the impression must be stored in a dry environment until the cast is poured.

The set polyether material has a very high stiffness that may pose clinical difficulties, although the use of the body modifier reduces the stiffness. Because polyethers are somewhat hydrophilic, they form a relatively low contact angle with gypsum and, hence, are easy to pour.

Polyethers are clean to handle, odor free, and easy to mix. They have very short working times, which can be extended by the addition of the body modifier or by reducing the amount of reactor used in making a mix.

One additional caution should be noted. The polyether chemistry has been reported to create hypersensitivity in both patients and dental staff who are allergic to the material. If a known allergy exists, this material should be avoided. Even brief skin contact can result in contact dermatitis.

TECHNCIAL CONSIDERATIONS AND MANIPULATION OF RUBBER IMPRESSION MATERIALS

Because the manipulation of the four types of elastomeric materials is comparable, they are discussed together. Any differences to be observed with each type are duly noted.

Manufacturers supply the materials in a number of consistencies, depending on how each material is used.

- A very thin fluid mix is required if the material is to be injected into the cavity preparation by means of a syringe.
- A stiffer material is desirable for filling the tray, which is then placed into position over the syringe material that has previously been injected into and around the cavity preparation.

- The final impression is a combination of the two consistencies of the impression material.
- In yet another technique, the putty material is used in quite a different manner—to form a primary impression, which is then relined or *washed* with low-viscosity material to produce the final impression.

Shelf Life

The stability of an unused dental material when it is stored is referred to as its *shelf life.* Certain materials are sensitive in this regard. Ingredients may tend to settle out, temperature fluctuations may influence the reactivity, or undesirable chemical reactions may take place as the material ages. These result in a loss in the required physical properties and inferior handling characteristics when the product is used.

For this reason, the manufacturer usually labels the material as to the date on which it was made. These labels often are part of the batch number, which is stamped on the box and the tubes of material. One should ask the manufacturer's local distributor how the date of manufacture can be determined from the batch number. For materials that are known to be susceptible to deterioration on storage, the dental auxiliary should mark the date of receipt on every package when it arrives at the office and use the oldest materials first.

Condensation silicone impression materials are the most sensitive to prolonged storage. Most of the addition silicones are now claimed to have a shelf life of at least 2 years. Regardless of the type, all rubber impression materials should be stored in a cool place. Silicones should be refrigerated if possible. When a new package of material is received, it should be tested immediately for setting time. If it does not handle properly, it should be returned to the dealer. Other especially sensitive materials are identified in later chapters.

Techniques

As noted, two basic techniques are used for taking impressions with rubber base materials. The equipment used is shown in Figures 8–4 and 8–5. In each technique, a syringe is used to inject small amounts of very fluid material directly into the cavity preparations in the mouth and any other areas in which precise detail is needed. An impression tray filled with the more viscous material then is seated over the syringe material. The two materials unite to form the impression.

The most commonly used technique involves a one-step, single impression process and usually uses mixes of impression materials with two different viscosities.

1. The lower-viscosity material is mixed first, loaded into the syringe, and injected in the mouth.
2. While this is taking place, the auxiliary mixes the higher-viscosity material and fills the impression tray.
3. The loaded tray is seated in the mouth and held passively until the material has set.

In the case of impression materials that are supplied in a single viscosity only, a double mix still should be used, particularly with materials that have short working times.

Some products are formulated for use with a single-mix technique. The increase in viscosity that occurs after the material is mixed provides a heavier body material for use in the tray.

The second basic technique uses a two-step impression process, often called a *putty-wash* technique.

1. A primary impression is taken in a stock impression tray using a putty viscosity–type material. This is not intended to provide a highly accurate impression. Some relief space must be provided in the area of the prepared teeth. This space may be created by cutting away some of the set impression material or by placing a spacer over the teeth before the primary impression is taken.
2. After the primary impression has been taken, a low-viscosity impression material of the same type is mixed and injected in the mouth by use of a syringe. The primary impression then is reseated in the mouth over the "wash" material and held steady until the syringe material has cured.

The result is an impression with accuracy

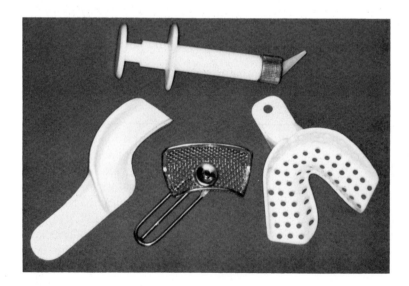

Figure 8–4. Stock impression trays and a syringe used with rubber impression materials.

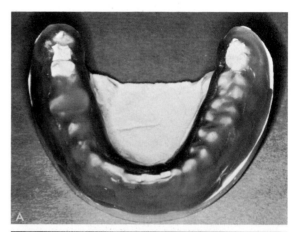

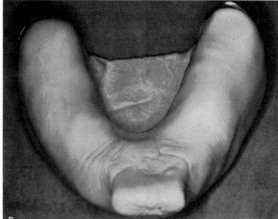

Figure 8-5. Steps in the fabrication of a custom impression tray for a rubber base impression. *A,* The cast is covered with a layer of wax to assure minimum and uniform thickness of impression material. *B,* A cold-cured resin tray is formed over the cast. *C,* After the resin tray is removed from the cast, the wax is peeled from the tray. (From Gilmore, H. W.: *Textbook of Operative Dentistry.* St. Louis, C.V. Mosby, 1967, pp 587–588, Figure 17–7.)

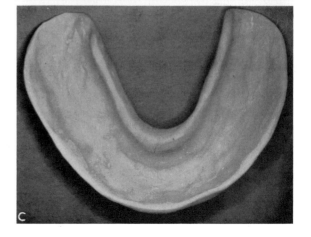

comparable to that of the single impression technique.

The Tray

Rubber impression materials can be used for almost any type of impression required by the dentist. They are intended primarily for obtaining impressions of the hard tissues where elasticity is an essential requirement. The following discussion is principally concerned with their use in the indirect technique for the construction of inlays, crowns, and bridges.

The tray used to hold the material while the impression is being obtained must be rigid. Flexible trays are invariably distorted when the impression is removed from the teeth.

If a single impression technique is used with polysulfide or condensation silicone materials, the tray *must* be adjusted to provide a moderate, uniform thickness of impression material. Because these materials undergo shrinkage during curing, the smaller the distance between the impression tray and the part to be duplicated, the more accurate the impression, provided the material is not strained too greatly during removal from the tooth. If the impression is withdrawn from deep undercut areas, then the elastic deformation may be quite high. The optimum thickness of material between the teeth and the sides of the tray is 2 to 3 mm.

Stock impression trays that can be contoured closely to the teeth are available from the manufacturer. A better method is to construct a custom tray for each individual arch from a dental plastic. Construction of a custom tray requires an additional patient appointment and is relatively expensive. The following steps are involved in constructing a custom tray:

1. Before the cavity preparations are made, the dentist obtains an impression of the mouth, typically using an alginate impression material.

2. A stone cast is constructed from that impression.

3. The areas in the cast that are to be included in the final impression are covered with one or two thicknesses of base plate wax or other spacer 2 to 3 mm thick (see Fig. 8–5A).

4. A cold curing resin (see Chapter 9) is placed over this cast (see Fig. 8–5B).

5. When the plastic has cured, it is removed from the cast and the wax peeled from the tray (see Fig. 8–5C).

6. If wax is used, it is covered with foil before forming the acrylic tray to prevent any residue of wax from remaining in the tray. The wax could interfere with the adhesion of the rubber to the tray.

This tray provides a suitable means for carrying the impression material into the mouth, where the rubber material will occupy the space that was formerly occupied by the wax spacer. This type of tray provides a uniform, minimum thickness of impression material.

Because of their low curing contraction, polyethers and addition silicones often are used in a stock tray. The putty-wash technique also makes use of stock trays—an inherent advantage of that system.

Adhesion to the Tray

As with hydrocolloid impression materials, complete adhesion of the rubber material to the tray is imperative. Otherwise, the impression material pulls away from the tray when it is removed from the mouth, resulting in a distorted impression. This adhesion usually is accomplished by application of an adhesive cement supplied by the manufacturer to the tray before the impression material is inserted. The cement is painted on 7 to 8 minutes before the tray is to be filled. The adhesive forms a tenacious bond between the tray and the impression material, particularly if the sides of the tray have been roughened slightly. Because the acrylic resin tray material may absorb the cement, several coats may be applied. Instructions supplied with the tray adhesive should be followed carefully.

Each kind of elastomer requires its own adhesive. A cement designed for use with a polysulfide should not be used with a silicone, for example. Some materials, especially the putty-like rubbers, do not adhere well to the adhesive. Mechanical retention is recommended, such as a perforated or mesh tray (see Fig. 8–2). Some addition silicones also do not adhere to their adhesives; mechanical retention is advisable then.

Spatulation

Mixing polysulfide polymers involves the following steps:

1. The correct lengths of the two pastes are squeezed onto the mixing pad (see Fig. 8–6).
2. The reactor paste (usually brown) is first smoothed flat with a flexible yet stiff spatula so that both sides of the blade are covered. This procedure provides for greater ease in cleaning the spatula later because the reactor paste is less adhesive than the base.
3. The reactor paste is incorporated into the base paste.
4. The mixture is spread over the mixing pad.
5. The process is continued until the mixed paste is of uniform color, without streaks.

A mix free of light and dark streaks should be attained in 1 minute or less, as shown in Figure 8–7. This process is somewhat difficult with the heavier viscosities and may require practice to obtain a streak-free mix.

The same procedure is followed in mixing polyethers and addition silicones, which are much easier to mix than polysulfides. The spatulation time, however, should be limited to 45 seconds; the mixed material will stiffen within 3 minutes or less. Putty-viscosity addition silicones should *never* contact latex gloves during mixing or handling. Even the use of vinyl gloves may interfere with the polymerization of these materials; this should be tested with the specific brand of glove and impression material used.

If both the base and the accelerator are supplied in paste form, the mixing procedure with condensation silicone impression

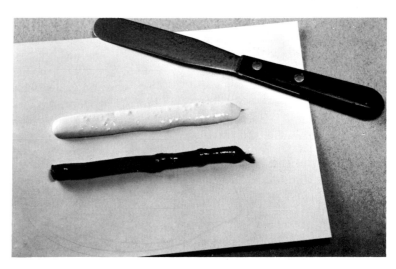

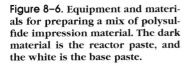

Figure 8–6. Equipment and materials for preparing a mix of polysulfide impression material. The dark material is the reactor paste, and the white is the base paste.

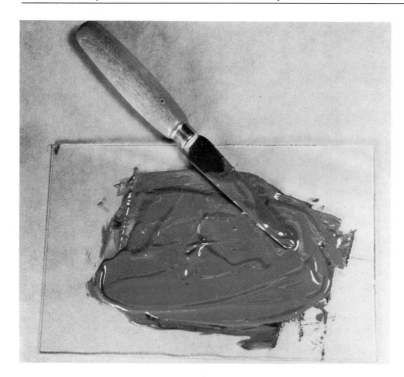

Figure 8-7. Correct mix of a poly-sulfide rubber impression material, free of streaks.

materials is the same as described for polysulfide polymers. The reactor usually is in a liquid form. The prescribed number of drops per unit length of base paste are placed on or beside the rope of extruded paste (Fig. 8–8). In either case, spatulation is continued until the mass is a uniform color.

Regardless of the type of rubber—whether polysulfide, silicone, or polyether—curing will not be uniformly complete if the mixture is not homogeneous. Then a distorted impression is likely to result.

One of the most significant developments in delivery systems for rubber impression materials has been the automatic dispensing and mixing device for addition silicones, shown in Figure 8–3. It commonly is used for low- and medium-viscosity materials, although one manufacturer markets a putty in this system. A low-viscosity polyether also has recently been made available for auto-mixing.

Automixing involves the following steps:

1. The two components of the impression material are contained in a dual cartridge, which is placed into the dispensing and mixing device.

2. As the trigger is pulled, the correct amounts of each component are metered into the spiral mixing nozzle where they are blended.

3. The thoroughly mixed material is ejected from the end of the nozzle ready to load into an impression tray or syringe and even to inject directly into the mouth if a syringe tip adapter is placed on the end of the mixing nozzle.

The advantages of this system are its uniformity of proportioning and mixing, ease of mixing, and reduced mixing time. Contamination of the impression material also is much less likely.

Although the material supplied in this delivery system is more expensive, manufacturers claim comparable cost per impression

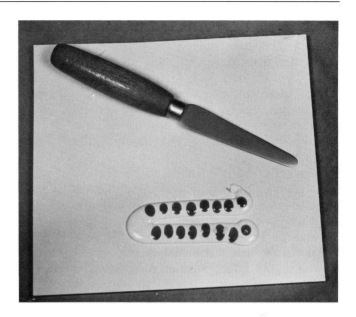

Figure 8–8. Mixing pad, spatula, and proportioned paste and liquid used for a silicone impression.

with hand-mixed material because less material is wasted. The dispensing and mixing devices are universal and interchangeable between brands of impression materials. However, the mixing nozzles, which are discarded after each mix, must not be interchanged. They are unique not only to the brand but also to the viscosity being mixed.

Working Time and Setting Time

The typical values for working and setting times are given in Table 8–1. Ways to adjust these times have been discussed for each kind of impression material. The next section explains the significance of these properties.

The clinical significance of the working time is that it represents the maximum amount of time available to mix and handle the material before the impression must be seated in the mouth. If the impression is not seated during this time period, the material may develop sufficient elasticity that a distorted impression results.

The setting time is the minimum time elapsed from the start of mixing until the material is sufficiently elastic that it can be removed from the mouth without clinically significant permanent deformation. Premature removal from the mouth results in significant deformation, a major contributor to failures encountered when using rubber base materials.

As can be seen from Table 8–1, the setting times for rubber impression materials vary considerably between different kinds of materials and even different brands of the same type. The manufacturers' instructions specify the minimum length of time the impression should remain in the mouth.

Although actual timing of the operation is recommended, the dentist can judge the appropriate time at which to remove the impression by lightly impressing the surface of the rubber with a blunt instrument. When the point no longer leaves an indentation on the surface of either the syringe or the tray material, the impression may be safely removed from the mouth.

Dimensional Stability

With rubber impression materials, changes in dimension caused by syneresis or imbibition during storage of the impression do not pose the problem they do with hydrocolloids. However, the cured polyether swells when stored in a high-humidity environment. The usual room atmosphere is suitable for storage of all four types of elastomeric materials. Storage in a humidor or desiccator should not be necessary and may be undesirable.

Storage of the polysulfide and condensation silicone impression is contraindicated. As previously mentioned, curing does not stop when the impression is removed from the mouth. The continued curing of the material before the stone cast is constructed produces distortion. Furthermore, some of the ingredients may volatilize, which results in additional shrinkage.

If a polysulfide or condensation silicone material is used, the stone die should be constructed within the first hour after removal of the impression from the mouth. The vivid effects of distortion upon storage of such an impression are shown in Figure 8–9. A discrepancy can be seen after storage of the impression for six hours. The inaccuracy after 24 hours of storage is more obvious.

If pouring of an impression must be delayed overnight or longer, an additional silicone or polyether impression material should be used, as shown in Figure 8–9. In some cases, manufacturers of addition silicone materials recommend delayed pouring to improve the surface of the stone die. This matter is discussed later in this chapter.

The Die

In most cases, the stone die should be constructed as soon as possible after the impression is removed from the mouth. The stone is mixed and vibrated into the impression, as described in Chapter 6. Vacuum mixing is highly recommended.

Because the surface of the silicone and polysulfide rubber impression materials is not easily wetted by the stone mix, considerable care is required in pouring the impression to avoid the trapping of air. Rinsing the impression with a suitable wetting agent before pouring may be beneficial. A blunt instrument also is helpful to assist in flowing the stone into the deeper areas. When handled correctly, rubber impression materials have a superior capacity to reproduce detail and provide maximum hardness on the surface of the stone die.

A number of die materials other than stone may be used with the rubber impression materials, although stone is the most common. If a plastic (resin) is used, the die material *must* be compatible with that particular brand of impression material. Otherwise, a reaction may occur between the die and the impression.

If certain addition silicone rubber impressions are poured immediately after they are taken, small bubbles appear in the surface of the stone die. The bubbles apparently are due to a gas that is not part of the addition-type reaction being produced during curing. This phenomenon depends on both the brand and the batch and may be aggravated if the base and reactor are incorrectly proportioned. As noted, many suppliers of addition silicones suggest delay of pouring for a specified time. These suggestions should be followed.

Because the polyether and addition silicone are stiff materials, fracture of the stone die or cast may occur during separation. Particular care given to proportioning the water and powder and to mixing and allowing sufficient time for the gypsum to set minimize this problem.

In some cases, multiple pours of an impression may be required. An impression occasionally needs to be poured again to make an additional cast or die. These situations require both dimensional stability and excellent recovery after deformation. Only

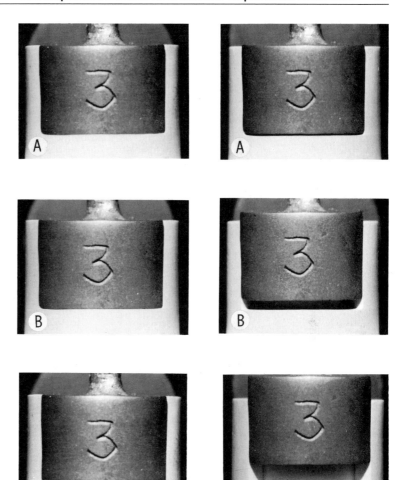

Figure 8-9. Fit of a master casting on stone dies constructed from an addition *(left column)* and a condensation silicone *(right column)*. Stone poured at *A,* 30 minutes; *B,* 6 hours; and *C,* 24 hours.

the addition silicone and polyether have elastic properties that permit multiple or delayed repouring of impressions. In the case of polyether, water absorption from the gypsum leads to some distortion of subsequent casts poured from the same impression.

INFECTION CONTROL

As with other impression materials, rubber impression materials must be able to with-

stand disinfection without clinically significant distortion or influence on the detail reproduction of the stone cast or die. All four chemical types of rubber impression material can be subjected to brief treatment in an appropriate disinfection agent if the contact time is short.

Polyether may sorb water from a water-based agent and swell with prolonged immersion. Polysulfide and condensation sili-

Type	Cause
Rough or uneven surface on impression	1. Incomplete polymerization caused by premature removal from the mouth, incorrect ratio or mixing of accelerator and base, or oil or other organic material on the teeth 2. Too rapid polymerization from high humidity or temperature or incorrect base-reactor ratios 3. Contamination of addition silicone by rubber gloves or other materials
Bubbles	1. Too rapid polymerization, preventing flow of impression material 2. Air incorporated during mixing 3. Incorrect injection technique, producing entrapment of air
Irregularly shaped voids	1. Moisture or debris on surface of teeth
Nodules (positive defects) on stone cast surface	1. Air trapped when making the impression
Rough or chalky stone cast	1. Inadequate cleaning of impression 2. Excess water left on surface of the impression 3. Premature removal of cast 4. Incorrect manipulation of stone 5. Excessively thin layer of impression material, resulting in the tray or adhesive being in contact with the stone 6. Gas liberated by addition silicone impression material
Distortion	1. Resin tray not aged sufficiently and still undergoing polymerization shrinkage 2. Lack of adhesion of rubber to the tray caused by not enough coats of adhesive, filling tray with material too soon after applying adhesive, or using wrong adhesive 3. Lack of mechanical retention for those materials with which adhesive is ineffective 4. Development of elastic properties in the material before tray is seated 5. Excess bulk of material 6. Insufficient relief for the reline material if this technique is used 7. Contiued pressure against impression material that has developed elastic properties 8. Movement of tray during polymerization 9. Premature removal from mouth 10. Incorrect removal from mouth 11. Delayed pouring of the polysulfide or condensation silicone impression

cone should not be subject to a prolonged delay in pouring because of their poor dimensional stability. Manufacturers' instructions should be consulted regarding the type of disinfection agent and the method and length of treatment.

CAUSES OF COMMON DIFFICULTIES

Failures that may occur in the use of rubber base impression materials and the causative factors are summarized above.

Selected Reading

Braden, M.: Characterization of the setting process in dental polysulfide rubbers. J. Dent. Res. 45:1066, 1966.

Braden, M., Causton, B., and Clarke, R. L: A polyether impression rubber. J. Dent. Res. 51:889, 1972.

Council on Dental Materials, Instruments, and Equipment: Infection control recommendation for the dental office and the dental laboratory. J. Am. Dent. Assoc. 116:148, 1988.

Craig, R. G.: Review of dental impression materials. Adv. Dent. Res. 2:51, 1988.

Cullen, D. R., and Sandrik, J. L.: Tensile strength of elastomeric impression materials, adhesive and cohesive bonding. J. Prosthet. Dent. 62:141, 1989.

Johnson, G. H., and Craig, R. G.: Accuracy of addition

silicone as a function of technique. J. Prosthet. Dent. 55:197, 1986.

Jorgensen, K. D.: Thiokol as a dental impression material. Acta Odontol. Scand. 14:313, 1956.

McCabe, J. F., and Carrick, T. E.: Rheological properties of elastomers during setting. J. Dent. Res. 68:1218, 1989.

McCormick, J. T., Antony, S. J., Dial, M. L., et al.: Wettability of elastomeric impression materials: Effect of selected surfactants. Int. J. Prosthodont. 2:413, 1989.

Munoz, C. A., Goodacre, C. J., Schnell, R. J., and Harris, R. K.: Laboratory and clinical study of a visible light-polymerized elastomeric impression material. Int. J. Prosthodont. 1:59, 1988.

Salem, N. S., Combe, E. C., and Watts, D. C.: Mechanical properties of elastomeric impression materials. J. Oral Rehabil. 15:125, 1988.

Stackhouse, J. A., Jr.: The accuracy of stone dies made from rubber impression materials. J. Prosthet. Dent. 24:377, 1970.

Sy, J. T., Munoz, C. A., Schnell, R. J., et al.: Some effects of cooling and chemical retarders on five elastomeric impression materials. Int. J. Prosthodont. 1:252, 1988.

Tjan, A. H. L.: Effect of contaminants on the adhesion of light-bodied silicones to putty silicones in putty-wash impression technique. J. Prosthet. Dent. 59:562, 1988.

Wilson, H. J.: Impression materials. Br. Dent. J. 164:221, 1988.

Reviewing the Chapter

1. Define the term *elastomer.*
2. Name four chemical types of rubber base impression materials.
3. Many brands of elastomeric impression materials are supplied in four viscosities. List the common terms used in referring to the four viscosity materials.
4. Define *polymer, polymerization,* and *curing* as these terms relate to the elastomeric impression materials.
5. For each of the four chemical types of elastomers, list the comparative advantages and disadvantages. How may the setting time be safely adjusted for each type?
6. Describe typical values for shelf life for these materials and how they should be stored.
7. Give two reasons why custom impression trays often are used with the elastomeric materials. How is the tray constructed?
8. Explain the function and use of a *tray adhesive.*
9. Describe the *multiple mix, single impression technique.* What is the *putty-wash technique?* List the advantages of each.
10. Why is it important that the material in the tray not develop elastic properties before seating of the tray?
11. Discuss the dimensional stability of the various kinds of elastomers. How long can such an impression be stored before pouring?
12. What special cautions should be taken when pouring a rubber elastomer impression?
13. List common difficulties seen with these materials and the handling errors probably related to these problems.
14. What precautions should be followed when subjecting a rubber impression to a disinfection process?
15. What is the *automixing system* for addition silicone impression materials? Compared with hand mixing, what advantages and disadvantages does it have?
16. Addition silicone impression materials are particularly sensitive to contamination by what other substances? What influence might this have on the clinical manipulation of these materials?

DENTAL POLYMERS: Synthetic Resins, Denture Base Materials

REQUISITES FOR A DENTAL RESIN
CLASSIFICATION OF RESINS
POLYMERIZATION
MOLECULAR WEIGHT
Requisites for Addition
   Polymerization
CROSS-LINKING
COPOLYMERIZATION
DENTAL RESINS

PHYSICAL PROPERTIES AND
STRUCTURE OF PMMA
Handling Dental Resins
CONSTRUCTION OF A DENTURE
Construction of the Mold
Care of a Denture
Allergic Reactions
DENTURE RELINERS
OTHER USES OF RESIN

Synthetic resins belong to the class of materials called *polymers*. A more commonly used term for this class of materials is *plastics*. The term synthetic indicates that a material is man-made, usually from carbon, hydrogen, and oxygen. The basic structures from which all life is composed are natural polymers. Although the trend is to replace naturally derived materials with man-made ones, some natural resins have been used in dental materials.

The term *plastic* includes not only synthetic resins but also synthetic fibers or threads, such as nylon and Acrilan. Natural fibers, such as cotton and wool, also are

polymers. Because it is made from regenerated cellulose, rayon is better classified as a natural resin.

By definition, a synthetic polymer is a nonmetallic compound, synthetically produced (usually from organic compounds), which can be molded into various useful forms and then hardened for use. The terms resin and plastic are used synonymously.

Clothing, building materials, household appliances, electrical equipment, and articles used in almost every type of human activity today are constructed in part or whole of a synthetic resin or plastic. Resins can be fabricated into thread for weaving cloth and carpeting or molded to form lamp bases, toys, airplane parts, and even car bodies. Even where great strength and toughness are needed, plastics today compete favorably with metals.

The use of plastics has simplified and improved the dentist's work. Dental resins can be formulated to simulate the oral soft tissues or molded into tooth forms that defy detection when used in artificial dentures. Dental resins are used in tissue treatment materials, orthodontic appliances, and cements and as restorative materials.

Probably no other area of research has greater importance to dentistry than the development of improved synthetic resins. As dentistry moves into the 21st century, the focus of dental materials research is shifting from the development of metallic dental materials to polymers. The requirement that dental restorative materials restore appearance as well as function is the basic force driving the move from metals to polymers.

REQUISITES FOR A DENTAL RESIN

For a number of reasons, not all plastics can be used in the mouth. Some of the requisites for a dental resin are as follows:

- The material should exhibit a translucence such that it can duplicate aesthetically the oral tissue that it replaces. It should be capable of being tinted or pigmented to blend into the adjacent natural structures, whether hard or soft tissue.
- The color and appearance of the plastic should be stable over its intended lifetime.
- The plastic must be capable of being shaped into an appliance or restoration that fits accurately over the natural tissues. It should not expand, contract, or warp during use by the patient.

- It should possess adequate strength, resilience, and wear resistance to withstand normal usage.
- It should be light in weight.
- It should be completely insoluble in mouth fluids or substances normally taken into the mouth.
- It should be impermeable to mouth fluids so that it does not become biologically contaminated or disagreeable in taste, odor, or appearance.
- It should be tasteless, odorless, nontoxic, and nonirritating and should not cause an allergic response.
- Food or other substances normally taken into the mouth should not adhere to the resin or result in degradation of its properties.
- Its softening temperature should be well above the temperature of any hot foods or liquids taken into the mouth.
- The resin should be easily repairable.
- Fabrication of the resin into a dental appliance should not require complicated, expensive equipment or an unreasonably long time.

No current plastic material completely meets all these requirements. The oral environment, described in Chapters 2 through 4, is very demanding. Only the most inert, stable plastics can withstand its challenges.

CLASSIFICATION OF RESINS

Because of the complexity of the chemistry and composition of resins, a simple system for their classification is difficult. One classification is made on the basis of *thermal behavior*. Plastics usually are molded under heat and pressure. If the resin is molded without a chemical change occurring—by simply using heat and pressure and then cooling it to form a solid shape—it is classified as *thermoplastic*. As pointed out in Chapter 6, impression compound can be classified as a thermoplastic material because it softens under heat and cools to form a solid without a chemical reaction occurring. Impression compound usually is not classified as a synthetic resin because it contains little or no synthetic plastic.

If a chemical reaction takes place during the molding process, the final product is chemically different from the original substance. The plastic is classified as *thermosetting*. This type of resin is not softened by heating after the chemical reaction has occurred. The curing of rubber dental impression materials, discussed in Chapter 8, is an example of thermoset polymers.

Thermoplastic resins usually are soluble in certain organic solvents, such as acetone and chloroform, whereas most thermoset resins are insoluble.

A more definitive way of classifying resins is in terms of their structural units.

POLYMERIZATION

Synthetic resins are *polymers*, formed by *polymerization*, as briefly discussed in Chapter 8. Assume that the polymerization reaction begins with a single molecule, designated as *A*. This single molecule is known as a *mer*, and the material in this form is called a *monomer*, meaning one molecule. If two monomer molecules react to form a single molecule containing two mers, the result

$$—A—A— \qquad 9-1$$

is called a *dimer*. These two molecules are linked by a strong chemical bond, and energy (exothermic heat) is given off in this reaction.

If three monomer molecules combine to form one molecule,

$$—A—A—A— \qquad 9-2$$

a *trimer* is formed. A *polymer* (many mers) is formed if several monomer molecules are joined to form one large molecule:

$$—A—A—A— \cdots —A—A—A— \qquad 9-3$$

Each *A* (or mer) in the polymer is the same original monomer molecule, joined together with other monomer molecules to form a chain, with the mer repeated time after time. The lines between the A's indicate primary chemical bonds that hold the molecules together.

Bonds are present at each end of the chain, indicating that the molecule or polymer may continue to grow in both directions because the number of mers is not fixed. A single polymer chain or molecule can have many thousands of mers. In the example above, the monomer *A* is repeated in the center of the polymer many times as indicated by $\cdots$. Because the number of mers joined together has significant influence on the properties of the polymer, knowing the number of mers that have been joined is important. A shorthand notation that shows this directly is

$$—A—[—A—]_n—A— \qquad 9-4$$

Here the mer, —A—, is repeated *n* times in the center of the molecule for a total of $n + 2$ monomer molecules. In this manner, the writing of the formula can be simplified.

As discussed in Chapter 8, this type of polymerization, known as *addition polymerization*, is the simplest of all mechanisms of polymerization. Most resins polymerized by addition are thermoplastic and soluble in certain organic solvents.

Thermosetting resins usually are formed by *condensation polymerization*. This type of reaction differs from addition polymerization in that the joining of the mers is accompanied by a chemical reaction and the formation of by-products.

$$A + A \rightarrow —A'—A'— + H_2O$$
$$—A'—A'— + A \rightarrow —A'—A'—A'— + H_2O \qquad 9-5$$
$$—A'—A'— \cdots —A'—A'— + A \rightarrow$$
$$—A'—A'— \cdots —A'—A'—A'— + H_2O$$

Water is the by-product in this example. In other cases, the by-product may be hydrochloric acid, ammonia, ethyl alcohol, or other simple chemical compounds. Unlike the polymer formed by addition polymerization, the mers in the polymer chain formed by condensation polymerization are not exactly the same as the mers of the monomer. This is indicated by the prime sign beside the mers *(A')* that are joined together. This change is due to the formation of the by-products. Each unit, or mer, in the chain, however, is identical to the others. The polymerization of polysulfide rubber impression material, described in Chapter 8, is a condensation reaction.

Because it is a repetitive reaction between molecules, polymerization theoretically is capable of proceeding until all monomer building blocks are exhausted. In practice, unreacted monomer usually is present and may have considerable influence on the properties of the polymer.

The polymer chains form into a three-dimensional structure, creating a tangled mass. The end result is not unlike a bowl of cooked spaghetti.

MOLECULAR WEIGHT

The length of the polymer chain is described by its molecular weight. Polymers for a denture base resin may have weights as high as 600,000. By comparison, the molecular weight of water is only 18, and table sugar is 342.

The molecular weight of a polymer formed by addition polymerization is equal to the molecular weight of the monomer multiplied by the number of mers in the polymer chain.

This fact is of considerable importance in connection with the strength and hardness of the polymer. Assume, for example, that the original monomer, *A*, is a liquid. The molecules apparently are small enough that they can roll over one another at will and, therefore, constitute a liquid. As soon as polymerization begins, the following process occurs:

1. The molecule lengthens.
2. Because the longer molecules can no longer roll over one another as readily, the viscosity of the liquid increases.
3. Weak secondary forces tend to hold these lengthening molecules to each other.
4. The molecule finally becomes so long that the polymer no longer is a liquid and becomes a solid.
5. The longer the polymer chain becomes, the more the polymer chains become entangled.
6. As a result, the solid becomes stronger and harder.

In other words, the longer the polymer or the greater the molecular weight, the stronger and harder the resin. Because the resin is thermoplastic, however, the resin decreases in strength and hardness as its temperature increases.

The molecular weight (and thus the strength) of the final polymer formed is influenced also by the amount of polymerization that occurs—that is, the percentage of original monomer liquid that can be converted to the solid polymer. As noted, polymerization never is complete, and the residual monomer remaining in dental resins may be as great as 5 per cent. For this and other reasons, the molecular weight of dental resins never approaches the 50,000,000 possible in certain industrial plastics. Even in dental resins, however, the polymer formed exceeds the minimum molecular weight of 5000 considered necessary for a substance to be classified as a *macromolecule.*

Requisites for Addition Polymerization

Because almost all dental resins are formed by addition polymerization, only addition polymers are discussed in detail. The structure of an addition polymer has been described.

Understanding how the polymerization

$$\text{Ethylene} \quad \begin{matrix} H & H \\ | & \| \\ C = C \\ | & | \\ H & H \end{matrix} \quad \text{Ethylene activated} \quad * \begin{matrix} H & H \\ | & | \\ C - C \\ | & | \\ H & H \end{matrix} * \qquad 9\text{--}6$$

process occurs is fundamental for understanding the manipulation of different dental resins. Addition polymerization is possible because the monomer molecule has at least two carbon atoms that possess a double bond or linkage to each other. A carbon atom has four chemical bonds. When two of these are used to bond to another carbon atom, as in the compound ethylene, in 9–6 above, each carbon atom has a bond available for further chemical reaction if the double bond is broken (* activated). Such a compound is said to be unsaturated. Margarines and cooking oils that claim to be *highly unsaturated* also are polymers. Highly unsaturated means that they have a large number of carbon atoms with double bonds. If these double bonds can be *activated*, they allow the carbon atoms to bond to other molecules—the requirement for addition polymerization to occur.

Ethylene monomer, which is a gas, will polymerize under proper conditions to form the solid polymer polyethylene, as in 9–7.

Many polymer chains are formed simultaneously, but for simplification, the formation of a single chain will be discussed. The polymerization reaction takes place in three stages:

1. *Induction.* The double bond of a sin-gle monomer molecule is opened, or *activated*, by adding energy.

2. *Propagation.* That energy is transferred to an adjacent monomer molecule, opening its double bond and pairing the two monomer molecules into a dimer. That dimer in turn transfers energy to the next nearby monomer molecule, opening its double bond and pairing with it. The polymer chain lengthens rapidly by this process.

3. *Termination.* Growth eventually is halted because there are no more adjacent monomer molecules with which to pair or the growing chain links with another chain growing toward it.

The reaction may be compared to a row of dominos standing on end. A flick of the finger supplies the energy to knock over the first domino (*induction* or *activation*) and starts the chain reaction. As it falls, it furnishes the energy to knock over the next domino, and that domino knocks over the next one (*propagation*) until all the dominos that are properly aligned have fallen (*termination*).

The activation energy may come from heat, light, or certain reactive chemicals. The latter break down or split up to form activated particles called *free radicals*, which open the double bond on the monomer and

$$\text{Polyethylene} \quad \begin{matrix} H & H \\ | & | \\ - C - C - \\ | & | \\ H & H \end{matrix} \left[\begin{matrix} H & H \\ | & | \\ - C - C - \\ | & | \\ H & H \end{matrix} \right]_n \begin{matrix} H & H \\ | & | \\ - C - C - \\ | & | \\ H & H \end{matrix} \qquad 9\text{--}7$$

thus activate or initiate the polymerization reaction.

The most common *induction system* used in dentistry uses the chemical initiator benzoyl peroxide $(C_6H_5COO)_2$. When benzoyl peroxide is heated to about 60° C (140° F) or is mixed with another chemical—usually a tertiary amine—the molecule splits to form two free radicals (I*) that can pair with adjacent monomer molecules. The pairing opens the carbon double bonds to initiate the polymerization reaction.

$$I^* + \begin{matrix} H \\ | \\ C \\ | \\ H \end{matrix} = \begin{matrix} H \\ | \\ C \\ | \\ H \end{matrix} \rightarrow I - \begin{matrix} H \\ | \\ C \\ | \\ H \end{matrix} - \begin{matrix} H \\ | \\ C^* \\ | \\ H \end{matrix} \qquad 9\text{--}8$$

Resin systems that use heat to activate the peroxide initiator are referred to as heat-activated, heat-polymerized, or heat-cured resins. Those that use a chemical to activate the initiator polymerize without application of external heat. They are referred to as *chemically activated, cold-cured, autopolymerized,* or *self-cured* resins.

The third type of polymerization induction system used in dentistry involves the use of light. These resins use photo initiators, such as camphoroquinone and amine activators, that react to form free radicals when exposed to light in the blue range of the spectrum (wavelengths between 400 and 500 nm). Such resins are referred to as *visible light–cured, light-polymerized,* or *light-activated* resins.

The simple monomer ethylene has been used here to demonstrate the addition polymerization mechanism. Although more complex, dental monomers, such as methyl

methacrylate (MMA), polymerize by the same addition mechanism, through the C = C as indicated by the arrow.

$$\text{Methyl methacrylate} \quad \begin{matrix} H & & CH_3 \\ | & \Downarrow & | \\ C & = & C \\ | & & | \\ H & & C=O \\ & & | \\ & & O \\ & & | \\ & & CH_3 \end{matrix} \qquad 9\text{--}9$$

CROSS-LINKING

In the addition polymerization reaction described, the individual linear molecules are not actually linked together. Each molecule builds individually, forming a long strand. Although the individual strands are intertwined, resembling a bowl of cooked spaghetti, they are not chemically bound together.

Dental manufacturers sometimes advertise that a dental resin is *cross-linked*, which means that two adjacent polymer chains have been joined. This condition can be diagrammatically indicated below in 9–10. Although this formula shows cross-linking in only one direction, it may be three-dimensional.

The requirement for cross-linking of polymer chains is a monomer with at least two C = C unsaturated groups.

$$\begin{matrix} \cdots-A-A-A-A-A-A-A-A-A-A-A-A-\cdots \\ |\quad|\quad|\quad|\quad|\quad|\quad|\quad|\quad|\quad|\quad|\quad| \\ \cdots-A-A-A-A-A-A-A-A-A-A-A-A-\cdots \end{matrix} \qquad 9\text{--}10$$

The cross-linking agent commonly used in dental resins is glycol dimethacrylate:

$$\left[\begin{array}{cc} H & CH_3 \\ | & | \\ C & = C \\ | & | \\ H & C = O \\ & | \\ & O \\ & | \\ & CH_2 \\ & | \end{array}\right.$$

Glycol dimethacrylate

$$\left.\begin{array}{cc} H & CH_2 \\ | & | \\ C & = C \\ | & | \\ H & C = O \\ & | \\ & O \\ & | \\ & CH_3 \end{array}\right]$$ 9–11

At first glance, this formula appears to be complicated, but if it is separated into two parts, as indicated by the square braces, the formulas contained within each pair are essentially those for MMA. As glycol dimethacrylate polymerizes, each section of the molecule within the braces can join a growing chain by opening its C=C double bond. Thus, the polymer chains of poly(glycol dimethacrylate) cross-link through the C—C groups. These materials are referred to as *cross-linked resins.*

Such resins are widely used for denture bases and acrylic teeth for prosthetic devices. The latticework of molecules produced through cross-linking inhibits penetration of water or other fluids between polymer chains and increases the polymers' resistance to cracking and crazing. The effect of cross-linking on certain other physical properties is not as marked; it depends on the composition and the concentration of the agent used.

COPOLYMERIZATION

The term *copolymer* indicates that two or more monomer molecules have been polymerized at the same time by a process known as *copolymerization.* Not all monomers can be copolymerized. The two monomers must be soluble in each other and must polymerize at about the same rate. The copolymer molecular chain is formed with both monomer units appearing in the chain, linked together.

In this example, two resin monomers, A and B, are mixed in equal amounts. If they both polymerize at the same time at the same rate, the copolymer might be as in 9–12 below. This copolymer possesses properties different from those of either the polymer of A or B. If the two monomers are mixed with one third monomer A and two thirds monomer B, the copolymer obtained has different properties from one with equal parts of each monomer.

As an example of copolymerization, methyl methacrylate can be copolymerized with a small amount of another acrylic resin monomer, such as ethyl acrylate, to provide a copolymer that is less brittle than poly(methyl methacrylate) (PMMA). In other cases, copolymerization can be used to form soft, flexible resins. These materials are useful as denture reliners and protective devices, such as mouth guards.

Another method for softening a resin is to add a *plasticizer.* A plasticizer can be in the form of a *comonomer,* as discussed above, or it can be an external additive to produce a lubrication effect between the resin molecules, decreasing the polymer's brittleness. Plastic raincoats and handbags often are made of resins that contain external plasticizers. Because of the loss of strength and hardness that occurs, plasticizers of this type are used sparingly in dental resins. The leaching out of the plasticizer into the oral fluids also results in a rather short useful lifetime for these dental polymers.

DENTAL RESINS

The resin most frequently used in prosthetic dentistry is called *acrylic,* a generic

—A—B—A—B—A—B—A—B—A—B—A—B—A—B—A—B—   9–12

term denoting a large family of compounds derived from acrylic acid.

$$
\text{Acrylic acid} \qquad
\begin{array}{c}
H \quad\;\; H \\
| \qquad | \\
C = C \\
| \qquad | \\
H \quad\;\; C = O \\
| \\
OH
\end{array}
\qquad 9\text{--}13
$$

To call a dental resin an acrylic resin does not indicate its real identity any more than to identify a certain person as Mr. Jones without specifying which Mr. Jones. PMMA, the acrylic resin most widely used in dentistry, is a polymer that has been polymerized from the monomer MMA.

The properties of PMMA can be modified and optimized for particular uses by cross-linking agents and by copolymerization with various monomers. This produces resins suitable for dentures, artificial teeth, denture liners, and other intraoral appliances.

Because of its high water absorption, the polymer of acrylic acid is unsuitable for use as a dental resin. It is, however, a component of polycarboxylate dental cements and some glass ionomer cements, as discussed in Chapters 21 and 22.

Most resins used as the matrix for composite resin restorations and resin cements have a backbone chain similar to that of an epoxy resin with a functional methacrylate group attached at each end of the molecule. They thus are *dimethacrylates*. The resin is referred to as *BIS-GMA*.

Another resin used in commercial composite resins is *urethane dimethacrylate*. In both cases, the monomers polymerize by addition, using the $C = C$ on the methacrylate groups.

PHYSICAL PROPERTIES AND STRUCTURE OF PMMA

MMA is a clear, transparent liquid that boils at $100.8°$ C ($213.4°$ F). It has a low vis-

cosity and a high vapor pressure, which can be observed from the marked odor that fills a room when a container of the liquid is opened. After polymerization, PMMA is a transparent resin with optical properties that resemble glass. It actually transmits light better than glass. PMMA is a moderately hard resin with a Knoop hardness of about 18 to 20. Its tensile strength is about 59 MPa (8500 psi), and its density is 1.19 g/ml. PMMA is extremely stable: it will not discolor when exposed to light and remains remarkably clean in the mouth.

PMMA, like all acrylic resins, exhibits a tendency to take up water and swell. Because both adsorption and absorption are involved, this is referred to as *water sorption*. PMMA absorbs less water than any other acrylic resin, however, and the resulting change in dimension is not critical in the normal use of dental appliances constructed from PMMA. The sorption of water or oral fluids does not soften the resin appreciably or render it foul.

Like most polymers, PMMA's structure is essentially noncrystalline.

Handling Dental Resins

Dental resins typically are supplied in the form of a powder and liquid. The powder consists of particles of the polymer and usually the initiator—benzoyl peroxide for heat and chemically activated resins. As shown in Figure 9–1, the polymer particles, called *beads*, appear round and iridescent under the microscope.

The polymer beads are transparent. Some are covered with a pigment to match the color of the oral soft tissue or tooth structure. As light penetrates the polymerized resin, the pigment reflects the light to provide the proper color and shade. At the same time, the resin exhibits a translucence that matches that of the human tooth or soft tissue to an extent that defies detection.

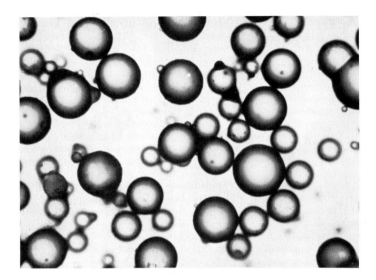

Figure 9–1. Polymer beads of PMMA in a denture resin.

The liquid is MMA monomer. A small amount of *inhibitor*, such as hydroquinone, is added to prevent polymerization of the monomer during storage. The liquid component of chemically activated resins contains the amine activator.

The monomer liquid and polymer powder are mixed together in certain proportions. These proportions are not critical, but every polymer bead must be wetted by the monomer. As the mixture stands, the monomer liquid begins to dissolve the outside of the polymer beads. During this stage, the mix is quite sticky and adheres to the container, spatula, and anything else it touches.

As the monomer becomes saturated with the PMMA, the mass becomes increasingly doughy. At this point, the soft, plastic mass is molded easily into the shape of a denture base or tooth. After molding, the monomer in the dough is polymerized into a solid. Although this process often is referred to as *curing*—a term inherited from the rubber industry—*polymerization* is a more acceptable term.

As described in the next section, the mold for the dental appliance usually is constructed of plaster or stone. The monomer-

polymer dough is packed into this mold, which is closed tightly.

In the heat polymerization method, the closed mold is placed in water, and the temperature gradually increased until the polymerization begins. When the temperature of the dough reaches 60° C (140° F), the benzoyl peroxide is activated and polymerization starts. The reaction rate increases as the temperature rises and is particularly rapid between 60° and 70° C (140° and 158° F). The closed mold is allowed to stand at room temperature until the polymerization reaction has ended.

Specially formulated heat-activated denture resins have been marketed for processing in microwave ovens. The fit and properties of these dentures are comparable to those of dentures processed in the conventional heat-water bath. The advantages are rapid processing and elimination of the need for a large water bath. The microwave-activated resins cannot be processed in the metal flask used for water-bath processing, as shown in Figure 9–2, but require a special fiberglass resin flask.

Among the chemically activated denture resins are those known as *pour-type* or *fluid*

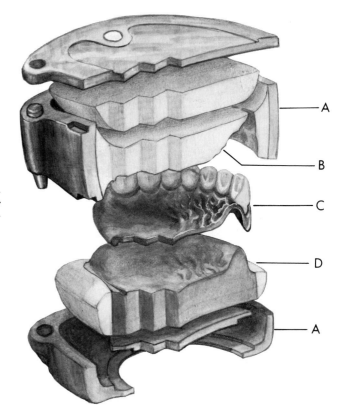

Figure 9–2. Cross section through a metal denture flask, showing the metal flask *(A)*, plaster investing material *(B)*, wax denture and denture teeth *(C)*, and the stone cast *(D)*.

resins. A very fine particle size of polymer is used, and the mixed dough has a very low viscosity. The dough is poured into the mold through an opening, or vent, and held in a pressure chamber at room temperature until polymerized.

Heat-activated resins commonly are used for constructing denture bases. Although the chemically activated resins have less polymerization shrinkage and dimensional change during curing, they create a more porous denture surface than the heat-activated resins. Chemically activated resins, however, have a distinct advantage for repairing or relining an existing denture: the repair is simple and quick, and the denture can be returned to the patient in a short time. These materials are used almost exclusively for procedures done in the dental office.

Light-activated materials are the most re-

cent innovation in denture base materials. Supplied in lightproof packages, these resins are single-component resins using acrylic beads suspended in urethane dimethacrylate, a viscous monomer. They use a camphoroquinone-amine photo initiator, which is activated by high-intensity visible light in the blue part of the spectrum (400- to 500-nm wavelength). Resin encased in a flask and gypsum mold cannot be polymerized by light activation, so the denture fabrication technique is quite different from that used with conventional heat- and cold-cured resins.

CONSTRUCTION OF A DENTURE

Dental auxiliaries usually are not involved in the construction of a full or partial denture. Some knowledge about the fabrication of dentures still is important because they work with patients who have such appliances and advise and assist in cleaning and maintaining the appliances.

As previously noted, heat-activated PMMA most commonly is used in the construction of denture bases. Other resins, such as polystyrene, vinyl copolymers, or even nylon, have been marketed for this purpose, but none has proved superior.

The portion of the denture that rests directly on the soft tissues is known as the *denture base*. The following steps are involved in constructing a denture base:

1. The dentist obtains an impression of the edentulous mouth.

2. A stone cast is poured from this impression. The stone cast is an accurate model of the area to be covered by the denture. The fabrication procedures for the denture are performed on this cast.

3. The denture base pattern is constructed on the cast with wax.

4. Artificial teeth—either porcelain or resin—are placed in the wax in the position they will occupy in the finished denture.

5. The wax model of the denture with teeth in place is tried in the patient's mouth to check for proper fit and alignment.

Construction of the Mold

The following steps are used to construct the mold.

1. The wax denture and the cast are placed in the lower half of a metal denture flask, shown in Figure 9–2.

2. The flask is separated into its three parts—a lid, a top half, and a bottom half.

3. A mix of plaster is poured into the bottom half.

4. The cast with the wax denture is placed into the plaster. Care is taken not to cover the wax but to anchor the cast in place.

5. After the plaster has hardened, a separating medium, such as petrolatum, is applied to the plaster.

6. The top half of the flask is seated and filled with plaster or stone (called the *investing material*).

7. The lid is placed on the flask.

8. After the plaster sets, the flask is placed in hot water for about 15 minutes to soften the wax.

9. The two halves of the flask are separated. The hardened plaster holds the teeth in the upper half of the flask.

10. The wax is removed, forming a mold space that duplicates the wax portion of the denture.

11. This space is filled with the acrylic resin dough.

12. The flask is gradually closed, molding the resin dough into the space left by the wax denture base.

13. Pressure is applied, squeezing out any excess resin until the mold halves completely close (Fig. 9–3).

14. The denture then is subjected to an appropriate heat-curing cycle to activate polymerization of the resin.

15. After the flask has cooled, the finished denture can be removed from the mold.

16. As shown in Figure 9–2, the components of the flask must be separated. The plaster is carefully chipped from the cast and resin denture, and the denture is removed from the cast, cleaned, and polished.

17. The denture is ready for insertion into the patient's mouth.

Figure 9–4 shows a finished upper and lower denture.

Care of a Denture

An acrylic resin denture base material exhibits a number of unavoidable dimensional changes. The shrinkage during polymerization produces a contraction. Thermal shrinkage occurs as the heat-processed resin cools

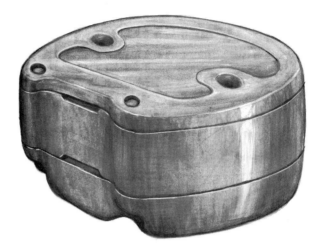

Figure 9–3. Completely closed denture flask, ready for processing.

in the flask. During that time, stresses that may eventually relax to produce a distortion are induced into the material. After the denture is placed in the mouth, the acrylic resin absorbs water from saliva and expands slightly.

These dimensional changes are small and probably not significant. The total dimensional change that occurs in an acrylic denture base during processing and after 2 years

of clinical service, for example, is only about 0.1 to 0.2 mm.

Thus, it is not likely that the major cause for an ill-fitting denture is dimensional instability of the material. It is far more likely to be the result of changes that have occurred in the tissues on which the denture is seated.

To avoid unnecessary distortion, the patient should avoid the use of very hot water in cleansing the denture. The temperature at

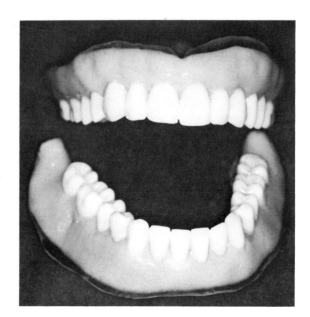

Figure 9–4. An upper and lower complete denture.

which PMMA begins to soften is only 80° C (180°F). If the denture is taken out of the mouth for any extended period, it should be placed in a container filled with water to prevent dehydration of the resin and an accompanying contraction.

A wide variety of agents are used by patients for cleaning artificial dentures—dentifrices, commercial denture cleansers, soap and water, household cleaners, and bleaches. With the exception of abrasive household cleaners, most of these have little harmful effect on the surface or color of the denture. Prolonged use of abrasive agents produces a rough surface that makes maintenance of a clean denture difficult and may even affect the fit. Any cleanser that will scratch a plastic countertop will damage an acrylic denture.

As discussed in Chapter 16, partial denture frameworks commonly are constructed from base metal alloys. The framework and the clasps are made from a chromium-based alloy on which the teeth and acrylic resin are mounted.

Chlorine bleaches should not be used for cleansing such partial dentures. The base metal alloys are attacked chemically by the chlorine. Bleaches also should be avoided in the cleaning of dentures that contain colored fibers. These fibers often are added to simulate the tiny blood vessels in the gingival tissue. The bleach will not harm the denture base material itself, but the fiber color will bleach out.

Although most acrylic denture base resins are partially cross-linked, they are still classified as thermoplastic materials and are somewhat soluble in organic solvents such as acetone and chloroform. Exposure of an acrylic appliance to such a solvent can result in rapid, severe damage. Crazing of the denture base can occur if it is immersed in or wiped with concentrated alcohol (Fig. 9–5). If a denture needs to be disinfected, a chemical disinfectant that does not contain an or-

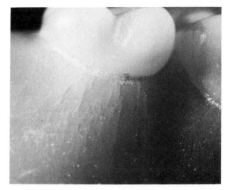

Figure 9–5. Crazing of the denture base material around denture teeth. (From Phillips, R. W.: *Skinner's Science of Dental Materials*, 9th ed. Philadelphia, W. B. Saunders Co., 1991.)

ganic solvent should be used. A denture must never be autoclaved or dry-heat sterilized.

Allergic Reactions

Irritated tissue under a denture base, referred to as *denture sore mouth*, often is attributed to an allergy to one of the ingredients of the resin—the monomer, polymer, activator, or coloring agent. The monomer is considered the most likely source for the irritation. In a chemically activated acrylic resin, as much as 5 per cent monomer may remain unpolymerized. Even when polymerization is properly accomplished, the heat-polymerized resin contains about 0.5 per cent of monomer, which has not been converted to polymer. This unpolymerized monomer may leach out in the saliva and be a source of irritation to the soft tissues.

Evidence shows, however, that monomer is not a cause for concern because it is rapidly leached from the surface of the denture by saliva. True allergic reactions to the commonly used acrylic resins are seldom seen in the oral cavity. Careful clinical evaluation of large numbers of so-called allergies to acrylic resins shows that the cause of denture sore mouth more likely is a result of poor denture hygiene or an ill-fitting denture producing excessive pressure on regions of the soft tissue. The dental auxiliary often plays an important role in educating the patient about the routine cleaning of any removable dental appliance.

As with many substances, a relatively small percentage of people can be sensitized by an acrylic resin. Such a true allergy should be diagnosed by a physician, and the dentist then can examine alternative materials, such as cast metal denture bases.

DENTURE RELINERS

As soft tissue changes occur during the lifetime of a denture, it usually is necessary to adjust the tissue surface of the denture so that it conforms to the new contours and occlusal relations. This readaptation may be accomplished by either *rebasing* or *relining* the denture.

In rebasing, an impression of the soft tissue is obtained using the existing denture as an impression tray. A stone cast is then constructed in the corrected denture. After the denture teeth are correctly indexed, the old denture base material is removed and a new denture base resin processed around them. In other words, a new denture is constructed using the original denture teeth.

In a reline procedure, an impression of the soft tissue is obtained using the existing denture as the impression tray. In this case, however, new resin is cured against the old denture resin.

Relining materials used by the dentist may be classified as either hard or soft. A hard reliner may be a conventional heat-processed denture resin, but a chemically activated resin typically is used because it is simple and fast to use and does not require heating the old denture to temperatures that might result in distortion.

As a temporary measure, the dentist can use a chemically activated resin to reline a denture directly in the oral cavity. Such materials usually are acrylic resins that contain solvents or low-molecular-weight polymers, which are added to obtain the fluidity needed to reproduce tissue detail. These resins liberate considerable heat during polymerization and retain a high percentage of residual monomer—both tending to produce tissue irritation. Furthermore, the reline resins are porous, discolor rapidly, and may separate from the old denture base. Thus, these chemically activated resins are appropriately termed temporary relining materials.

In some instances, the patient cannot tolerate a rigid surface on the denture. Using a soft or resilient relining material in the expectation that it will need to be replaced within a short time may then be desirable. Such soft resins may be formulated in a number of ways, such as by the addition of copolymers to act as plasticizers, the addition of external plasticizers, or even the use of silicone rubbers, which are elastomers like those discussed in Chapter 8.

Resilient liners are far from ideal, however, and must be considered temporary. They should be examined regularly by the dentist and replaced when unsatisfactory.

- Water sorption often produces a loss in the bond between the liner and the denture base.
- The softness of the lining may be only short-lived with certain materials, especially those that use external plasticizers.
- Silicone rubber remains soft, but it supports the growth of yeasts that are present in the mouth and is difficult to bond to the acrylic denture base.

Soft treatment liners sometimes are placed in the denture for a few days to allow the soft tissues to regain their health and form before a final impression is made. An example of such a material is a powder, such as

PMMA, mixed with a liquid that contains various plasticizers, such as ethyl alcohol and ethyl acetate. Although quite soft initially, these materials harden rapidly as the volatile plasticizers leach out in oral fluids. For this reason, they are serviceable for only a short period.

An additional distinction between a soft liner and a tissue conditioner should be noted. The soft liner can be elastically deformed with very low applied stress but recovers its original shape when stress is removed. The tissue conditioner is expected to plastically deform or flow, and thus readapt to the shape of the underlying soft tissues as they recover to their healthy form.

Various types of over-the-counter plastic materials are available to patients for adjusting a denture that no longer fits correctly. Many of these materials contain solvents that are injurious not only to the denture base but also to the oral tissues. The heat generated as these materials polymerize in the mouth can burn soft tissues. Home relining by the patient also may produce an incorrect fit of the denture, resulting in physical trauma to the underlying tissues.

Denture wearers should be encouraged to visit their dentists regularly so that the fit of the denture can be evaluated and adjusted as needed. Only materials available to the dentist, used professionally, should be used for denture relining.

OTHER USES OF RESIN

In addition to their use in the fabrication of dentures, resins of various types serve many other dental purposes. Custom-made impression trays (see Fig. 8–5) are constructed from acrylic resin. Space maintainers and orthodontic retainers are fabricated from denture resins, usually chemically activated PMMA.

These resins should be handled with caution. Incorrect handling of these dental materials has resulted in the citation of dental practices for violating occupational safety rules.

MMA monomer can cause allergic reaction and irritates the skin of people not particularly sensitive to it. The vapor from the monomer is flammable and can be hazardous if inhaled in large concentrations. Direct skin contact should be avoided. The hands can be covered with petroleum jelly to minimize skin absorption. The monomer should be handled in a well-ventilated area, and prolonged exposure to the vapor should be avoided.

Resin systems based on nonvolatile monomers like those used in composite resins (see Chapter 10) are available and may replace the PMMA system for use in the dental office. Those intended for the fabrication of custom impression trays are either chemically activated or light-activated and are fast and convenient to use. They are considerably more expensive than PMMA tray resin.

Other types of resins are used to make *mouth protectors* for athletes engaged in contact sports, such as football, hockey, and boxing. The mouth protector fits over the teeth of the maxillary arch and is intended to absorb the energy of a blow to the mouth. The resin used is soft and flexible. Important physical properties for such a material are resilience, to absorb energy, and toughness, to resist tearing and chewing.

Because of superior fit and greater comfort, most athletes prefer custom-made mouth protectors to the stock items purchased over the counter. Thermoplastic resins are sold in sheet form for this purpose. A popular one is poly(vinylacetate)-poly(ethylene). Construction of such an appliance includes the following steps.

1. Using an alginate impression, the dentist makes a gypsum model of the maxillary arch.
2. The resin sheet is softened in boiling

water and then adapted, usually with the aid of a vacuum, over the gypsum model of the arch.

3. Vacuum forming devices that hold and soften the resin sheet and then press it down over the model, which rests on a perforated platform with vacuum applied, are available.

4. After the material has cooled, the borders are trimmed to the desired shape.

Such a procedure also is used to fabricate night guards for patients who grind their teeth in their sleep. Similarly, custom trays are fabricated for use in vital bleaching of teeth.

Preformed thermoplastic mouth inserts, which can be softened in hot water and placed into the mouth and adapted to make a custom-fitted appliance, also are available.

Resins are increasingly used in maxillofacial prosthetics for the replacement of portions of the facial anatomy that are congenitally missing or have been damaged by disease or accident. Various resins are used to fabricate realistic noses, ears, eyes, parts of the mandible, and other portions of the face. The resins used have included acrylic and vinyl resins, highly plasticized to provide a soft, flexible material.

The demands made on such a material are formidable. It must be flexible, tear-resistant, nontoxic, capable of being accurately molded, aesthetic, and resistant to sunlight, the elements, and facial cosmetics. It also must be dimensionally stable. A resin that completely meets these requirements has not as yet been developed. The current material of choice is a silicone elastomer similar to the silicone impression materials described in Chapter 8.

Selected Reading

Bates, J. F., Stanford, G. D., Huggett, R., and Handley, R. W.: Current status of pour-type denture base resins. J. Dent. 5:177, 1977.

Bowen, R. L.: Crystalline dimethacrylate monomers. J. Dent. Res. 49:810, 1970.

Braden, M.: Tissue conditioner. I. Composition and structure. J. Dent. Res. 49:145, 1970.

Caswell, S. W., and Norling, B. K.: Comparative study of the bond strengths of three abrasion-resistant plastic denture teeth bonded to a cross-linked and a grafted, cross-linked denture base material. J. Prosthet. Dent. 55:701, 1986.

Chaing, B. K. P.: Polymers in the service of prosthetic dentistry. J. Dent. 12:203, 1984.

Chalian, V. A., and Phillips, R. W.: Materials in maxillofacial prosthetics. J. Biomed. Mater. Res. 5:349, 1974.

Clancy, J. M. S., and Boyer, D. B.: Comparative bond strengths of light-cured, heat-cured, and autopolymerizing denture resins to denture teeth. J. Prosthet. Dent. 61:457, 1989.

Cowie, J. M. G.: *Polymers: Chemistry and Physics of Modern Materials*. Glasgow, International Textbook Co., Ltd. Printed by Bell and Bain Ltd., 1973.

Devlin, H., and Watts, D. C.: Acrylic "Allergy"? Br. Dent. J. 157:272, 1984.

Grant, A. A., and Atkinson, H. F.: Comparison between dimensional accuracy of dentures produced with pour-type resin and with heat processed materials. J. Prosthet. Dent. 26:296, 1971.

Heath, J. R., Davenport, J. C., and Jones, P. A.: The abrasion of acrylic resin by cleaning pastes. J. Oral Rehabil. 10:159, 1983.

Kapur, K. K., and Somarn, S. D.: Masticatory performance and efficiency in denture wearers. J. Prosthet. Dent. 14:687, 1964.

Levin, B., Sanders, J. L., and Reitz, P. V.: The use of microwave energy for processing acrylic resins. J. Prosthet. Dent. 61:381, 1989.

McCabe, J. F., and Wilson, H. J.: The use of differential scanning calorimetry for the evaluation of dental materials. II. Denture base materials. J. Oral Rehabil. 7:235, 1980.

Means, C. R., Rupp, N. W., and Paffenbarger, G. C.: Clinical evaluation of two types of resilient liners on dentures. J. Am. Dent. Assoc. 82:1376, 1971.

Monsenego, P., Baszkin, A., deLourdes Costa, J., and Lejoyeaus, J.: Complete denture retention, wettability studies on various acrylic resin denture base materials. J. Prosthet. Dent. 62:308, 1989.

Nyquist, G.: Study of denture sore mouth. An investigation of traumatic, allergic, and toxic lesions of the oral mucosa arising from the use of full dentures. Acta Odontol. Scand. 10:154, 1952.

Paffenbarger, G. C., Woelfel, J. B., and Sweeney, W. T.: Resins and technics used in constructing dentures. Dent. Clin. North Am. March 1965, pp. 251–262.

Rosen, S. L.: *Fundamentals and Principles of Polymeric Materials*. New York, John Wiley & Sons, 1982.

Sheldon, R. P.: *Composite Polymeric Materials*. New York, Applied Science Publ., 1982.

Schlosberg, S. R., Goodacre, C. J., Munoz, C. A., and Moore, B. K.: Microwave energy polymerization of poly (methyl methacrylate) denture base resin. Int. J. Prosthodont. 2:453, 1989.

Smith, D. C., and Baines, M. E. D.: Residual methyl methacrylate in the denture base and its relation to denture sore mouth. Br. Dent. J. 98:55, 1955.

Takamata, T., and Setcos, J. C.: Resin denture bases: Review of accuracy and methods of polymerization. Int. J. Prosthodont. 2:555, 1989.

Takamata, T., Setcos, J. C., Phillips, R. W., and Boone, M. E.: Adaptation of acrylic resin dentures influenced by the activation mode of polymerization. J. Am. Dent. Assoc. 119:271, 1989.

Tan, H. K., Brudvik, J., Nickolls, J., and Smith, D. E.: Adaptation of visible light-cured denture base material. J. Prosthet. Dent. 61:326, 1989.

Tulacha, G. J., and Moser, J. B.: Evaluation of viscoelastic behavior of light-cured denture resin. J. Prosthet. Dent. 61:695, 1989.

Vermilyea, S. G., Powers, J. M., and Koran, A.: The rheological properties of fluid denture-base resins. J. Dent. Res. 57:227, 1978.

Woelfel, J. B., Paffenbarger, G. C., and Sweeney, W. T.: Clinical evaluation of complete dentures made of 11 different types of denture base materials. J. Am. Dent. Assoc. 70:1170, 1965.

Wright, P. S.: Soft lining materials: Their status and prospects. J. Dent. 4:247, 1976.

Reviewing the Chapter

1. Define *synthetic resin*, *plastic*, and *polymer*.
2. What are the requisites for a dental resin?
3. Explain the difference between a thermoset resin and a thermoplastic resin. Give dental examples of each.
4. Define *mer* and *monomer*.
5. How are the properties of a resin affected by the molecular weight of the polymer?
6. Explain a condensation polymerization reaction.
7. Describe and illustrate an addition polymerization reaction. What is a requisite for the structure of any monomer molecule that polymerizes by means of an addition reaction?
8. What is *copolymerization*?
9. Describe the various stages of the polymerization process. Define *initiator* and *activator* and give dental examples.
10. Describe *cross-linking*, give an example of a monomer that will cross-link, and list the advantages of a cross-linked resin.
11. How does the composition of heat-activated (heat-cured) resins differ from that of chemically activated (cold-cured) resins?
12. Compare the properties of heat-cured and cold-cured resins.
13. Discuss the procedure used in constructing a denture. What is a microwave denture resin? A light-activated resin?
14. What is *denture sore mouth?* What is its most common cause?
15. List the cleansing agents that can be used to clean dentures safely. Which cleansing materials and procedures could damage the denture?
16. What precautions should be used in cleaning partial dentures with base metal frameworks?
17. What is a soft denture liner? A tissue conditioner? How do these differ in composition, properties, and clinical function?
18. What materials are used to fabricate mouth guards and similar appliances? How are these custom devices made?
19. What is maxillofacial prosthodontics? What materials are used? What requirements are placed on these materials?
20. What health risks may be associated with the use of acrylic resins in the dental office?
21. Which materials can be safely used to disinfect a denture? Which materials or techniques should not be used?

SYNTHETIC RESINS

RESTORATIVE MATERIALS

Chapter 9 covered dental resins used in the indirect fabrication of restorations and prosthetic appliances. This chapter discusses the various restorative resins.

Their excellent aesthetic properties make resins well suited for the restoration of lost-tooth structure. After the dentist prepares the cavity in the usual manner, the resin mixture is inserted into the cavity and polymerized at mouth temperature. These resins are referred to as *direct filling resins*. Because polymerization must be carried out in the oral cavity, either chemically activated or light-activated resins, as described in Chapter 9, are used.

After the development of chemically activated polymer systems, the first direct filling resins, based on poly(methyl methacrylate), were introduced in the late 1940s. The system consisted of a liquid (monomer) and a

TABLE 10–1. Properties of Restorative Resins

	Unfilled Acrylic	Conventional	Microfilled	Small-Particle	Hybrid
Inorganic filler (vol %) (weight %)		60–65 70–80	20–55 35–60	65–77 80–90	60–65 75–80
Compressive strength (MPa) (psi)	69 10,000	250–300 36,250–43,500	250–350 36,250–50,750	350–400 50,750–58,000	300–350 43,500–50,750
Tensile strength (MPa) (psi)	24 3,500	50–65 7250–9425	30–50 4350–7250	75–90 10,875–13,050	70–90 10,105–13,050
Elastic modulus (GPa) (10^6 psi)	2.4 .34	8–15 1.16–2.18	3–6 44–.87	15–20 2.18–2.90	7–12 1.02–1.74
Thermal expansion coefficient (10^{-6}/°C)	92.8	25–35	50–60	19–26	30–40
Water sorption (mg/cm²)	1.7	0.5–0.7	1.4–1.7	0.5–0.6	0.5–0.7
Knoop Hardness (KHN)	15	55	25–30	50–60	50–60

powder (polymer). Similar to chemically activated denture resins, these resins usually were referred to as direct filling acrylic resins. Although they resembled tooth structure and were insoluble in oral fluids, they had a number of serious liabilities that limited their use.

- The strength, stiffness, and hardness were low compared with those of other restorative materials.
- One of the greatest problems was a volumetric polymerization shrinkage of 7 to 8 per cent.
- Because acrylic resin does not bond to tooth structure, the material tended to pull away from the walls of the cavity preparation as the material polymerized.
- The problem was further compounded by a coefficient of thermal expansion seven to eight times greater than the tooth, resulting in expansion and contraction of the restoration with the ingestion of hot and cold foods.
- This can lead to microleakage of the restorations and subsequent marginal dis-

coloration, sensitivity, and secondary caries.

Typical properties are listed in Table 10–1.

Although direct filling acrylic resins are no longer in use, their insolubility and initial aesthetics stimulated research that led to development of the direct filling composite resins widely used today.

In addition to the direct filling materials, this chapter also discusses the resins used as pit and fissure sealants, coatings for eroded areas, or provisional or temporary restorations and in the fabrication of crowns and bridges.

COMPOSITE RESINS

Materials classified as *composites* are formed from two constituents that are insoluble in each other so that a definite interface exists between them. The rationale for combining two materials is to provide properties that are superior or intermediate to those of each constituent. The composite resin fiberglass, for example, consists of a resin matrix reinforced by glass fibers. The resulting composite is harder and stiffer than the resin matrix but less brittle than the glass fibers.

The three major constituents of modern dental composite resins are as follows:

- An organic resin matrix
- An inorganic filler
- A coupling agent that chemically bonds the filler to the resin matrix

Fillers reinforce the matrix. The filler's strength and hardness influence the properties of the composite.

As illustrated by tooth structure, the amount of filler also has a profound effect on properties. Both enamel and dentin are natural composites in which collagen is the matrix and hydroxyapatite the filler. The difference in the properties of the two tissues is due, at least in part, to the ratio of matrix to filler. Enamel contains a much higher percentage of hydroxyapatite than dentin and is harder, stiffer, and more brittle.

Composite resins that have higher percentages of filler usually have better properties. This can be seen by comparing the properties in Table 10–1 for unfilled acrylic resins and microfilled resins with those of the more highly filled conventional, small-particle, and hybrid composites. (A range of values is presented for each type because commercial products vary among themselves.) In almost all instances, the physical and mechanical properties of the more highly filled resins are superior.

In addition to the improvement in mechanical properties, composite resins have less polymerization shrinkage than unfilled resins. This is due to the reduced resin content. Unfilled acrylic restorative resins shrink 7 to 8 per cent by volume when they polymerize, whereas the shrinkage of most composite resins is less than 2 per cent. Likewise, the coefficient of thermal expansion is reduced as a result of the decreased resin content.

COMPOSITION OF DENTAL COMPOSITES

Resin Matrix

The BIS-GMA and urethane dimethacrylate resins discussed in Chapter 9 commonly are used as matrix material in composite resins. Both have relatively large molecules, and their monomers are quite viscous. To decrease viscosity and improve handling characteristics, they are diluted with lower-molecular-weight dimethacrylate monomers.

Fillers

Inorganic fillers used in the composite resins include quartz, glasses, and colloidal silica particles. Metals such as lithium, barium, or strontium are used in some glasses to impart radiopacity.

Quartz and glass fillers are ground to sizes ranging from 0.1 to 100 μm. A large range of particle sizes is incorporated in the resin matrix to achieve the highest level of filler loading. As illustrated by a box filled with identical marbles (Fig. 10–1), this could not be achieved with filler particles that are all the same size. Much vacant space can be filled by adding smaller sizes of marbles.

Colloidal silica particles range from 0.02 to 0.04 μm in size. Called *microfillers,* they are too small to be seen without extremely high magnification. They also are referred to as *pyrolytic* or *precipitated silica* in reference to processes by which they are produced.

Coupling Agent

To strengthen the composite, the inorganic filler particles must be adhesively bonded to the organic resin matrix. The fill-

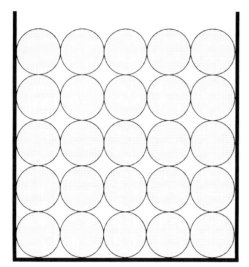

Figure 10–1. Box filled with identical marbles. Note the large amount of empty space between the marbles, which could be filled with smaller-diameter marbles.

ers are coated with an organosilane compound. The silane portion of the molecule bonds to the quartz, glass, and silica filler particles and the organic portion bonds with the resin matrix, thus bonding the filler to the matrix. The bond of the resin and filler transfers stress to the filler particles and reduces infiltration of fluids along the filler-matrix interface.

POLYMERIZATION SYSTEMS

Chemically activated resins (Fig. 10–2) are supplied as two containers of composite paste, one containing the benzoyl peroxide initiator and the other, the tertiary amine activator. When the two pastes are mixed together, the amine reacts with the benzoyl peroxide to form free radicals that initiate polymerization of the resin matrix.

Visible light–activated resins (see Fig. 10–2) are supplied as a single paste that contains both the photo initiator and the amine activator. This paste is furnished bulk in lightproof syringes or prefilled into single-

dose tips used with a composite resin syringe. This resin does not polymerize until it is exposed to light of the proper wavelength. Both chemical- and light-activated induction systems contain amines that in time form colored products when exposed to ultraviolet light (UV). UV-blocking agents are incorporated in the resins to reduce discoloration of resin restorations caused by exposure to UV.

Dual-activated restorative resins also are marketed. They are furnished in two light-proof containers that contain the activation chemicals described for both chemical- and light-activated resins. When the two pastes are mixed, a slow chemical activation begins. Exposure of the mixed material to a curing light results in a rapid photoactivation. The chemically activated reaction continues as well, ensuring complete curing of any portions of the restoration that might not have received adequate light activation.

Light Devices

Typical curing lights are shown in Figure 10–3. All transmit light of the proper wavelength to the site of the restoration by means of a light guide. Two basic types of curing lights are used in the dental office. Hand-held light-curing devices contain the light

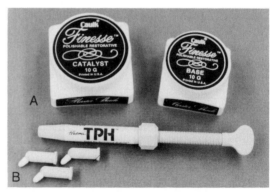

Figure 10–2. Commercial products representative of available resin systems. A, Chemically activated composite and B, light-activated composite supplied in single-dose syringe tips and in bulk in lightproof syringes.

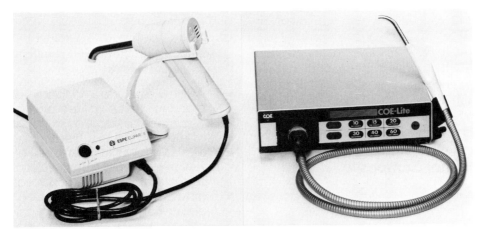

Figure 10–3. Examples of commercial visible light–curing units. (From Phillips, R. W.: *Skinner's Science of Dental Materials*, 9th ed. Philadelphia, W. B. Saunders Co., 1991.)

source and are equipped with a rigid light guide made up of fused optical fibers. In the other type, the light source is remote, and a long, flexible fiberoptic cord is used to transmit light to the mouth.

The light source usually is a tungsten halogen light bulb. The light generated by the bulb passes through filters that remove the infrared and visible wavelengths that are greater than about 500 nm. Wavelengths shorter than 400 nm (UV) also are removed.

Proper care of these lights is important. A reduction in light output results in an inadequately polymerized restoration, which has poor properties and probably will fail prematurely. The output of the bulb falls off with age. In devices that use flexible fiberoptic bundles to transmit light, careless handling can fracture some of the fibers and reduce the output from the light guide. The end of the light pipe can become contaminated by composite resin, which must be removed carefully to assure maximum light output.

Light meters designed to measure the output of curing lights are available commercially. Routine checking of light output by such a device is the best way to assure that the optimum level is being maintained.

CLASSIFICATION OF COMPOSITE RESIN RESTORATIVE MATERIALS

A number of classification systems have been proposed for composite resin restorative materials. One workable system is to categorize the materials according to the mean particle size of the major filler.

Category Type	Average Particle Size (μm)
Conventional	8–12
Microfilled	0.04–0.4
Small-particle	1–5
Hybrid	1

Subgroups and overlap may exist for some categories, especially hybrids. A hybrid composite can use ground filler from either the small or the conventional categories, in combination with a microfiller. Resins that contain any combination of ground filler and microfiller theoretically could be considered hybrids. Such a broad definition would not be useful because most modern dental composites that use ground fillers also contain small amounts of microfiller (less than 5 per cent by weight) as thickeners to attain the desired viscosity for the paste. This amount is too small to contribute to the physical properties.

The term *hybrid composite* usually refers to materials that contain ground fillers that have an average particle size of 0.6 to 1.0 μm in combination with 10 to 15 weight per cent of microfiller. This definition for the term *hybrid* composites is used in this book.

Conventional Composite

Conventional composites also are called *traditional* or *macrofilled* composites. The most commonly used filler is quartz, which has wide particle size distribution. Although the average size is 8 to 12 μm, particles as large as 50 to 100 μm may be present. Filler loading is 70 to 80 per cent by weight or 60 to 70 per cent by volume. The structure of the conventional composite resin is evident in the photomicrograph of the polished specimen shown in Figure 10–4.

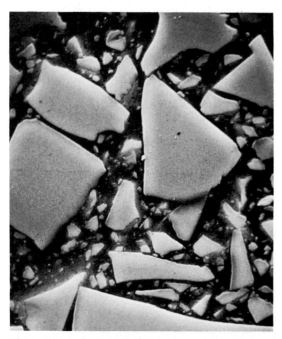

Figure 10–4. Scanning electron micrograph of the surface of a conventional composite resin after finishing (original magnification 1800 ×).

The properties of typical conventional composites are listed in Table 10–1. As can be seen, they are improved significantly over the unfilled acrylic.

- Strength is about four to five times greater than that of the unfilled acrylic.
- Elastic modulus is four to six times greater.
- Tensile strength is doubled.
- Water sorption, the coefficient of thermal expansion, and polymerization shrinkage are appreciably reduced.
- The Knoop Hardness Number (KHN) is about 55, compared with 15 KHN for unfilled acrylic. Conventional resins suffer from surface roughening, however, as a result of more rapid wear of the soft resin matrix compared with that of the quartz filler. This is a major clinical disadvantage because the surface of the restoration becomes rough with finishing, tooth brushing, and wear in the oral cavity. As shown in Figure 10–5, the soft resin matrix wears away, leaving the more resistant quartz particles elevated. The restorations tend to discolor because the rough surface is susceptible to stain.

Fracture of resin restorations is not a common problem. If, however, resins are used for restoration of the occlusal surfaces of posterior teeth, their poor resistance to wear is an important consideration.

Although its polymerization shrinkage is substantially lower than that of the acrylic resins, the resin matrix does not bond to tooth. Therefore, insertion techniques must be used to reduce the effects of dimension change stemming from this source. This principle holds true for all categories of composite resins.

Microfilled Composite

In an effort to overcome the problems of surface roughness associated with conventional composites, researchers developed a class of materials that use colloidal silica par-

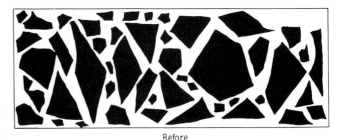

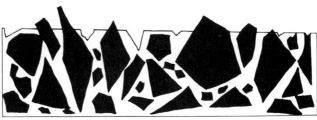

Figure 10–5. Diagram of the surface of a conventional composite resin before and after finishing. Note that the resin matrix has been worn away by the finishing procedure while the filler either projects above the surface or has fallen out, leaving a rough surface. (From Phillips, R. W.: *Skinner's Science of Dental Materials,* 9th ed. Philadelphia, W. B. Saunders Co., 1991.)

ticles as the inorganic filler. The inorganic particles are 0.02 to 0.04 μm in size—200 to 300 times smaller than the average quartz particle in conventional composites. The design of the microfilled composite was intended to reinforce the resin by means of a filler while retaining a surface smoothness similar to that of an unfilled acrylic restoration.

Large amounts of the colloidal silica filler must be added to the resin matrix to gain significant improvements in physical properties. The addition of even relatively small amounts of microfiller, however, rapidly increases the viscosity of the paste. Long before sufficient amounts have been added, the paste becomes an unmanageable solid.

The common method for increasing the filler loading is to make a new filler from a prepolymerized composite resin that is highly filled with colloidal silica particles. The monomer resin is thinned to permit the addition of 60 to 70 per cent by weight of silane-coated colloidal silica. This composite paste is heat-cured, and the solid composite is ground into particles of the size used in conventional composites. Although these prepolymerized particles also are called organic fillers, the name is not technically correct because the particles contain a high percentage of inorganic colloidal silica.

The *ground composite resin particles,* along with additional silane-coated colloidal silica, are mixed into unpolymerized matrix resin to form the composite paste. A diagram representing the structure of microfilled resins of this type is shown in Figure 10–6.

The total volume of inorganic filler in microfilled resins is much less than in other types of composites. Because of the presence of the prepolymerized resin particles, however, the amount of unpolymerized resin in the paste is not much different from that in other composites, and the polymerization shrinkage is about the same.

Except for compressive strength, microfilled composites have physical and mechanical properties that are inferior to those of conventional composites (see Table 10–1). This is to be expected because about 50 per cent of the volume of the restorative material is made up of resin. The larger amount of resin compared with filler results in greater water sorption and a higher coefficient of

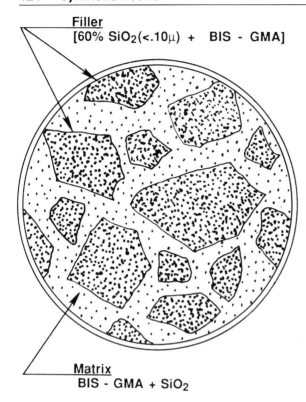

Filler
[60% SiO$_2$(<.10μ) + BIS - GMA]

Matrix
BIS - GMA + SiO$_2$

Figure 10–6. Diagram showing the structure of a microfilled resin. (From Phillips, R. W.: *Skinner's Science of Dental Materials,* 9th ed. Philadelphia, W. B. Saunders Co., 1991.)

thermal expansion. The bond of the resin matrix to the prepolymerized filler particles may be weak, possibly contributing to the low tensile strength.

As can be seen in the photomicrograph of the polished microfilled resin in Figure 10–7, the surface of the resin is very smooth. Note that no filler particles are visible. The individual colloidal silica particles are too small to be visible—even at a magnification of 10,000 ×. The filler particles are so tiny that they are removed with the resin by the finishing tools. Thus, as diagrammed in Figure 10–8, the finished surface is smooth.

The decreased physical properties do not create a problem for many applications. The potential for fracture is greater, however, in stress-bearing situations, such as Class IV and Class II restorations. Chipping at the margins of restorations—attributed to debonding of the prepolymerized composite

filler—has been observed on occasion. Because of their smooth surface, microfilled resins often are the resin of choice for aesthetic restoration of anterior teeth in non–stress-bearing locations.

Small-Particle Composites

Small-particle composite resins were developed in an attempt to approach the surface smoothness of microfilled composites and yet retain the physical and mechanical properties of conventional composites. The inorganic fillers are ground to a smaller size than that used in conventional composites. The average filler size is in the 1- to 5-μm range, but the size distribution is fairly broad, as can be seen in the photomicrograph of a polished small-particle composite (Fig. 10–9). This broad particle size distribution facilitates high filler loading. Small-

Figure 10–7. Scanning electron micrograph of the surface of a microfilled composite resin after finishing. Note the smooth surface.

Some small-particle composites use quartz particles as fillers, but most use glasses that contain radiopaque metals. As previously noted, colloidal silica usually is added in a small amount to adjust the paste viscosity.

The best physical and mechanical properties are identified with this category of composites. With the increased filler content, virtually all properties improve (see Table 10–1).

- Compressive strength, elastic modulus, and tensile strength exceed that of conventional composites.
- The coefficient of thermal expansion is less than that of the other composites.
- The surface smoothness of these resins is improved compared with conventional composites but is inferior to the microfilled resins.
- The wear resistance also is improved.
- Polymerization shrinkage is comparable to or less than that of conventional resins.
- Resins filled with radiopaque glasses are more radiopaque than dentin, an important property for materials used for restoration of posterior teeth.

particle composites contain more inorganic filler (70 per cent by volume or higher) than do conventional composites. This is particularly true of those designated for use in posterior restorations. The high loading of filler particles is evident in the polished specimen.

Figure 10–8. Diagram of the surface of a microfilled resin before and after finishing. Note that the finishing procedure produces a smooth surface because the filler is removed at the same rate as the resin matrix.

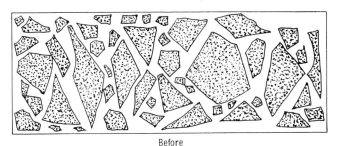

Before

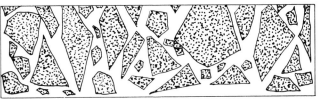

After

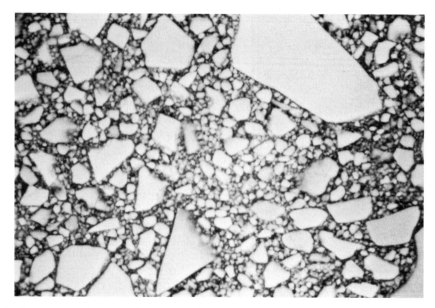

Figure 10–9. Scanning electron micrograph of the polished surface of the small-particle composite (× 1500). (Courtesy of W. H. Douglas.)

Because of their improved strength and higher filler loading, these composites are suggested for applications in which large stresses and abrasion might be encountered, such as Class IV and Class II restorations. The particle sizes of some products make it possible to attain reasonably smooth surfaces for anterior applications, but they are not as good as microfilled materials or the more recently developed hybrid composite materials.

Hybrid Composites

The newest category of composite materials is the hybrid. These materials were developed in an effort to obtain better surface smoothness than that provided by the small-particle composites and still maintain their physical properties.

As the name implies, hybrid composites have two kinds of filler particles: ground radiopaque glasses and colloidal silica with a total filler content about 60 to 65 per cent by volume. The glasses have an average particle size of 0.6 to 1.0 μm. Colloidal silica represents 10 to 20 per cent by weight of the total filler content. In these amounts, the microfiller contributes significantly to the properties. The smaller filler particles—as well as the greater amounts of microfiller—increase the filler surface area. Thus, the overall filler loading is not as high as for the small-particle composites.

A polished surface is shown in Figure 10–10. Compared with the conventional and small-particle composites, the ground particle size is smaller. The smoothness of this surface is competitive with the microfilled resins.

Physical and mechanical properties for these resins range between those of the conventional and small-particle composites but are superior to the microfilled composites. Because the radiopaque glasses are used for the ground filler particles, the hybrids possess the desired radiopacity for posterior applications.

Because of their smooth surface and good strength, these composites are widely used for anterior restorations, including Class IV.

Although the mechanical properties are

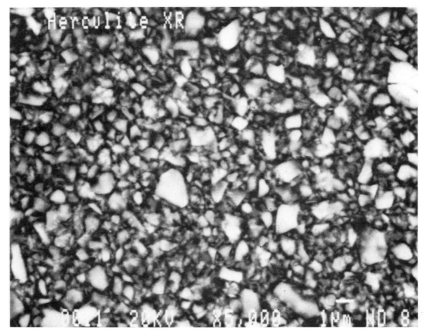

Figure 10–10. Scanning electron micrograph of the polished surface of a hybrid composite (5000 ×). (Courtesy of R. L. Erickson.)

somewhat inferior to those of small-particle composites, the hybrids are being widely used for stress-bearing restorations. The hybrid resins often are referred to as general or all-purpose resins.

COMPOSITE RESINS FOR POSTERIOR RESTORATIONS

Amalgam has been the standard direct filling material for restoration of posterior teeth. Its attributes are ease of placement, good mechanical properties and wear resistance, and the unique characteristic of decreasing microleakage as the restoration ages. With the increasing demand for aesthetic dentistry and concerns about the toxic effects of mercury, usage of composite resins for Class I and Class II restorations has increased.

Radiopacity is an important property for any posterior restorative material. Although not all composite resins are radiopaque, many of the hybrid and small-particle composites are satisfactory in this respect.

Most small-particle and hybrid composites have adequate strength for conservative posterior applications, and fracture is not a major cause of failure.

Composite resin is more difficult to place than amalgam. In many instances, the gingival margins of a restoration are located in dentin or cementum with the other margins firmly anchored to etched enamel. As the resin polymerizes, it pulls away from the gingival margin, creating a gap and the resultant clinical problems associated with leakage. This is one of the greatest problems in the use of composites in Class II cavities; it also is a problem in Class V cavities. Measures to maintain the integrity of gingival margins by the use of dentin bond agents and glass ionomer liners are discussed later in this chapter and in Chapter 21.

In addition to polymerization shrinkage,

occlusal wear has been the most frequent clinical problem. The first generation of conventional composites wore over the entire occlusal surface at rates as high as 150 μm per year. In these composites (see Figs. 10–4 and 10–5), a relatively large amount of soft resin matrix is exposed between the filler particles. When sufficient matrix is abraded away, the hard filler particles are dislodged, exposing more resin matrix, and the process continues. Figure 10–11 shows a clinical composite resin that has undergone occlusal wear as a result of abrasion.

The small-particle and hybrid composites with higher filler levels have greatly reduced the amounts of resin exposed at the surface and markedly improved wear resistance.

Today, some products wear less than 20 μm per year, approaching the wear resistance of amalgam, which is in the 10-μm range. Wear rates for composite restorations have been established over relatively short periods, such as 5 years. Whether this same wear relation compared with amalgam will hold true over longer intervals has not been determined.

Highly filled composites in which filler particles are small and well bonded to the resin matrix are the most wear-resistant. Large restorations also wear more than smaller ones, as do restorations in molars compared with premolars.

BIOCOMPATIBILITY

The BIS-GMA and urethane dimethacrylate monomers irritate the dental pulp so that chemical insult occurs if unreacted monomer leaches from the restoration and penetrates the dentinal tubules. For this reason, a protective layer of a $Ca(OH)_2$ cement should be placed on the pulpal wall of deep cavities before insertion of the resin paste. Zinc oxide–eugenol preparations are not recommended because the eugenol can interfere with polymerization of the resin.

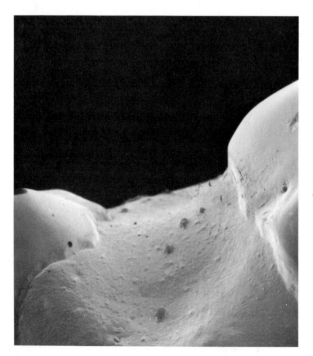

Figure 10–11. Scanning electron micrograph of a 9-year-old posterior composite demonstrating general wear. (From Phillips, R. W.: *Skinner's Science of Dental Materials,* 9th ed. Philadelphia, W. B. Saunders Co., 1991.)

MANIPULATION OF RESINS

The dentist can choose from several types of composite resins. The choice depends to a large degree on the intended use and on a personal preference for the handling properties of particular materials. Regardless of the choice of resin, proper manipulative techniques are essential.

Chemically Activated Composites

As noted, chemically activated resins are supplied as two pastes. The pastes are identical, except that one contains the amine activator and the other the peroxide initiator. Equal quantities of each paste, as judged by eye, are proportioned onto a nonabsorbent mixing pad. Special care is required in mixing the pastes:

- The two containers of paste must not be cross-contaminated. Opposite ends of the mixing stick should be used when proportioning the pastes.
- Mixing of the pastes is accomplished by a 30-second spatulation with the plastic mixing stick supplied. Care should be taken to avoid incorporating air during mixing because voids in the restoration can result. Air also inhibits polymerization of the resin.
- Immediately on completion of the mix, the composite is inserted into the cavity. It may be wiped in with a dental plastic instrument or injected by means of a composite resin syringe designed for this purpose.
- The working time with chemically activated resins is short because the polymerization reaction starts once the pastes are mixed. The resin must be placed in the cavity while it is sufficiently plastic to adapt to the cavity walls. Most resins harden sufficiently to be finished within 15 minutes after mixing.
- If a matrix was not used to contour the resin restoration, the external surface may be somewhat sticky because of air inhibition of the polymerization. This inhibited layer is only a few microns thick and is readily wiped away.

Light-Activated Composites

Light-activated resins have several advantages over chemically activated systems, which they have virtually replaced. As already noted, light-activated materials are single-component pastes supplied in syringes or unit dose syringe tips.

- No mixing is required, eliminating several variables.
- Working time is virtually unlimited and can be determined by the clinician.
- The materials harden rapidly once they are exposed to the curing light.
- The depth of cure is limited. It is *not* recommended that a thickness greater than 2 mm be cured. Therefore, restorations must be built up in increments. This is an advantage. As each increment is inserted and polymerized, it shrinks, but much of that shrinkage is filled in by the next increment as the restoration is built up. As each increment of resin is inserted, it is formed to the desired contour and cured.

To attain maximum properties, the resin must be properly polymerized. This is important from a biological standpoint also because the light-cured composite resins polymerize starting at the surface exposed to the light and continuing toward the depth. In a poorly polymerized light-cured restoration, the resin in contact with the pulpal wall contains a high percentage of irritating monomer.

The exposure time required to achieve maximum polymerization varies with the shade and with the resins themselves. Because darker shades of resin do not transmit light as well as lighter shades, they require longer cure times to achieve maximum polymerization. Exposure of the resin to the light for 40 to 60 seconds is a good general rule.

The factors that reduce output of curing lights have already been discussed. A reduction in light emission as small as 10 per cent can significantly reduce depth of cure of certain composites. A 60-second exposure to the light (compared with 30 seconds) can compensate, to some degree, for small reductions in light output.

Several other precautions should be observed in the use of light-cured resins.

- Operatory lights produce some light in the critical wavelengths for curing. If the resins are exposed to operatory light for an extended period, some polymerization, accompanied by a reduction in plasticity, may occur. Therefore, they should not be dispensed until the dentist is ready to place the restoration.
- The light emitted by the curing lights can potentially damage the eyes if one looks directly at the end of the light guide. Protective eyeglasses and various types of shields that filter out the harmful rays are available and should be used.

Acid Etch

Marginal leakage probably is a more acute problem with resin restorations than with other restorative materials. As noted in Figure 2–2, the amalgam restoration is self-sealing through the formation of corrosion products along the tooth–restoration interface. Other dental materials contain leachable fluorides that protect the restored tooth from secondary caries. Composite resins shrink on polymerization and do not form corrosion products or leach fluoride. Hence, resin restorations are vulnerable to leakage and the associated problems of stain, sensitivity, and secondary caries.

An effective way to improve the seal of resin restorations is to treat the enamel mar-gins with acid before inserting the resin filling material. This procedure—called the *acid etch technique*—also is the basis for several other modern dental procedures, including the attachment to enamel of laminate veneers, resin-bonded bridges, and orthodontic appliances.

A proper treatment of enamel by acid results in a selective and discrete dissolution of the surface that produces microporosities, as seen in the photomicrograph in Figure 10–12. When the resin is placed on this etched surface, it flows into the porosities and forms tags 15 to 25 μm in length, as shown in Figure 10–13. Compared with a smooth surface, the rough enamel surface also provides a larger area for contact between the enamel and the resin. These factors markedly increase the mechanical bond between the resin and the enamel. Acid etching results in better retention and an intimate contact between the resin and the tooth structure, thus reducing marginal leakage.

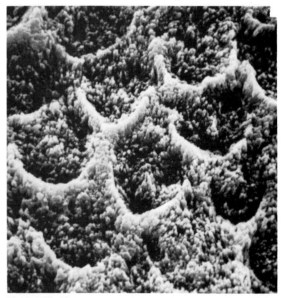

Figure 10–12. Scanning electron micrograph of an enamel surface that has been etched by phosphoric acid (original magnification 5000 ×).

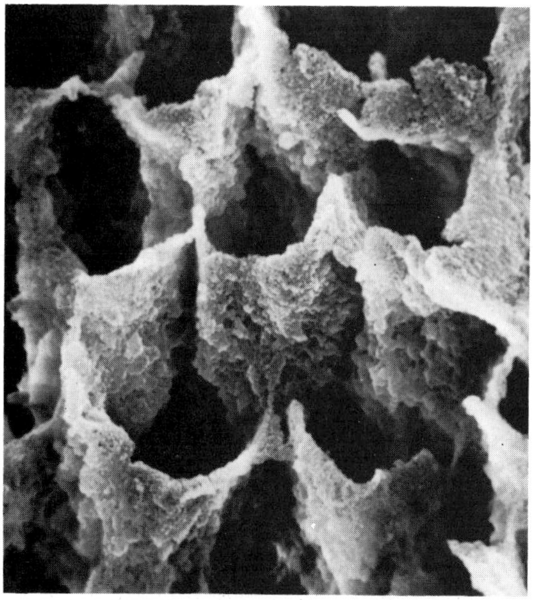

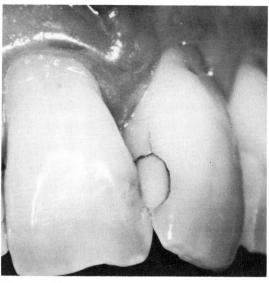

Figure 10–13. Scanning electron micrograph of resin tags formed by penetration of resin into etched areas of enamel. The resin was applied to the etched enamel and the enamel then dissolved to reveal the tags (original magnification 5000 ×).

Figure 10–14 shows an example of a resin restoration with severe marginal stain indicative of microleakage. In contrast, resin restorations placed by a well-executed procedure using the acid etch technique are shown in Figure 10–15. Even after 6 years, the restorations have no detectable stain at the margins.

Phosphoric acid solutions in concentrations ranging from 30 to 50 per cent are used for etching enamel. The most common concentration is 37 per cent. The acid is supplied in both liquid and gel form. The gels have become more popular because they are easier to confine to the desired area of the tooth.

The acid etch technique involves several steps.

- The acid is applied with a brush or a syringe. A 15-second application of the acid usually is adequate to produce the desired degree of etch. Some teeth—those with high fluoride content, for example—may require longer etch time.
- The acid treatment is followed by rinsing with a stream of water for 15 seconds.
- The tooth is then dried. The etched surface must be kept clean and dry until the resin restoration has been placed. If it should become contaminated by saliva, it must be washed, dried, and re-etched by a 10-second application of the acid.
- A correctly etched enamel has a white, frosty appearance.

The bond strength of composite resin to etched enamel is quite high, ranging from 22 to 25 MPa (2500 to 3200 psi). Bond strength can be further improved by use of the bond agents discussed in the next section.

Bond Agents

The original enamel bond agents were diluted, unfilled composite resin matrix monomers marketed for coating the etched

Figure 10–14. Clinical restoration with severe marginal discoloration, which resulted from poor adaptation and subsequent leakage. (Courtesy of J. Osborne.)

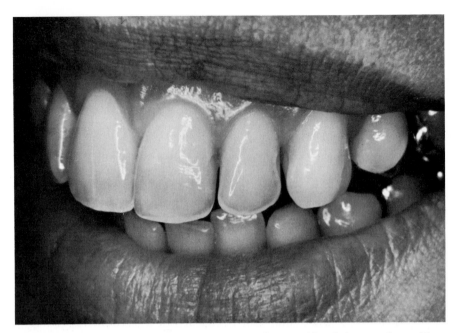

Figure 10–15. Anterior Class III resin restorations that are 6 years old and show no detectable marginal stain. (Courtesy of H. W. Gilmore.)

enamel before insertion of the resin. The low-viscosity unfilled resin would better penetrate into the enamel irregularities than the more viscous composite, thus enhancing the bond. These largely have been replaced by the newer dentin bond agents, which also improve the bond to enamel. Many of the newer products are designated as *universal bond agents,* indicating that they are suitable for use on both enamel and dentin.

The acid etch technique largely alleviated problems associated with the retention and marginal leakage of restorations whose margins are solely in enamel. It did not solve the leakage problem in those restorations that have margins in dentin or cementum, such as the gingival margins of many Class II and V restorations.

Adhesive bonding to dentin has many more obstacles than bonding to enamel. Dentin is heterogeneous. It has a high water content that can interfere with bonding an adhesive to the tooth. It also has a high col-

lagen content and a tubular structure through which dentinal fluids can flow.

A further complication is the *smear layer,* which is formed on the cut dentin surface by cavity preparation (Fig. 10–16). The rotary instruments produce a tenacious layer of debris on the surface that is 5 or 10 μm thick. This layer prevents contact between the intact dentin and the adhesive. Although an adhesive bond to the mineral component of the smear layer is possible, the bond of the smear layer to the underlying intact dentin is in question.

Practical dentin adhesives have emerged only during the past few years. The development has seen several generations of types of bonding agent, and improvements still are being sought.

Most dentin bond agents consist of three or more components (Fig. 10–17).

● All systems contain a *dentin surface cleaner,* which is a weak acidic solu-

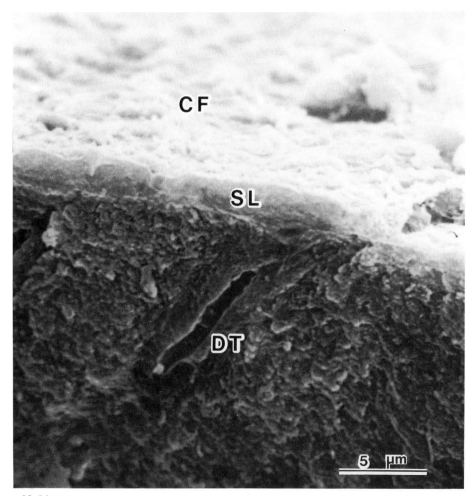

Figure 10-16. Scanning electron micrograph of the smear layer (SL) lying on the prepared cavity floor (CF). Dentinal tubules (DT) are apparent in this cross section. (Courtesy of M. Fukushima.)

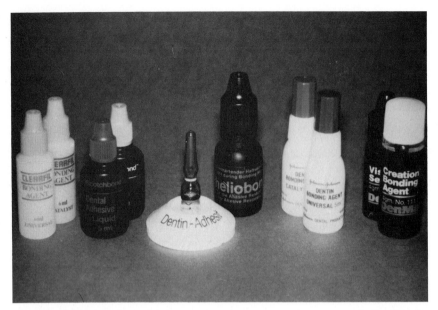

Figure 10–17. Commerical dentin bonding agents. Many of these are sold as universal bonding agents for dentin and enamel. (From Phillips, R. W.: *Skinner's Science of Dental Materials*, 9th ed. Philadelphia, W. B. Saunders Co., 1991.)

tion—nitric, maleic, or EDTA (ethylene-diaminetetraacetic acid). The solution may be designated as a cleaner, a conditioner, or an etchant. Some universal bond agent systems use etchants, which purportedly are applicable to etching both enamel and dentin. These solutions remove the smear layer and produce a subtle opening of the dentinal tubules and a discrete etching of the surface and the dentinal tubules.

• This treatment is followed by application of a *primer* that wets the surface and may contain molecules that have the potential to chemically bond to the dentin. These molecules vary with the product but include NPG (*N*-phenylglycine), HEMA (hydroxyethylmethacrylate) for bonding to the hydroxyapatite portion of dentin and glutaraldehyde, and 4-META (4-methyloxyethyltrimellitic anhydride), which can react with collagen.

• The *bonding resin* then is applied to the primed surface. It consists of a low-viscosity polymerizable monomer that contains adhesive molecules (HEMA, for example). This bonding resin readily wets and flows into the irregularities in the primed dentin surface, apparently providing mechanical bonding. This mechanical interlocking is thought to provide the major contribution to the bond of resin to dentin.

Sensitivity of the dentin bond agents to manipulative variables cannot be overemphasized. It is imperative that the manufacturer's instructions for the particular product be scrupulously followed.

A wide discrepancy exists in reported bond strengths for dentin bond agents, making it difficult to present exact figures. Each new generation of bond agent has resulted in an improvement in bond strength, but the bond's long-term stability in the oral cavity is yet to be determined. Studies also have shown that bond strengths do not necessarily correlate with microleakage data, suggesting that both need to be considered when evaluating a new dentin bonding system.

COATINGS FOR ERODED AREAS

Erosion and toothbrush abrasion frequently lead to unsightly sensitive cervical lesions with exposed areas of dentin and cementum. An example of such a lesion is seen in Figure 10–18A. Traditionally, a Class V restoration has been used for the treatment of such conditions. A technique now being advocated involves mechanical bonding by acid etching of the enamel margins and placement of a BIS-GMA resin to recontour and seal the exposed surfaces without the aid of retention by way of the traditional cavity preparation (Fig. 10–18B).

Although this conservative concept has virtue, reservations exist about the therapy as sometimes applied. If all margins of the restored area lie in enamel, retention should be acceptable, with virtually any resin providing an adequate mechanical bond.

The gingival margins, however, typically involve dentin or cementum, where the bond of the resin to the tooth is extremely poor. This results in a high percentage of the restorations being lost soon after insertion. For this reason, it usually is advisable to provide modest mechanical retention by cutting a small groove just inside the gingival border of the lesion along the gingival margin. A slight bevel also can be placed in the occlusal enamel to improve the etching pattern and, hence, retention of the restoration (Fig. 10–19).

Even in those cases in which the restoration is retained, a completely satisfactory result may not have been accomplished. Microleakage still may occur at the gingival margin. Whenever a portion of the cavosurface margin lies in dentin or cementum, a dentin bond agent should be used. The alternatives of using a glass ionomer cement liner with the composite resin (sandwich technique) or restoring the lesion with a glass ionomer filling cement are discussed in Chapter 21.

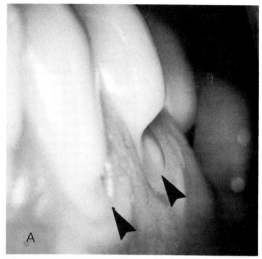

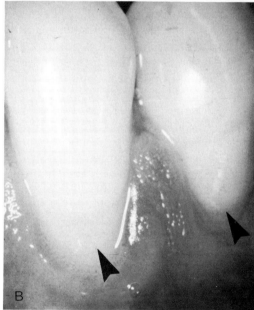

Figure 10–18. *A,* An example of the so-called eroded area with exposed dentin or cementum. (Courtesy of B. Matis.) *B,* The lesion restored using an acid etch technique and a composite resin. (Courtesy of B. Matis.)

RESIN INLAY SYSTEMS

The problem of wear of posterior resin restorations has been considerably reduced with newer formulations, but difficulties still

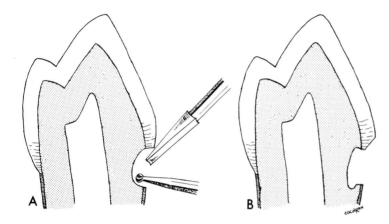

Figure 10–19. Eroded lesion *(A)* with beveled enamel for acid etching and mechanical gingival retention. *B,* Completed preparation. (From Baum, L., Phillips, R. W., and Lund, M. R.: *Textbook of Operative Dentistry,* 2nd ed. Philadelphia, W. B. Saunders Co., 1985.)

exist in high-stress situations. The problem is thought to be related to both mechanical and chemical degradation of composite resins. Polymerization shrinkage, technique sensitivity of dentin bond agents, and difficulty in obtaining a predictably reliable bond to margins in a dentin or cementum also have made potential leakage of Class II restorations a concern.

The composite inlay systems that are polymerized outside the mouth and then luted to the tooth with a compatible resin cement are an attempt to overcome some of the limitations of direct-filling posterior composite resins. If the restoration is first polymerized and then cemented into the tooth, the space created by polymerization shrinkage of the resin is filled largely by the resin cement.

Several systems for resin inlay construction have been marketed. These include both direct and indirect fabrication and polymerization by light, heat, pressure, or a combination of these curing systems. Commercial resins designed for inlays are hybrid and microfilled composites.

With the direct inlays systems, a separating medium (agar solution or glycerine) is applied to the prepared cavity. The resin is inserted into the tooth preparation, and the inlay is contoured and light-cured. It then is removed from the tooth and subjected to further curing by light and/or heat. The enamel margins of the preparation are then etched and the inlay cemented with a dual-cure resin cement (Chapter 22).

With the indirect resin inlay technique, an impression is taken of the prepared tooth and a stone die poured. The resin inlay is formed on the stone die. The inlay is polymerized on the die by light-curing and then is subjected to a heat cure. Some systems use both heat and pressure.

Overall, the physical properties of these inlay resins do not appear to be superior to those of most direct filling composite resins. Laboratory studies, however, indicate that the seal of the critical gingival margins of Class II inlays is superior to that of Class II direct composite restorations. Long-term clinical data are lacking with respect to performance of composite resin inlays, but a number of studies have reported satisfactory performance after 3 and 4 years.

PIT AND FISSURE SEALANTS

The pit and fissure areas of the occlusal surfaces of molar teeth of children are particularly susceptible to caries. Fluoride applications have not been nearly so effective in preventing caries on occlusal surfaces as on other surfaces of the teeth.

Through the years, various materials and techniques have been advocated to prevent pit and fissure caries without resorting to the conventional Class I restoration. Resin pit and fissure sealants have proved the most successful. The rationale for this technique is that when the resin is correctly applied to the surface, it penetrates into the pits and fissures, polymerizes, and seals these areas against the oral environment. A cross section of a tooth to which a pit and fissure sealant has been applied is shown in Figure 10–20.

Most commercial pit and fissure sealants are unfilled composite resin matrix materials or resins with only a small amount of filler. The sealants are polymerized by the conventional peroxide-amine system or are light-activated systems.

The success of the sealant technique depends on obtaining intimate adaptation of the resin to the tooth surface, thereby sealing it.

- The resins used must have a low viscosity so that they flow readily into the fissure and wet the tooth surface.
- As discussed previously, the tooth must first be etched with acid to clean the surface, enhance wetting, and provide mechanical retention.
- The etched surface must be kept clean and free of moisture until the sealant has been applied and cured.

Sealants are susceptible to occlusal wear, but this should not pose a serious problem if the material is retained in the pits and fissures. The results of clinical studies indicate impressive reductions in occlusal caries by the careful use of the material.

Because the application of sealants by dental auxiliaries is permitted in some areas, a thorough understanding of the correct manipulation of this material is important.

When sealants are used, the dental staff should be oriented toward preventive dentistry. The patient should be on a 6-month recall so that the sealant can be examined and reapplied as necessary. Likewise, the patient must be educated to understand that a pit and fissure sealant program is not a substitute for other caries control measures, including fluoride application, oral hygiene, and diet.

COATINGS TO MASK ENAMEL DEFECTS

Unsightly appearance of anterior teeth caused by developmental defects or discoloration of the enamel often is a problem, particularly in the young patient. A resin coating can be applied to the facial surface of the impaired tooth to cover or mask the defect. Basically, the technique consists of etching the enamel of the facial surface of the tooth and then applying a layer of composite resin over the etched surface. Laminate resin veneers also have been used for this purpose. They consist of a prefabricated

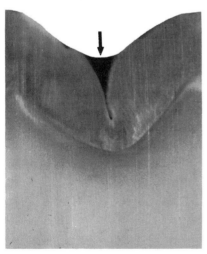

Figure 10–20. Cross section of a tooth showing penetration of a sealant into an occlusal fissure.

thin resin facing that is cemented onto the etched facial surface of the defective tooth by means of a resin cement.

Laminated porcelain veneers, to be discussed later, are more durable and have largely replaced the prefabricated resin veneers. To mask dark discoloration, an opaquing material or an opaque cement may need to be used beneath the veneering material.

CROWN AND BRIDGE RESINS

Resins are used in the construction of restorations that are cemented onto the tooth, primarily as an alternative to porcelain for veneering cast metal crowns and bridge components in aesthetic restorations. Poly(methyl methacrylate) once was used for this purpose, but highly cross-linked composite resins, either heat- or light-polymerized, designed specifically for this purpose now are available.

The resin originally was mechanically retained to the metal by wire loops or cast metal beads. Recent improvements include the development of resin metal bonding agents and a process for applying a coating of silicon dioxide to the metal by flame spraying. The latter is followed by an application of an organosilane *coupling agent* similar to those used to coat the inorganic fillers in composite resins. For appliances cast from base metals, the surface of the metal may be etched to provide a mechanical bond similar to the resin-etched enamel bond.

The advantages of resin-metal veneers compared with ceramic restorations are ease of fabrication and repair in the oral cavity. Resin-metal veneers are vulnerable to microleakage at the resin-metal interface, which can result in discoloration. Compared with porcelain, they are less resistant to wear, including that produced by a toothbrush. They

should not be used on occlusal surfaces or on surfaces engaged by a partial denture clasp.

Although aesthetic resin jacket crowns that have no metal substructure have been used clinically, the inherent properties of the resin make such restorations greatly inferior to ceramic crowns. Resin is used, however, for provisional (temporary) crowns and bridges in fixed prosthodontics. A time lapse exists between tooth preparation and cementation of cast metal and ceramic restorations. Provisional resin restorations provide protective coverage of the prepared teeth while maintaining the position of the teeth during the interval required to fabricate the permanent restorations.

Chemically activated resins designed for this application are used. Most are some type of acrylic, such as poly(methyl methacrylate), poly(ethyl methacrylate), and poly(vinylethylmethacrylate). The resins are supplied as a liquid (monomer) and powder (polymer) that are mixed together into a fluid consistency.

The technique for constructing provisional restorations consists of the following steps:

1. Before tooth preparation, an impression is taken of the involved teeth.
2. After tooth preparation, the resin is mixed and placed in the impression of the prepared teeth.
3. The impression is reseated in the mouth and the resin allowed to polymerize. The polymerization time is about 5 minutes from the start of the mix.
4. The impression then is removed from the mouth.
5. The restorations are recovered, trimmed of excess resin, checked for fit, and polished.
6. The restorations are cemented with a zinc oxide–eugenol cement. This is one of few times that zinc oxide–eugenol is advocated for use with a resin.

Selected Reading

Academy of Dental Materials, International Congress on Dental Materials: *Transactions.* Houston, Academy of Dental Materials, Baylor College of Dentistry, 1990.

Albers, H.: *Tooth Colored Restoratives: A Syllabus for Selection, Placement and Finishing,* 7th ed. Catati, CA, Alto Books, 1985.

Asmussen, E., and Munksgaard, E. C.: Bonding of restorative resins to dentine: Status of dentine adhesives and impact on cavity design and filling techniques. Int. Dent. J. 38:97, 1988.

Avery, D. R.: The use of preformed acrylic veneers for aesthetic treatment of severely discolored permanent teeth. Int. Dent. J. 30:49, 1980.

Baum, L., Phillips, R. W., and Lund, M. R.: *Textbook of Operative Dentistry,* 2nd ed. Philadelphia, W. B. Saunders Co., 1985.

Bowen, R. L., Eichmiller, F. C., Marjenhoff, W. A., and Rupp, N. W.: Adhesive bonding of composites. J. Am. Coll. Dent. 56:10, 1989.

Brooks, J. D., Mertz-Fairhurst, E. J., Della Gustiana, V. E., et al.: A comparative study of two pit and fissure sealants: Three year results in Augusta, Ga. J. Am. Dent. Assoc. 99:42, 1979.

Buonocore, M. G.: A simple method of increasing the adhesion of acrylic filling materials to enamel surface. J. Dent. Res. 34:849, 1955.

Buonocore, M. G.: *The Use of Adhesives in Dentistry.* Springfield, IL, Charles C Thomas, 1975.

Chung, R., and Greener, E. H.: Degree of conversion of seven visible light-cured posterior composites. J. Oral Rehabil. 15:555, 1988.

Consensus Development Conference: Statement on dental sealants and the prevention of tooth decay. J. Am. Dent. Assoc. 108:233, 1984.

Douglas, W. H.: Clinical status of dentine bonding agents. J. Dent. 17:209, 1989.

Farrah, J. W.: Unfilled, filled and microfilled composite resins. Oper. Dent. 6:95, 1981.

Gallegos, L. I., and Nicholls, J. I.: In vitro two-body wear of three veneering resins. J. Prosthet. Dent. 60:172, 1988.

Hollinger, J. D., Moore, E. M., Jr., Brady, J. M., and Lorton, L.: Clinical and laboratory comparison of three adhesive resins for restoring noncarious cervical lesions. Gen. Dent. 29:504, 1981.

Horn, H. R. (Ed.): Symposium on composite resins in dentistry. Dent. Clin. North Am. 25:207, 1981.

Jacobsen, P. H.: The current status of composite restorative materials. Br. Dent. J. 150:15, 1981.

Lambrechts, P., Braem, M., and Van Herle, G.: Evaluation of clinical performance for posterior composite resins and dentin adhesives. J. Oper. Dent. 12:53, 1987.

Loeys, K., Lambrechts, P., Van Herle, G., and Davidson, C. L.: Material development and clinical performance of composite resins. J. Prosthet. Dent. 48:664, 1982.

Lutz, F., and Phillips, R. W.: A classification and evaluation of composite resin systems. J. Prosthet. Dent. 50:480, 1983.

Mertz-Fairhurst, E. J.: Current status of sealant retention and caries prevention. National Institutes of Health Consensus Development Conference. Dental Sealants in the Prevention of Tooth Decay. J. Dent. Res. 48:18, 1984.

Raptis, C. N., Fan, P. L., and Powers, J. M.: Properties of microfilled and visible light cured composites. J. Am. Dent. Assoc. 99:631, 1979.

Roulet, J. F.: The problems associated with substituting composite resins for amalgam: A status report on posterior composites. J. Dent. 16:101, 1988.

Silverstone, L. M., and Dogon, I. L. (Eds.): *The Acid Etch Technique: Proceedings of an International Symposium.* St. Paul, North Central Publishing Co., 1975.

Swartz, M. L., Moore, B. K., Phillips, R. W., and Rhodes, B. F.: Direct restorative resins—a comparative study. J. Prosthet. Dent. 47:163, 1982.

Swartz, M. L., Phillips, R. W., and Rhodes, B.: Visible light activated resins, depth of cure. J. Am. Dent. Assoc. 106:634, 1983.

Tsai, Y. H., Swartz, M. L., Phillips, R. W., and Moore, B. K.: A comparative study: Bond strength and microleakage with dentin bond systems. J. Oper. Dent. 15:53, 1990.

Vanherele, G., and Smith, D. S.: *Posterior Composite Resin Dental Restorative Materials.* St. Paul, Dental Products Division, 3M Co., 1985.

Wendt, S. L., Jr., and Leinfelder, K. F.: The clinical evaluation of heat-treated composite resin inlays. J. Am. Dent. Assoc. 120:177, 1990.

Reviewing the Chapter

1. Describe the difference in the composition of a composite resin compared with an unfilled acrylic direct filling resin.
2. What are the three major components of a composite resin? What is the function of each one?
3. What were the serious clinical problems with the unfilled acrylic restorative resins, and how do composites solve those problems?
4. Describe the different matrix materials

and fillers most commonly used in modern composite resins.

5. Describe the three types of composite resins based on their polymerization systems. What is the air-inhibited layer? How are each of these types supplied to the dentist? What are the advantages and disadvantages of each?

6. Describe the types of visible light–curing units available. What things can influence the light output of these units? Why is this important?

7. List the types of composite resin available based on differences in filler types and loading. Describe the filler used in each type.

8. What is a *conventional* or *macrofilled composite?* What are its advantages and disadvantages?

9. What is a *microfilled composite?* What are its advantages and disadvantages?

10. What is a *small-particle composite?* List its advantages and disadvantages.

11. What is a *hybrid composite?* List its advantages and disadvantages.

12. Compare the physical properties of unfilled acrylic resin with the four categories of composites in questions 8 through 11.

13. List the principal clinical applications for each type of composite.

14. What are the requirements for a composite resin to be used as an occlusal restorative material in posterior teeth? Which of the four types is best suited to this application? Does clinical evidence support the replacement of dental amalgam with composite resin in all cases?

15. Discuss the biocompatibility of composite resin. What precautions should be taken to protect a vital tooth from possible chemical insult?

16. Discuss the correct manipulation of chemically activated composite resins. Include any special precautions that should be taken for this type of restorative resin.

17. Discuss the correct manipulation of light-activated composite resins. Include any special considerations in the placement of this type of restorative.

18. Does exposure to the light from a visible light–curing unit pose any risk for dental personnel or the patient? What precautions are suggested?

19. Describe the acid etch technique for bonding to enamel. Explain the rationale for this process.

20. What precautions should be taken when using the acid etch technique?

21. What are *enamel bond agents?* How are they used?

22. What are *dentin bond agents? Universal bond agents?* How are they used?

23. What is the *smear layer?* Why do most dentin bonding systems use an etchant to at least partially remove the smear layer?

24. Why is the bond between restorative resin and enamel stronger than the bond to dentin? Are these bonds mostly mechanical, or chemical in nature?

25. How are restorative resins used to protect cervical eroded areas? Is a cavity preparation needed? What are the potential problems with this technique? What other restorative materials can be used to restore cervical erosion lesions?

26. What are *resin inlays?* What are their advantages compared with direct filling composite restorations? Describe the indirect and direct resin inlay technique.

27. What are *pit and fissure sealants?* What has been the clinical success record for this material? Describe the technique for application of pit and fissure sealants. Why is this topic particularly relevant for dental auxiliaries?

28. Describe the use of resin materials to mask enamel defects. What other restorative materials also are used for this purpose?

29. Describe the resins used in fixed prosthodontics (crown and bridge) for both permanent and provisional restorations. What is the clinical experience with this material for permanent restorations?

30. What material would be used to cement a provisional resin crown? Why is this material normally not used with composite resins?

CHAPTER 11

METALLURGY: Solidification, Wrought Metals, and Direct Filling Gold

SOLIDIFICATION OF METALS
How Solidification Occurs

WROUGHT METALS
Deformation of Metals
Strain Hardening
Annealing
    Effect of Grain Size

DIRECT FILLING GOLD RESTORATIVE MATERIALS

What is a metal? Although metallic substances are commonplace in daily life, giving a simple definition of a metal is difficult. One might say that it is a solid—but mercury and hydrogen are both metals. Mercury is a liquid at room temperature, and hydrogen is a gas. One characteristic of a metal that is difficult to imitate with any other substance is its metallic luster when highly polished. A metal also usually is a good electrical and thermal conductor and is more ductile than nonmetals. In comparing the relative conductivities and ductilities, however, defining the value that separates metals from nonmetals is not easy. Probably the best definition is chemical in nature. *Any chemical element that loses one or more valence electrons to form a positive ion in a chemical reaction or in solution is a metal.* If one considers the listing of pure elements shown in the Appendix, about 85 per cent of the elements meet this definition of a metal.

At this point, a distinction should be made. Metals exist as chemical elements, called *pure metals*, and as combinations of a pure metal and one or more other elements, called *alloys*, which are described in Chapter 12. Both pure metals and alloys are referred to simply as metals. Pure metals seldom are used in dentistry or any structural application because they lack adequate strength and resistance to corrosion.

Almost all metals are crystalline solids at room temperature, and many of the metals used in dentistry have crystal lattices that belong to the cubic systems (see Fig. 3–2).

One characteristic of a pure metal is that it possesses distinct freezing and melting temperatures that are identical and characteristic of that particular metal. This is a characteristic of any pure crystalline material.

SOLIDIFICATION OF METALS

Whenever a pure metal solidifies, certain effects occur. Assume that a metal is heated to the temperature at which it is molten or liquid. If the temperature of the metal is recorded as it cools, a peculiar thing can be observed. When the temperature of the metal is plotted in terms of the time elapsing, a curve such as that shown in Figure 11–1 is obtained. This curve is referred to as a *time-temperature cooling curve*. Each metal ex-

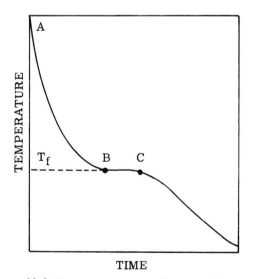

Figure 11–1. Time-temperature cooling curve for a pure metal. At any temperature above *B*, the metal is molten. Below temperatures at *C*, the metal is solid. Temperature T_f is the fusion temperature.

hibits its own time-temperature cooling curve, which is characteristic of that metal.

The interpretation of this curve is of practical importance. When a substance is heated to a temperature higher than that of its environment, it starts to cool immediately after the heating has ceased and continues to cool until it reaches the temperature of its surroundings. If a pure metal is heated to temperature point A as shown on the graph, one might expect that it would cool at a uniform rate to room temperature even though it was liquid at the temperature at point A. Initially, it does cool quite regularly, as shown by the curve AB. Then the temperature remains constant between B and C even though the metal must continue to lose heat. The temperature at BC, indicated as T_f on the graph, is called the *freezing temperature* or *solidification temperature*. At this temperature, the metal freezes or becomes solid. As the metal cools below temperature C, the temperature decreases with time as might be expected, but the metal is entirely solid after point C.

If the same experiment is done by slowly heating the metal from room temperature, a similar curve is obtained. The temperature remains constant for a period of time while the metal is passing from a solid to a liquid. This is called the *melting temperature* or *fusion temperature*. If the temperature changes are relatively slow, the melting and freezing temperatures are the same for pure metals.

Because the metal must be losing heat during the time elapsing between B and C and the temperature does not change, the heat given off is called the *latent* (hidden) *heat of solidification*. The source of this heat is the energy given up when a liquid changes to a solid. *The latent heat of solidification is defined as the number of calories of heat liberated from 1 gram of a substance when it changes from the liquid to the solid state.*

When a crystalline material freezes, it gives off an amount of heat that is characteristic for the particular substance. Thus, when water changes to ice at 0° C (32° F), 80 calories of heat are given off for every gram of water changed to ice. If one lives near a large body of fresh water, such as the Great Lakes, the temperature near the shore during the winter is likely to be higher than that a few miles inland. As the water freezes, 80 calories of heat are given off for every gram of water solidified. Conversely, when the ice melts in the spring, the temperature near the body of water is likely to be lower than that further inland. For every gram of ice melted, 80 calories of heat must be taken from the surroundings to melt the ice. In the latter case, the heat absorbed is called the *latent heat of fusion.*

This knowledge is important because many dental structures, such as inlays and crowns, are *cast.* That is, they are formed into their final shapes by pouring liquid metal into an accurately shaped container or mold and allowing it to freeze. The mold is an exact reproduction of the missing tooth structure. This procedure is described in detail in Chapter 19. Knowledge of the theory involved is needed for one to thoroughly understand the technique of casting. Because of the processes required to refine metals from the ores (minerals) found in nature, even metal objects that are not shaped in this manner start out as cast metals.

How Solidification Occurs

The question of just how solidification occurs is of considerable practical importance because the physical properties of the solid material often can be predicted on the basis of the method of crystallization from the fusion temperature.

The metal crystals form on a nucleus of crystallization in a manner similar to that described for plaster of Paris. As in the case of plaster, the greater the number of nuclei present, the larger the number of crystals

formed during solidification. This process can be best illustrated diagrammatically, as shown in Figure 11–2.

In Figure 11–2A, at least one nucleus of crystallization is shown as a square figure. Other nuclei are present, but branching crystallization is starting. These tree-like branches are called *dendrites*. In Figure 11–2B, the branching has increased, as is the case in the succeeding Figures 11–2C and 11–2D. Again, like the crystals of plaster, the crystals in Figure 11–2E are growing out and beginning to touch one another. They grow toward one another until the space is fairly well filled, as shown in Figure 11–2F. Only the outlines of the boundaries at which they met one another are present because they have crowded together so tightly. The crystals in a solid metal are called *grains* (after grains of corn), and their boundaries are called *grain boundaries.*

Each grain started from a different nucleus of crystallization and is, therefore, an independent crystal formation with the same space lattice but having an orientation different from that of its neighbor. The crystals did not join at their meeting point because their space lattices did not match because of their different orientations. If they did match exactly as they approached one another, they would join to form a larger single grain or crystal. (Large "single crystals" are important in the fabrication of modern electronic devices.) Most metals used for structural applications contain a large number of small crystals and are referred to as polycrystalline. The number of grains per square centimeter (or the size of the grain, which is the same thing) is important because the smaller the grain size (the greater the number of grains), the greater the yield strength of the metal.

Again—using the crystallization of plaster as an analogy—the greater the number of nuclei of crystallization during solidification, the smaller the size of each grain. In turn, the number of nuclei of crystallization is

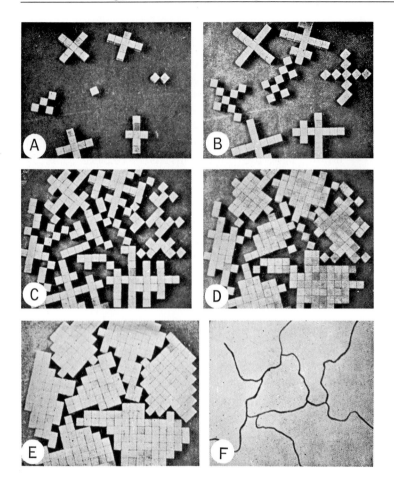

Figure 11–2. Diagrammatic representation of the formation of grains during solidification. *A,* The crystals begin to form on nuclei of crystallization. *B* and *C,* Crystals are growing in all directions. *D* and *E,* Individual crystals approach one another. *F,* Individual crystals finally crowd together to form the metallic grains. (Rosenhain, W.: *Introduction to Physical Metallurgy.* 3rd ed. London, Constable and Co. Ltd., 1935.)

largely determined by the speed with which the metal is cooled from its molten to its solid state. The faster it is cooled, the more nuclei are present and, therefore, the greater the number of grains.

The grains can be seen with a microscope if the metal surface is correctly prepared. If the metal surface is highly polished and then chemically attacked by some reagent that dissolves the metal, the grain structure can be seen. A *photomicrograph* of the grain structure of pure gold prepared in this manner is shown in Figure 11–3. The dark lines are the grain boundaries and the enclosed areas are the grains. The fact that the grain boundaries are preferentially attacked has

significance when considering corrosion resistance, as seen in Chapter 13.

WROUGHT METALS

Up to this point, the metals used for illustration were assumed to be in the "as cast" condition: they had been heated above their fusion point and allowed to solidify.

Many metal objects are made from metal that has been greatly altered in shape after casting—for example, pipes, wires, rods, sheets, most cooking utensils, and similar articles. These are fabricated from metal that has been cast and then extensively deformed

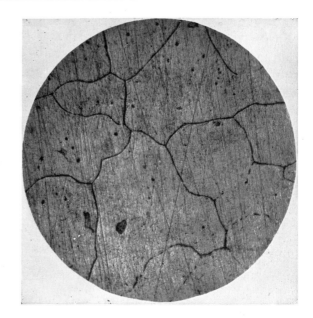

Figure 11-3. Microstructure of an ingot of pure gold. Note the similarity to Figure 11–2F (100 ×). (Courtesy of S. D. Tylman.)

or worked by rolling between cylindrical rolls or by drawing (pulling) or extruding (pushing) through a hole. Metal can be rolled into a sheet, which in turn can be bent and pressed into different shapes. The cast metal also can be extruded to form pipes and rods or drawn into the shape of a wire. After a casting has been worked or shaped, it becomes what is known as a *wrought* metal and exhibits a somewhat different grain structure. Certain other properties also differ from those of the casting.

The fundamental requirement for a wrought material is that it has been subjected to stress in excess of the elastic limit, resulting in plastic deformation (strain).

Although many metals used in dentistry are castings, the dentist or dental technician usually alters the surface or contour. During mastication, the patient produces further changes in the metallic restoration or appliance. Certain dental appliances, such as orthodontic springs, are wrought structures. Thus, a few principles concerning the behavior of wrought metals need to be considered.

Deformation of Metals

Reviewing the stress-strain curve (see Fig. 3–4) is useful in understanding deformation of a metal. For stresses below the proportional limit, all atoms in the space lattice merely move apart and produce an elastic strain. Relative to the neighboring atoms, the movement is small. When the stress is released, the lattice returns to its original size and the strain is gone.

If the stress exceeds the proportional limit, a permanent deformation occurs; that is, some of the atoms are so far removed from each other that they cannot readily return to their original positions. A permanent strain then exists. The separation of the atoms eventually becomes so great that a fracture results.

A simple mechanism that explains the possible changes in the space lattice for this permanent deformation is that one layer of atoms in the space lattice slips over the layer below. This situation is represented diagrammatically in Figure 11–4. A simple cubic space lattice is shown in two dimensions.

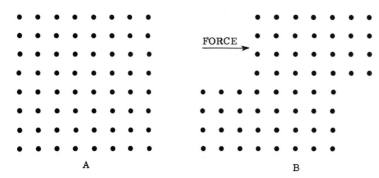

Figure 11-4. How slip may occur in a space lattice. The dots in *A* represent the original positions of the atoms. When the stress is greater than the proportional limit, one layer of atoms may slip or slide over the other layers, as shown in *B*. A permanent deformation exists because the atoms have been displaced too much; they cannot return to their former positions.

The original space lattice is represented by the dots (Fig. 11–4*A*). Assume that a stress exceeding the elastic limit has been induced and that the top four layers of atoms simply slide over the bottom four layers of atoms, as diagrammed in Figure 11–4*B*. The first four layers of atoms are said to *slip* over the bottom four layers. Because the atomic displacements are so great, the atoms cannot return to their original positions after slip, and a permanent deformation occurs.

The upper four rows of atoms have slipped three atomic spacings, but they could have slipped one or a thousand atomic spacings, depending on the stress present. Once slip has taken place, the metal becomes a wrought metal instead of a cast metal.

Slip, as diagrammed in Figure 11–4, requires a large applied stress in a perfect metal crystal lattice that contains no *lattice imperfections*. Such crystals are rare research curiosities. All practical metals slip at surprisingly low stresses. A particular type of defect in the crystal lattice, called a *dislocation*, permits easy slip to occur. Such a defect is shown in Figure 11–5. Easy slip occurs as illustrated when the applied stress moves the extra plane of atoms across the crystal one position at a time. This process is analogous to moving a large rug across the floor by forming a wrinkle at one edge of the rug and simply walking the wrinkle across the floor.

A single crystal of a pure metal typically is too soft to withstand any significant applied stress. Consequently, various hardening methods to inhibit slippage are important. These are discussed in the next and subsequent sections.

Strain Hardening

To produce plastic deformation of a polycrystalline metal, the slip that occurs in one grain, as shown in Figure 11–3, must be transferred to adjacent grains. Slip occurs in one grain and crowds against the adjoining grain. If the stress is great enough, slip also occurs in the adjoining grain but in a different direction because the direction of the atom rows is different. This grain crowds the next one and so on. The difficulty in transferring slip from one grain to the next explains, in part, the increase in yield strength with increased number of grains per unit volume (decreased grain size).

As the grains become distorted, more and more stress is required to cause additional slip. The grains finally become so mixed up that no further slip can occur. If the stress continues to increase in magnitude, the atoms must separate entirely—the structure breaks or fractures.

As slip increases, the amount of stress needed to produce additional slip also increases. Because the atoms become more difficult to displace, the metal must become stronger and harder. The proportional limit also increases but, as might be expected, the ductility decreases. This method of changing the properties of a metal is known as *strain hardening*. A paper clip, for example, can

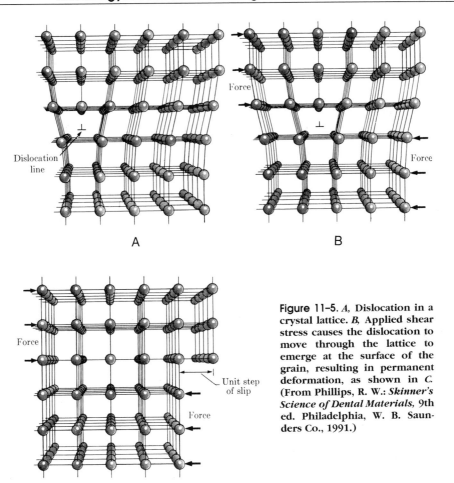

Figure 11–5. *A*, **Dislocation in a crystal lattice.** *B*, **Applied shear stress causes the dislocation to move through the lattice to emerge at the surface of the grain, resulting in permanent deformation, as shown in** *C*. **(From Phillips, R. W.:** *Skinner's Science of Dental Materials*, **9th ed. Philadelphia, W. B. Saunders Co., 1991.)**

be broken by bending it back and forth several times. Each time it is bent it becomes more difficult to bend again until finally it fractures.

To summarize, strain hardening increases the yield strength, hardness, and ultimate tensile strength, but it decreases the ductility and does not significantly change the elastic modulus. Strain hardening usually occurs when the metal is plastically deformed at room temperature. For this reason, the process of producing strain hardening is called *cold working*, as opposed to working the metal at high temperatures, called *forging*.

Because forging does not result in work hardening, a metal can be shaped more easily with lower applied stresses. The blacksmith heats bars of iron to red heat before beating them into horseshoes for exactly this reason. The temperature limit that divides cold working and forging depends on the melting point of the metal. Pure metals with low melting points, such as lead, do not work harden appreciably at room temperature.

Annealing

A ductile metal that has been extensively cold worked loses most of its ductility and can become brittle. Such a material usually is not a good choice for structural use. In many cases, a metal object also does not have sufficient ductility to be shaped into a complex shape by cold working.

After a metal has been strain hardened, it can be treated to reduce or eliminate the strain hardening and substitute a small, regular grain structure. The theory of such a treatment is related to the phenomenon of relaxation, discussed in Chapter 4. When the space lattices are entangled as described, the atoms are out of position and want to return to a normal regular position. This can be accomplished by heating the metal to a temperature below the melting point and holding it at that temperature for some length of time. This process is called *annealing*. At this temperature, the atoms move about or diffuse to form a small, regular grain structure, and the effects of strain hardening begin to disappear.

The temperature required, called the *recrystallization temperature*, may be quite critical. If the metal is heated to too high a temperature or for too long a time at a lower temperature, the grains actually coalesce or join together and thereby increase in size. Such a phenomenon is known as *grain growth*. If the grains become too large, the strength and proportional limit of the metal may be reduced considerably and the metal may lose its usefulness. In annealing a wrought structure, it is necessary to prevent overannealing so that grain growth does not take place.

Effect of Grain Size

As mentioned in the previous section, the ductility and strength are greater when smaller grains are present. The reason for this condition is that the greater the number of grains, the greater the amount of slip that can occur. Because ductility depends on the amount of slip or permanent deformation, it

is, therefore, increased. The annealing time and temperature depend on the amount of strain hardening. Cold working reduces the grain size, decreases the recrystallization temperature, and increases the rate at which annealing changes the mechanical properties.

Many wrought metals rely on strain hardening to give them adequate yield strength for particular application. The stainless steel wire used to fabricate springs in orthodontics is a good example. If these materials are subjected to a significant amount of annealing, they become too soft to deliver the required forces and their utility is destroyed.

DIRECT FILLING GOLD RESTORATIVE MATERIALS

Only pure metallic elements have been discussed to this point. Only one pure metal is used to any extent for dental purposes, and that is gold. When used as a restorative material, it is referred to as *direct filling gold*. The various forms in which pure gold may be used for a dental restoration are shown in Figure 11–6.

The use of pure gold as a direct restorative material depends on several unique properties of this pure metal.

- Gold is the most resistant of all metals to corrosion.
- Gold is the most ductile and malleable of all metals.
- Gold forms cohesive bonds at room temperature and relatively small applied stresses.
- Although annealed gold is very soft, it work hardens rapidly to a strength and hardness adequate for small restorations subjected to minimal stresses.

Gold can be rolled into very thin sheets, which can in turn be thinned by hammering to such a point that light can be transmitted through the metal. In this condition, it is

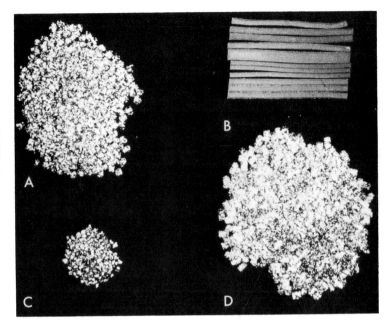

Figure 11–6. Forms of pure gold used for dental restorations. *A,* Hand-rolled pellets; *B,* mat gold; *C,* powdered gold pellets; *D,* machine-rolled cylinders. (Baum, L.: Gold foil in dental practice. Dent. Clin. North Am. March 1965, p. 200.)

known as *foil.* The foil is supplied to the dentist as a flat sheet or in the form of rolled ropes or cylinders. Pure gold is the noblest of metals; it neither tarnishes nor corrodes under normal environmental conditions.

When the surface of the foil is absolutely clean, two pieces of foil may be welded together by simply bringing them into contact. If the surfaces are very clean and no oxide coating is present on the gold, the atoms of one piece join cohesively to those of the other to form a solid structure. Many metals can be welded in this manner, but they must be heated to a very high temperature and subjected to a considerable amount of pressure. Pure gold is unusual in that it can be "cold welded" with modest applied pressure.

The surface of the gold must be free from absorbed gases or impurities. To remove surface impurities, the pieces of foil are heated immediately before being placed into the cavity preparation. This step often is referred to as *annealing.* The objective of this step, however, is to volatilize any contaminants collected on the surface. A better term for this step is *degassing.* The degassing may be done with an electric heating tray or, more commonly, by passing each increment of gold through a clean-burning alcohol flame.

A number of gases can contaminate the foil, including sulfur dioxide, oxygen, and ammonia. Sulfur is particularly bad because it is virtually impossible to remove from the surface by degassing. For this reason, the foil should be kept in tightly closed containers and never stored in contact with matches or rubber products that usually contain free sulfur.

After the cavity has been prepared, the pieces of gold are heated individually to drive off any contamination and then placed in the tooth one piece at a time. Each piece is welded against the previous piece under pressure exerted by hand or using some type of mechanical mallet.

The point of a special instrument, known as a *condenser,* is placed against the piece of foil and the other end of the instrument is

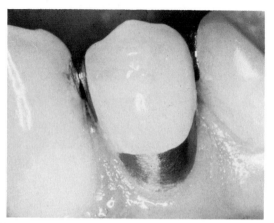

Figure 11–7. Class V gold foil restoration showing excellent clinical performance and tissue tolerance. (Courtesy of J. Osborne.)

struck with a small mallet. Some types of equipment deliver condensation blows automatically. The process of welding the small pieces of gold into a solid mass is called *condensation* or *compacting*.

As the gold foil is condensed, it is strain hardened, and a marked increase in hardness and strength takes place as the restoration is constructed. The Brinell Hardness Number of pure gold in cast form is about 27, whereas the Brinell Hardness Number of a well-condensed gold foil restoration may be as high as 65 with a tensile strength of 310 MPa (45,000 psi).

A correctly placed gold foil restoration can provide excellent, long-term service. The nobility of gold and its ability to be finished to a very smooth surface result in good tissue response in the case of restorations with subgingival margins (Fig. 11–7). The greatest disadvantages of this restorative material are the demand placed on the dentist's technical skill and the time required for placement.

Selected Reading

Baum, L., Phillips, R. W., and Lund, M. R.: *Textbook of Operative Dentistry.* Philadelphia, W. B. Saunders Co., 1981, ch. 14.

Mahan, J., and Charbeneau, G. T.: A study of certain mechanical properties and the density of condensed specimens made from various forms of pure gold. J. Am. Acad. Gold Foil Oper. 8:6, 1965.

Nielsen, J. P., and Tuccillo, J. J.: Grain size in dental gold alloys. J. Dent. Res. 45:964, 1966.

Phillips, R. W.: *Skinner's Science of Dental Materials,* 9th ed. Philadelphia, W. B. Saunders Co., 1991, chs. 13, 14–19.

Richter, W. A., and Cantwell, K. R.: A study of cohesive gold. J. Prosthet. Dent. 15:722, 1965.

Xhonga, F.: Direct Golds, Part I. J. Am. Acad. Gold Foil Oper. 13:17, 1970.

Xhonga, F.: Direct Golds, Part II. J. Am. Acad. Gold Foil Oper. 14:5, 1971.

Reviewing the Chapter

1. What is a *metal?*
2. Using a cooling curve, describe the solidification process of a pure metal.
3. Define *cast structure, freezing temperature, fusion temperature,* and *latent heat of fusion.*
4. Explain how grains form in the solidification of a pure metal. What is meant by *grain boundary* and *dendritic structure?*
5. Define *wrought structure.* Name some ways wrought metals are shaped. List some dental uses for wrought materials.
6. How does deformation affect the stress–strain curve and mechanical properties of a metal? The grain size?
7. Define *dislocation.* Explain its role in easy plastic deformation.
8. Define *strain hardening;* give a dental example.
9. Define the annealing heat treatment. How does this process affect the mechanical properties? Grain size?
10. What is the recrystallization phenomenon?
11. What is the only pure metal used in dentistry? In what forms is it available?
12. Explain *annealing* as related to gold foil.
13. Describe the preparation of direct gold for use as a restorative material. What does condensation do?

CHAPTER 12

DENTAL METALLURGY: Alloys

TYPES OF ALLOYS **Solid Solutions** **Eutectic Alloy** **PHYSICAL PROPERTIES OF SOLID** **SOLUTION ALLOYS**	**HEAT TREATMENT** **CONTROL OF PHYSICAL PROPERTIES**

As noted in Chapter 11, gold is the only pure metal used in dentistry. The metals usually used—both in dentistry and in everyday life—are not pure metals but rather combinations of two or more metals. When the combined metals are mutually soluble in the molten state, the resulting metal is known as an *alloy*. Certain metals are not soluble when melted together. Instead, they separate into distinct layers, depending on the specific gravities of the individual metals. Such a mixture of metals is not classified as an alloy.

Many pure metals do combine to form alloys with properties that are superior to those of the individual metals. Bronze, an alloy of copper and tin, was the first metal used to any great extent. Brass, an alloy of copper and zinc, is used in everyday life much more frequently than either copper or zinc. Copper itself is a rather soft, ductile metal and not very strong, and zinc, a brittle metal, seldom is used alone. Brass is stronger than either copper or zinc and more ductile than zinc.

TYPES OF ALLOYS

In dentistry, pure gold is used only in the form of foil. Gold normally is too soft to be used for a cast crown in the mouth. The stresses of mastication would severely deform it, and the crown would soon be useless. On the other hand, an alloy of gold and 5 per cent copper is a much harder and stronger material that can be used in positions in the mouth not subject to great stress. More copper and other metals usually are added to give the alloy sufficient hardness and strength for it to function in almost any dental application. This point is discussed at greater length in Chapter 16 on dental casting alloys.

If one of the metals or constituents of an

alloy is mercury, the alloy is called an *amalgam*. Dental silver amalgam, one of the most commonly used dental alloys, is discussed in detail in Chapters 14 and 15. *An amalgam is an alloy.*

Distinguishing between an alloy and a pure metal often is difficult. For example, the microstructure of an alloy that contains 90 per cent gold and 10 per cent copper is shown in Figure 12–1. When compared with the photomicrograph of pure gold in Figure 11–3, little structural difference between the two can be seen. The difference in the shading of the grains in Figure 12–1 is due to the manner in which the light was reflected from the surface of the metal and not to a difference in structure.

One difference between a pure metal and most alloys is that the time-temperature cooling curve of the alloy usually is different. The cooling curve for the alloy does not have a horizontal line or plateau at the melting temperature, but rather the alloy solidi-

fies over a range in temperature, as shown in Figure 12–2. A pure metal has a *melting point*, but most alloys have a *melting range*.

Such a time-temperature cooling curve is characteristic of a particular alloy, just as the similar curve for a pure metal is characteristic and distinct (see Fig. 11–1). In Figure 12–2, the metal begins to solidify at temperature B and is completely solidified at temperature C. The metal is liquid or molten at all temperatures above B and solid at all temperatures below C. Between temperatures B and C, it will be both liquid and solid—comparable to a slush of salty water and ice, as often is found on the streets in winter. Temperature B is the upper limit of the melting range, called the *liquidus*, and temperature C is the lower limit of the melting range, called the *solidus*.

Alloys can be classified several ways, including the following:

- *The number of metals present.* The sim-

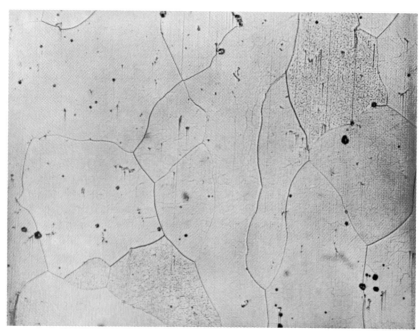

Figure 12–1. Photomicrograph of an alloy containing 90 per cent gold and 10 per cent copper (60×).

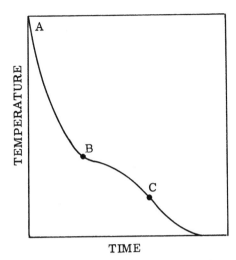

Figure 12–2. Time-temperature cooling curve for a solid solution alloy. Points B and C indicate upper and lower limits of melting range.

plest would be the alloy that contains two metals, known as a *binary alloy.* If three metals were present, it would be a *ternary alloy,* and so forth. This type of classification becomes cumbersome because many dental alloys contain six or more constituent metals.

● *Their crystal lattice forms.* The atoms of copper, for example, are randomly distributed throughout the space lattice of gold in the alloy shown in Figure 12–1. It is impossible to determine from the photomicrograph whether copper is present. This type of alloy is known as a *solid solution* alloy. At the other extreme are alloys in which the metals separate from one another when the alloy solidifies from the molten state. Each grain then is composed of one of the nearly pure metal constituents. Eutectic alloys are an example of this structure.

● *Their chemical formula.* When other alloys solidify, the atoms arrange themselves in definite proportions to each other. This type of alloy can be given a chemical formula. For example, one of the most important alloys in the formation of dental amalgams has the for-

mula Ag_3Sn. Most of these alloys possess a complex space lattice and are extremely hard and brittle. They are called *intermetallic compounds.*

● *Combinations of types.* A fourth type of alloy may be composed of combinations of two or more types. As a matter of convenience, this alloy is known as a *mixed-type alloy.*

Two types, solid solution alloys and mixed-type alloys, are important in dentistry.

Solid Solutions

By far the greatest number of alloys that are useful as dental restorations are solid solution alloys. Certainly almost everyone knows what a liquid solution is. When sugar is dissolved in water, for example, a solution of sugar and water is obtained. The water is known as the *solvent* and the sugar is termed the *solute.*

When an alloy is liquid by definition, the metals must be soluble in one another. In the alloy shown in Figure 12–1, for example, in the liquid condition, the copper atoms mingle with the gold atoms at random in the same manner that the dissolved sugar molecules mingle with those of the water. When the two solutions solidify or freeze, each reacts differently.

● When the solution of water and sugar freezes, the sugar molecules immediately separate from the water or ice molecules and are no longer in solution.

● Metals may solidify differently. When the two metals copper and gold, in the proportions indicated, solidify or freeze, the solution structure persists. The copper atoms remain distributed randomly throughout the space lattice of the gold atoms. The analogy of solvent and solute persists; the gold is known as the solvent and the copper as the solute.

In the space lattice of a solid solution,

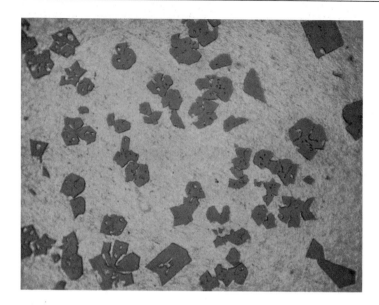

Figure 12–3. Microstructure of the gold-silicon eutectic (540 X). (Courtesy of J. Tuccillo.)

those atoms that are most numerous usually are designated as the solvent and the least numerous are known as the solute.

Solid solutions may form in two ways. If the two metals have similar atomic sizes, the atoms of the solute substitute for solvent atoms in the solvent space lattice. This type of *substitutional solid solution* is formed by gold and copper. If the solute atoms are significantly smaller than the solvent atoms, they may occupy spaces between the normal lattice positions for the solvent metal, called an *interstitial solid solution.* An important alloy is an interstitial solid solution of carbon in iron called steel.

Most solid solution alloys have higher yield strengths, tensile strengths, and hardnesses than the pure metals from which they are made. They also have adequate corrosion and tarnish resistance in the mouth and, therefore, are important types of alloys for dental use.

Eutectic Alloy

Eutectic alloys melt at a distinct temperature rather than over a range of temperatures like solid solution alloys. Eutectic means lowest melting. The eutectic alloy formation is closer to what one would expect in comparison to liquid solutions. Although they were soluble in the molten state, metals of the eutectic alloys separate on freezing, just as the sugar molecules crystallize separately from the water molecules during freezing.

The microstructure of such alloys is somewhat complex, as illustrated by the microstructure shown in Figure 12–3. The composition of this alloy is 6 per cent silicon and 94 per cent gold. The lighter particles are grains of gold, and the dark areas are silicon grains.

The practical importance of such alloys to the dentist is that the eutectic alloy has a melting temperature far below that of any of the constituent metals. For example, the alloy shown in Figure 12–3 fuses at 370° C (698° F), whereas the melting temperatures of gold and silicon, respectively, are 1063° C (1944° F) and 1420° C (2588° F). The alloy with the eutectic composition has the lowest melting temperature of any alloy of gold and silicon and commonly is known simply as the *eutectic.*

Eutectic alloys are used in dentistry mainly in solders. Solders are alloys with low melting points that are used to mechanically hold two metal structures together. Because the soldering process requires heating the structures to a temperature higher than the solder's melting point, low fusion temperatures are important to avoid damaging the components being soldered. Most eutectic alloys are brittle and lack tarnish and corrosion resistance. Another eutectic alloy is the silver-copper component of certain types of amalgam alloys, which are described in Chapter 14.

PHYSICAL PROPERTIES OF SOLID SOLUTION ALLOYS

Metals usually are alloyed to obtain some properties that permit the alloy to function most advantageously under the conditions of use. In dentistry, the most important property is the degree of resistance to chemical attack, tarnish, and corrosion in the mouth, where conditions are conducive to deterioration by corrosion. To achieve this objective, one must use either of the following:

- A noble metal alloy (based on gold, platinum, and palladium) or
- An alloy that protects itself by forming an impenetrable oxide skin, such as stainless steel.

Gold alloys fall into the first category.

Once this primary objective of resistance to corrosion is realized, the physical properties pertaining to resistance to stress without permanent deformation or fracture are important.

As previously noted, the addition of copper to gold, even in relatively small amounts, greatly increases the hardness, proportional limit, and strength of the gold. The solute atoms (copper, in this case) of a solid solution alloy displace the solvent or gold atoms in the gold space lattice, just as the sugar

molecules displace the water molecules in a liquid solution.

The sugar molecules go into solution in the water because the water molecules exert more attraction for the sugar molecules than do the sugar molecules for one another. In other words, the *adhesive* forces between the water and the sugar are stronger than the *cohesive* forces of the water or the solid sugar. Also, objects have a natural tendency to become mixed rather than to remain separated.

The same rules apply in the case of the solid solution alloy. A solid solution of two or more metals cannot be formed unless the adhesive forces between the solvent metal and the solute metal are greater than the cohesive forces of the individual metals. Otherwise, the solute metal would not be present in the space lattice of the solvent.

One step further in reasoning indicates that when the copper atom is present in the gold space lattice, its attraction is greater for the gold atoms than the attraction of the gold atoms for one another. Consequently, the copper atom attracts the surrounding gold atoms, and they are displaced slightly from their normal, regular lattice positions.

Figure 12–4 shows this effect in an idealized manner—as it might appear when a simple cubic space lattice is the lattice of the solvent metal. The solid dot represents a solute atom. As can be noted in the figure, the atoms of the solvent become somewhat disarranged from their normal positions by the attraction of the solute atom.

This localized irregularity of the space lattice caused by the copper atom makes it difficult for slip to occur. Dislocations tend to be attracted to the solute atoms, and additional applied stress is required to break this attraction. The more areas of this sort in the solvent (gold) lattice, the greater the slip interference. In other words, the more solute (copper) added to the solvent (gold), the greater the proportional limit, strength, and

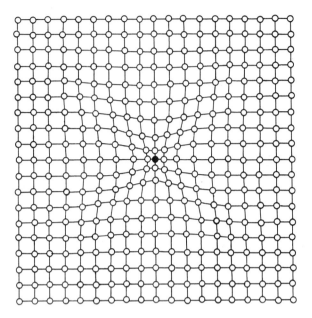

Figure 12-4. The attraction of solvent atoms to the solute atom causes a localized distortion of the space lattice. The circles represent the solvent lattice.

hardness and the less the ductility (percentage of elongation). The general result is similar to the effect of strain hardening.

The effect of the solute atoms on strength may be greatly increased by allowing them to cluster into small platelets. This can be accomplished by aging the alloy at a low temperature. The resulting strengthening is called *age hardening*. If the clusters get too big and hence fewer in number, the hardening decreases. Metals that exhibit solid solubility at all compositions do not form alloys that age harden, so this process, unlike strain hardening, is applicable to certain alloys only.

Other metals that commonly are added to the gold to produce such an effect in a dental gold alloy are platinum, palladium, and silver.

During either solidification or subsequent heat treatment, some solute metals and other contaminants concentrate along the grain boundaries, resulting in a brittle alloy by inhibiting slip across the grain boundary.

A slight contamination of gold foil with arsenic, for example, may render it so brittle that it fractures when handled. When impurities segregate, the oxides that they form during the melting process solidify in the grain boundaries. As a result of these grain boundary films, the ductility may be markedly decreased, although the strength and similar properties may not be greatly changed. As discussed for the case of strain hardening, excessive embrittlement results in an unusable structure material.

HEAT TREATMENT

In some dental gold alloys, the physical properties can be altered by the method of heating and cooling the alloy. If a gold alloy containing about an equal number of gold and copper atoms is cooled rapidly from slightly below its solidus temperature by dropping it into water—a process called *quenching*—its strength, proportional limit, and hardness are lower than if it were allowed to cool slowly in air. If cooled slowly, the physical properties mentioned are increased, but the ductility of the alloy is decreased. When the alloy is cooled rapidly, the gold and copper atoms are distributed randomly in the solid metal, forming a typical solid solution. If the same alloy is cooled slowly, the gold and copper atoms move (diffuse) in the solid in an attempt to surround each copper atom with gold atoms— a *superlattice* is thus formed.

The reaction is reversible. If the alloy is now heated to 700° C (1292° F) and held at that temperature for 10 minutes, the superlattice disappears and the atoms diffuse to their former solid solution condition. Note that this temperature is below the lower limit of the melting range. If the alloy is then quenched, the solid solution is preserved at room temperature because there is not sufficient time for the atomic diffusion to take place. Because the hardness is reduced, this heat treatment followed by quenching is technically known as a *softening heat treatment.*

Again, if the alloy is cooled slowly in air from 700° C (1292° F), the superlattice again forms. This treatment is known as a *hardening heat treatment.*

Metals other than gold, such as platinum and palladium, can react with copper to form a superlattice. Silver also can react with copper to produce a hardening effect. The composition of dental gold alloys often is adjusted by the manufacturer to produce an alloy that will be receptive to solid state reactions.

The practical importance of heat treatment is included in Chapter 16, which discusses the gold casting alloys used in dentistry.

CONTROL OF PHYSICAL PROPERTIES

In summary, three ways to control the physical properties of a metal have been described in the last two chapters. They are as follows:

- Alloying with other metals
- Strain hardening
- Heat treatment

The last two methods are under the control of the dentist or auxiliary. Examples of all three are included in the study of specific applications of metallic systems in dentistry.

Reviewing the Chapter

1. Define *alloy.* Can any two metals combine to form an alloy?
2. Define *binary alloy, solid solution,* and *eutectic.* Give a dental example of a substitutional solid solution and a eutectic alloy.
3. Draw a cooling curve for a solid solution. Indicate the upper and lower limits of the melting range.
4. Does a pure metal have a melting point or a melting range? What about a solid solution alloy?
5. List the classes of alloys according to their lattice forms.
6. Why are solid solution alloys used more often than pure metals?
7. List the properties that are characteristic of a eutectic alloy. Explain how and why eutectic alloys are used in dentistry.
8. What heat treatment would be used to soften a casting gold alloy? To harden it? Explain why.
9. List three ways in which the physical properties of a dental gold alloy can be controlled. Which can the dentist utilize?

CHAPTER 13

DENTAL METALLURGY: *Corrosion*

A primary requirement of any metallic restoration is that it should not corrode when placed in the mouth. *Corrosion* may be defined as a chemical or electrochemical attack of the environment on a pure metal or an alloy. If the corrosion is slow and uniformly distributed over the surface, it may not be objectionable. Corrosion can, however, lead to an unsightly restoration. Whether extensive or localized, degradation of the physical properties of the metal may occur to such an extent that the restoration or appliance fails. Unsightly restorations and failures caused by corrosion frequently are observed in dental practice.

As noted in Chapter 2, the conditions present in the oral cavity are conducive to corrosion. One can hardly envision a situation that is more demanding on metallic restorative materials. Dental manufacturers must make alloys that ensure maximum resistance to this corrosive environment. The dentist and dental auxiliary also must handle these

materials in a manner that does not reduce their resistance to corrosion.

Tarnish is a special term used for a uniform corrosive attack that produces a film or a layer on the surface of the metal. This tarnish film is not necessarily detrimental to the metal and may in fact retard the overall corrosion process. The layer often is augmented by deposited materials, however, and may become thick enough to be seen. The mouth is particularly vulnerable to hard and soft deposits on the surface of restorations. *Calculus* is the main hard deposit. The soft deposits are *plaques* and films composed mainly of bacteria and mucin. These hard and soft deposits may be found anywhere in the mouth, but they usually are located on surfaces that are protected from the abrasive action of foods and from toothbrushing.

As noted, *corrosion* is a chemical reaction of a metal with nonmetallic elements. The chemical compounds formed, known as *corrosion products*, may either retard or accelerate subsequent corrosion of the surface of effects of the corrosion process. In such cases, the metal disintegrates, owing to the action of air, moisture, acid or alkaline solutions, and certain chemicals.

On the other hand, some metals form *oxide skins* that are very protective. Aluminum, a reactive metal, is quite resistant to corrosion in the air. When exposed to air, a clean aluminum surface rapidly forms a tough, protective oxide film. Nonuniform surface films, however, often are the beginning of serious corrosion. In time, a film that is deposited may form or accumulate elements or compounds that can chemically attack the underlying surface of the metal. Chlorine and oxygen, which always are present in saliva, for example, can aid in the corrosion of silver, copper, tin, and similar elements used in dental amalgam and casting alloys. Other elements, such as sulfur, are present in the mouth only on occasion but are particularly reactive with metals such as silver.

Of all the elements, oxygen probably is the most important in the corrosion of dental metallic restorations. Although sulfur may be responsible for tarnish films on the surface of amalgam restorations, the deep pitting corrosion is associated with the formation of tin oxide and tin oxychloride corrosion products. With some of the newer amalgam alloys, the corrosion of copper forms oxides and chlorides. This corrosion and its significance are discussed in greater detail later. An example of a severely corroded amalgam restoration is seen in Figure 13–1.

Patients differ in the susceptibility of restorations to corrosion, even when the same materials are used and good oral hygiene is being practiced. These differences may be due to such factors as pH of the saliva, composition of foodstuffs, and nature of the plaque.

TYPES OF CORROSION

Most corrosion is *electrochemical* in nature. As the name implies, this is a combina-

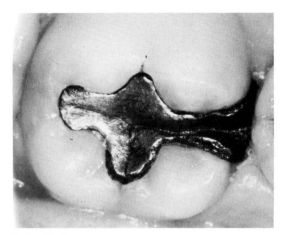

Figure 13–1. Corrosion on an amalgam restoration. The process probably contributed to the severe deterioration at the margins. (Courtesy of J. Osborne.)

tion of a chemical reaction and the flow of an electric current. The common situation occurs when a metal oxidizes.

Electrons are liberated from the metal to form positive metal ions. The liberated electrons must be carried to another place—usually a metal surface in contact with a liquid *electrolyte*—where a second chemical reaction that consumes the electrons can occur. This second reaction is called *reduction*. For electrochemical corrosion to occur, the following four things are required:

- A corroding metal surface
- An electrical conductor to carry electrons
- A second surface for the reduction reaction
- The electrolyte, usually a water solution

The wet-cell battery is an example of this. Two dissimilar metals are connected by a wire and immersed in an electrolyte. The most active of the two metals goes into solution, and a disintegration of the surface occurs. Depending on one's view, this is either an example of harmful corrosion or a useful battery.

In the oral cavity, several types of metallic materials often are present at the same time.

One situation in which *galvanic currents* are produced is when opposing dissimilar metals come into contact, as shown in Figure 2–4. There are other situations, such as those involving a bridge or an orthodontic appliance. The individual components of such devices are joined by a solder (discussed in Chapter 24). Because the alloy used as a solder differs in composition from that of the castings or wires, corrosion may occur at the interface between the dissimilar metals.

The clinical significance of galvanic currents, other than their influence on corrosion, is discussed later.

Another type of dissimilar metal corrosion is due to variation in *composition* of the metals on the surface of a single restoration.

A good example of this is the eutectic alloy. As pointed out in Chapter 12, the corrosion resistance of a eutectic alloy is poorer than that of a solid solution. The reason should now be obvious. When the eutectic alloy is immersed in an electrolyte, current is created between the individual grains, which are different in chemical reactivity. The most active metal then corrodes.

All types of alloys—even solid solution alloys—have differences in the concentration of the metals in various areas. Although the surface of an amalgam may appear to be uniform, differences in composition exist throughout the filling. These nonuniform areas can produce small batteries (corrosion cells), resulting in active corrosion.

Uneven composition within the alloy can occur if any impurity is present. The area in which the impurity collects forms a small battery with the uncontaminated area. For this reason, extreme care must be taken to prevent contamination of dental alloys. Gold alloys should never be placed in a drawer with other types of alloys or with amalgam scrap, which contains mercury. The gold may become contaminated by contact with these metals. The contaminated gold alloy restoration may then corrode in the mouth.

Another condition that produces electrolytic corrosion is any *nonuniform surface structure*. This type is associated primarily with internal strain hardening in the alloy or metal. Even in a pure metal, stress is created when the metal freezes. Any work done during fabrication of a dental structure, such as bending or finishing, produces strain hardening in parts of the restoration or appliance. A small battery then forms between the stressed metal, the saliva, and the unstressed metal. The stressed area is more readily attacked and corrodes or tarnishes.

On most dental appliances, the harmful effects of stress and corrosion are most apt to be accelerated because of metal *fatigue*. Repeated removal and insertion of a partial denture with metal clasps may build up in certain alloys a severe stress caused by strain hardening. Combined with a particular mouth condition that would promote corrosion, the stressed appliance develops corrosion fatigue. Any slight surface irregularity, such as a notch or pit, can accelerate the process, resulting in early failure. For this reason, extreme care must be exercised in finishing and polishing appliances to prevent surface defects.

The last type of electrolytic corrosion is called *concentration cell corrosion*. This situation exists whenever metals are exposed to two solutions, or electrolytes, at the same time. For example, food debris often accumulates between the teeth, particularly if the oral hygiene is poor. This debris then produces one type of electrolyte in that area. Normal saliva at the other surfaces of the same restoration represents another electrolyte. The two electrolytes form another type of small battery with the metal restoration. The current produced by that battery can then cause corrosion.

Sometimes corrosion seems to be concentrated at the margin of an amalgam restoration, even discoloring the adjoining tooth structure. Such a condition may be caused by a difference in the concentration or nature of the electrolytes. If food debris and acid accumulate in the open margin of the restoration, the electrolyte in that crevice is different from that of the saliva that surrounds the outer surface of the restoration. In particular, the oxygen concentration differs and is low at the bottom of the opening where the area is covered by debris and high in saliva. A corrosion cell is produced, with the greatest activity occurring around the areas with the least oxygen. The schematic drawing in Figure 13–2 shows the phenomenon. The significance of this phenomenon in the marginal deterioration of amalgam restorations is discussed in Chapter 14.

Possibly the most common cause for concentration cell corrosion is a small pit or scratch on the surface of the metal. The pit on the surface of an amalgam restoration traps debris. Because the pH and oxygen concentration of the debris at the bottom of the pit is different from that of the saliva, a concentration cell is created, as shown in Figure 13–2. The resulting corrosion produces further disintegration of the amalgam, enlarging the pit and propagating the process. If such an area is placed under masticatory stress, combined fatigue and concentration cell corrosion accelerate the destruction of the underlying metal.

The importance of proper polishing of metallic restorations now becomes apparent. The polished surface has fewer defects that lead to this type of corrosion. *The metallic restoration is not finished until properly polished.*

Certain metals develop a coating that protects them from corrosion. Aluminum is one of the best examples, as noted earlier. Chromium and titanium also are important in dentistry. The superior resistance of these metals to corrosion is due to the protective film of oxide that forms on the surface. Such a metal is said to be *passive*, and the process that protects it is called *passivation*.

THE DENTAL RESTORATION

Corrosion resistance is an important consideration in evaluating an alloy for intraoral use. There are basically only two ways to protect a dental alloy from corrosion. The first is to ensure that its composition contains sufficient noble metal content. Noble metals,

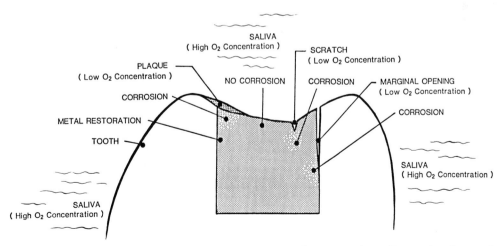

Figure 13–2. Schematic drawing depicting the various types of concentration cell corrosion that can be associated with a metallic dental restoration. (Courtesy of R. A. De Castro.)

such as gold and platinum, are unreactive chemically and do not tend to oxidize. Such alloys are referred to as *noble metal alloys.* (These are discussed in greater detail in Chapter 16.) The other way is to use sufficient amounts of passive elements, such as aluminum and chromium, to protect the alloy by passivation. Alloys that depend on passivation are referred to as *base metal alloys.*

The reader might wonder at the omission from this list of the most common corrosion prevention technique practiced outside the mouth: the use of a resin-type protective coating or paint. The oral environment is extremely aggressive to such a coating, and the problems discussed in Chapter 3 related to adhesion to tooth structure also act against its success. The use of protective coatings can provide temporary reduction in corrosion but does not serve as an effective long-term measure. Protective coatings that are damaged or scratched may accelerate localized corrosion and result in severe damage.

In addition to proper composition in the alloy, the surface condition of the restoration must be considered. The surface should be smooth and lustrous. This type of surface is not only aesthetically desirable but, as illustrated earlier, can minimize subsequent corrosion. A smooth, polished surface can be cleaned more easily during toothbrushing and flossing and does not readily pick up debris. No step is more important in preventing discoloration of metallic restorations than the elimination of surface irregularities at the time the restoration is placed or in the restoration of that smooth surface during prophylaxis.

In summary, the oral environment and dental structures present complex conditions that can promote corrosion and discoloration. Differences in discoloration often are noted between individual patients with the same dental alloy, handled in exactly the same manner.

CLINICAL SIGNIFICANCE OF GALVANIC CURRENTS

From the previous discussion of types of corrosion processes, it should be apparent that small galvanic currents generated by these various batteries are continually present in the mouth.

Although postoperative sensitivity and pain caused by galvanic shock are not common occurrences, they can be a source of real discomfort to a patient. Such postoperative pain usually occurs immediately after insertion of a new restoration and disappears in a few days after the pulp heals. Not much can be done to prevent this except to coat the outside of the restoration with a varnish or resin (Chapter 21), thus isolating the restoration from saliva. As long as the varnish remains intact, the restoration is insulated from the saliva and the current is reduced. By the time the varnish wears away, the irritation to the pulp caused by caries and placement of the restoration often has subsided and the patient no longer feels galvanic sensitivity.

If any evidence of corrosion exists on the surface of the amalgam restoration, it should be polished. The production of a more uniform surface may reduce the magnitude of the current and thus the sensitivity.

Galvanic currents often have been cited as a possible cause for various diseases, such as oral cancer, ulcers, and kidney dysfunction. The matter remains somewhat controversial, but little evidence supports the theory.

Whenever possible, avoid situations that exaggerate the condition. The placement of an amalgam restoration adjacent to a gold inlay seems to be contraindicated. Discoloration is likely to occur on both restorations. Likewise, whether harmful or not, the corrosion may produce a continuing unpleasant metallic taste. The resulting corrosion also can limit the service life of both restorations.

Selected Reading

Burse, A. B., Swartz, M. L., Phillips, R. W., and Dykema, R. W.: Comparison of the in vitro and in vivo tarnish of three gold alloys. J. Biomed. Mater. Res. 6:267, 1972.

Lain, E. S., Schriever, W., and Gaughnon, G. S.: Problems of electrogalvanism in the oral cavity caused by dissimilar dental materials. J. Am. Dent. Assoc. 27:1765, 1940.

Marshall, G. S., Jr., Jackson, B. L., and Marshall, S. J.: Copper-rich and conventional amalgam restorations after clinical use. J. Am. Dent. Assoc. 100:43, 1980.

Mills, R. B.: Study of incidence of irritation in mouths having teeth filled with dissimilar metals. Northwest. Univ. Bull. 39:18, 1939.

Mueller, H. J.: Tarnish and corrosion of dental alloys. In *Metals Handbook,* 9th ed., vol. 13. Materials Park, OH, ASM International, 1987, pp 1336–1366.

Nachlin, J. J.: A type of pain associated with the restoration of teeth with amalgam. J. Am. Dent. Assoc. 48:284, 1954.

Phillips, R. W., Schnell, R. J., and Shafer, W. G.: Failure of galvanic current to produce leukoplakia in rats. J. Dent. Res. 47:666, 1968.

Sandrick, J. L., Bapna, M. S., and Rysiejko, M. R.: Demonstration of corrosion of dental alloys. J. Dent. Educ. 38:106, 1974.

Schriever, W., and Diamond, L. E.: Electromotive forces and electric currents caused by metallic dental fillings. J. Dent. Res. 31:205, 1952.

Tuccillo, J. T., and Nielsen, J. P.: Observations of onset of sulfide tarnish on gold-base alloys. J. Prosthet. Dent. 25:629, 1971.

Reviewing the Chapter

1. Define *corrosion* and *tarnish.* Is tarnish necessarily detrimental? Why? Name the elements present in the oral environment that may cause corrosion.
2. Name two metals used in the mouth that passivate.
3. What protects a gold alloy restoration from corrosion?
4. Would dental amalgam be a good choice as a restorative material adjacent to a gold foil? Why?
5. What components are needed for electrochemical corrosion?
6. Name three types of electrochemical corrosion.
7. Is the use of protective films an effective corrosion prevention device in dentistry? Why?
8. Describe the potential effects of dissimilar metal corrosion currents. What can be done to minimize the postoperative sensitivity?

CHAPTER 14

Ag
Cu

DENTAL AMALGAM: Microstructure and Properties

Ag Silver
Cu Copper
Sn tin
Hg mercury

THE AMALGAM RESTORATION	**SETTING REACTIONS**
COMPOSITION	Low-Copper Alloys
High-Copper Amalgam	High-Copper Alloys
Admixed Alloys	**PHYSICAL PROPERTIES OF AMALGAM**
Single Composition	Dimensional Change
MANUFACTURE	Strength
Lathe-Cut (Filing) Alloys	Creep
Spherical Alloys	

Amalgam is one of the oldest of all recorded materials used for restoring the carious lesion. Its first reported use was in A.D. 659 in China. It remains the most commonly used restorative dental material. Millions of amalgam restorations are placed each year. These represent the majority of all single-tooth restorations. Other metallic or resin systems are unlikely to provide a significant replacement for this material in the immediate future.

Dental amalgam is one of the more controversial dental materials. Public awareness about the toxicity of mercury—along with questions raised within the dental profession—periodically bring the "amalgam con-

troversy" to the forefront. All available evidence suggests that dental amalgam is both a safe and an effective restorative material for the vast majority of the dental population. Dental auxiliaries should expect questions from patients about this material and should be prepared to answer them intelligently. Auxiliary personnel also must be knowledgeable concerning the occupational safety of the use of mercury in dentistry.

The dentist usually has assistance in preparing amalgam before its insertion in the tooth. This part of the technique is just as important as the steps done by the dentist in preparing the cavity and placing the amalgam. If the restoration fails, the preliminary work may have been the cause. In some states, the dental auxiliary may be directly involved in placing amalgam into the prepared cavity and in some of the finishing procedures.

As noted in Chapter 12, any alloy that contains mercury is called an *amalgam*. In dentistry, the mercury is combined—or *amalgamated*—with an alloy of silver, tin, and copper. This alloy, known as the *amalgam alloy*, is formulated by the manufacturer and shaped into small particles. The amalgam itself is manufactured in the dental office just as the manufacturer makes a casting gold alloy, impression material, or other dental material. The mechanical mixing of these particles with mercury is known as *trituration*. The composition of the amalgam—and consequently its physical properties—are determined at this time.

Using specially designed instruments, the dentist forces the plastic amalgam mass into the cavity preparation by *condensation*. The mercury and alloy particles react to form new chemical compounds that bring about the *setting*—or hardening—of the amalgam.

THE AMALGAM RESTORATION

It has been said that "an amalgam restoration is often much better than it looks." Many amalgam restorations eventually display obvious deficiencies yet continue to provide a useful service to the patient. Probably the most common defect inherent in amalgam restorations is the slow but continuous tendency to deteriorate at the margins, the so-called ditching of the material at the interface with the tooth. The crevices seen in the clinical restorations in Figure 14–1 illustrate marginal breakdown. Factors that contribute to this breakdown are discussed later.

One would suspect that caries would invariably be present at such an exposed margin because of the penetration of fluids, de-

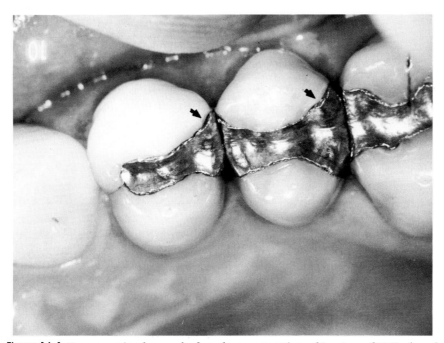

Figure 14–1. Open margins (*arrows*) of amalgam restorations. (Courtesy of M. Cochran.)

bris, and microorganisms. This usually is not the case. Surveys have shown that the percentage of failures among amalgam restorations is smaller than with any other restorative material.

The explanation lies in a uniqueness of amalgam. As the restoration ages in the oral cavity, corrosion products form along the tooth-restoration interface (see Chapter 2). These compounds then act as a mechanical barrier against penetration of deleterious agents. Although the margin may visually appear suspect, a self-sealing mechanism has occurred immediately below the surface. This reduction in microleakage as an amalgam ages may be the significant characteristic that accounts for amalgam's excellent clinical performance through the years.

Daily observations in the dental office do reveal amalgam failures, which may occur in the following forms:

- Secondary or recurrent caries around the restoration
- Bulk fracture
- Marginal breakdown
- Excessive dimensional change
- Excessive tarnish and corrosion

Since the adoption of American Dental Association (ADA) Specification no. 1 for amalgam alloy many years ago, the number of inferior commercial alloys has steadily decreased. Consequently, failures are more frequently due to improper design of the cavity preparation and faulty manipulation of the material. One survey has suggested that 40 per cent of all failures may be attributed to improper manipulation of the alloy.

Amalgam is susceptible to manipulative variables. Every step, from the time the alloy is selected until the restoration is polished, has a definite effect on the physical properties and potentially on the success or failure of the restoration.

The factors that govern the quality of the amalgam restoration can be divided into two groups: those controlled by the manufacturer and those controlled by the dental team.

- The manufacturer controls such factors as composition, the form in which the alloy is supplied, particle size and shape of the alloy, and the rate of its reaction with the mercury.
- The dentist and/or auxiliary govern such matters as final mercury content, trituration method and time, condensation technique, anatomical characteristics, and finishing procedure. The dental team also has the responsibility of selecting the particular brand of amalgam alloy to be used. An alloy certified by the ADA should be used. In addition, the choice should be based on the preference for particular handling characteristics, such as setting time and certain factors related to composition and properties.

The clinical success of amalgam depends on meticulous attention to detail at each stage of its formulation, preparation, and insertion.

COMPOSITION

Although amalgam has provided an excellent service as a restorative material for many years, efforts to improve its clinical performance have not ceased. This research has led to dramatic changes in the composition of amalgam alloys over the past 20 years.

The current ADA Specification no. 1 requires that amalgam alloy be composed predominantly of silver and tin. Other elements, such as copper, zinc, palladium, and mercury, may be present in lesser amounts. Copper has become an important constituent of modern amalgam alloys.

Silver and mercury react to form compounds that determine the dimensional change of the amalgam during hardening. Silver increases both setting expansion and strength. Amalgam alloys traditionally have contained 67 to 70 per cent silver, but many of today's alloys contain silver in considerably smaller amounts.

The tin content, in the range of 25 to 27 per cent, influences properties in a manner opposite to that of silver. Because tin has a high solubility in mercury, it facilitates amalgamation, decreasing setting expansion. The tin-mercury compound that forms when amalgam alloy reacts with mercury is weaker and more susceptible to corrosion than the silver-mercury reaction product.

Copper acts in much the same manner as silver: it increases strength, hardness, and setting expansion. The ADA Specification formerly limited the copper content of amalgam alloy to a maximum of 6 per cent. Research to improve the properties of amalgam revealed that amalgams prepared from alloys that contain more than 6 per cent copper generally are superior and perform better clinically. The composition restrictions with respect to copper and other elements in the alloy have been deleted from the amalgam specification.

Amalgam alloys that contain copper in amounts of 6 per cent or less are designated as *low-copper* or *traditional alloys*. Those that contain copper in greater amounts are referred to as *high-copper* amalgam alloys.

Zinc may or may not be present in an amalgam alloy. Alloys that contain zinc in excess of 0.01 per cent must be designated as *zinc-containing*, whereas those that contain less than 0.01 per cent Zn are designated as *nonzinc*. Even zinc-containing alloys seldom contain more than 1 per cent zinc.

Zinc is included as an aid in minimizing the oxidation of the other metals present in the alloy. When the metals are melted together during the manufacture of the alloy, the danger of oxidation always exists. Zinc readily reacts with any oxygen to prevent it from combining with silver, tin, or copper. Oxides of these metals would weaken the amalgam and interfere with amalgamation.

Moisture contamination of a zinc-containing alloy can result in a serious clinical problem, as discussed in Chapter 15.

Preamalgamated alloys are available. Particles of the alloy may contain as much as 3 per cent mercury. The mercury, added by the manufacturer, provides more rapid amalgamation but has little other effect on the working qualities of the alloy.

High-Copper Amalgam

As stated earlier, the most common clinical problem with the amalgam restoration is *marginal breakdown*. High-copper amalgam restorations have a much lower incidence of marginal failure than restorations made from low-copper amalgams. Thus, the high-copper alloys are almost universally used today. Because the increase in copper content in many of these alloys causes a reduction in the overall silver content, they also are referred to as *low-silver* alloys.

The copper content of commercial high-copper alloys varies considerably from one brand to another. A few alloys contain less than 10 per cent copper, whereas the copper content in others is as high as 30 per cent. In most cases, at least 11 per cent copper is required to gain the improved properties and clinical performance associated with high-copper amalgam.

There are two basic types of high-copper alloys: *admixed* and *single-composition*.

Admixed Alloys

The oldest type or form of the high-copper alloy is the *admixed* alloy. In the admixed alloy system, the alloy powder purchased from the manufacturer is a mixture of powders of two alloys. One is the traditional low-copper alloy, containing silver, tin, and less than 6 per cent copper. Adding a second powder—often a silver-copper eutectic prepared from a copper-rich alloy—

increases the overall copper content. The derivation of the term *admixed alloy* is obvious. Alloys of this type also are referred to as *dispersion* alloys, but this terminology is incorrect from a scientific standpoint.

The total copper content of commercial admixed alloys ranges from about 9 to 20 per cent. The alloy particles can be either spheres or filings. A common—but not universal—approach with these alloys is for the particles of one alloy to be filings and the particles of the second, spheres. The result is a mixture of filings and spheres.

Single Composition

The other approach to increasing the total copper content of amalgam alloys is to increase the amount of copper in the silver–tin–copper alloy particles. Because such an amalgam alloy contains powder particles of only one composition, this type is referred to as a *single-composition* high-copper alloy. Again, the copper content varies considerably from one manufacturer to another, ranging from about 13 per cent to as high as 30 per cent. Some of the single-composition alloys marketed today also contain small amounts of indium or palladium.

MANUFACTURE

More than 100 ADA-certified amalgam alloys are available, and new products appear constantly. The various brands differ in terms of ease of amalgamation, rate of hardening, character of the carved surface, and other factors that influence selection of a particular alloy. Such variations are produced by altering the composition and steps in the manufacturing process to achieve optimum properties and handling characteristics. A summary of the process follows.

Lathe-Cut (Filing) Alloys

Selected amounts of the various metals are carefully melted and cast into a solid rod or ingot that is heat-treated to produce a uniform composition. It then is cut into the small particles used by the dentist. Because the ingot of alloy is rather brittle, small shavings or *filings* can be produced by cutting on a lathe.

These particles are sifted through screens to grade the final size. The final powder usually is a blend of various-sized particles. The filings also are subjected to a heat-treatment procedure that regulates properties to some extent. Figure 14–2 shows an example of typical filing particles; Figure 14–3 shows the packaged powder. Because a lathe usually is used to prepare the filings, this type is called a *lathe-cut* alloy.

The alloy may be dispensed in the form of preweighed tablets or pellets (Fig. 14–3). The fine alloy particles are compressed

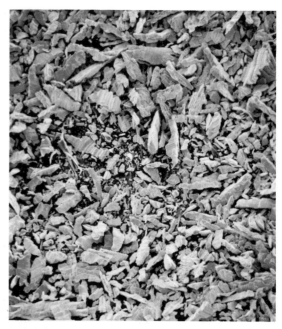

Figure 14–2. Particles of a conventional lathe-cut (filing) type of amalgam alloy.

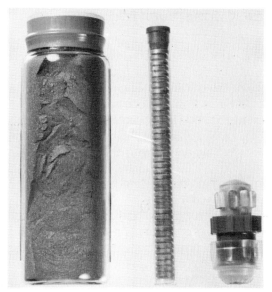

Figure 14-3. Various forms in which dental amalgam alloy may be supplied. *Left,* **powder;** *center,* **pellets;** *right,* **disposable preweighed capsule.**

lightly so that they adhere in tablet shape but still rapidly pulverize during amalgamation. The process is much like making an aspirin tablet. Either the powder or pellet form of the alloy is acceptable, although pellets are more commonly used because of their convenience.

Most brands of alloy have a small particle size, often characterized as *fine-cut* or even *microcut.* Such terms are misleading because one is really interested in the particle size distribution and the total surface area exposed to the mercury.

Regardless of terminology, if all other factors are equal, the smaller particles have better handling characteristics and provide a smoother carved and polished surface. This smoother surface is less readily tarnished or corroded. Any part of the amalgam procedure that reduces surface roughness minimizes eventual discoloration. Thorough trituration and proper polishing also produce a superior surface and maximum resistance to corrosion.

Spherical Alloys

Alloy particles also may be made in the form of small spheres. One method of preparing such an alloy is called an *atomizing procedure.* A fine mist of the molten alloy is sprayed into a cold, inert gas atmosphere. On solidification, tiny spherical or ovoid-shaped particles are formed, as shown in Figure 14–4. Referred to as *spherical alloys,* these alloys are available in powder and pellet form.

Spherical alloys amalgamate very readily. Amalgamation can be accomplished with a smaller amount of mercury than that required for filing-type alloys. The condensation pressure and technique used by the dentist in placing the restoration also are somewhat less critical—an advantage in difficult clinical situations where optimal access is limited and condensation difficult.

Spherical amalgam alloys have a different feel during condensation than conventional alloys. The dentist and auxiliary should fa-

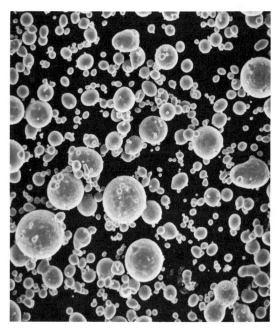

Figure 14-4. Particles of a spherical amalgam alloy.

miliarize themselves with the alloy before clinical restorations are placed. In this manner, the necessary experience may be gained with the different condensation and carving characteristics.

As noted earlier, some commercial alloys are blends of filing and spherical particles (Fig. 14–5). Their handling characteristics depend on the relative amounts of each type of particle in the blend.

SETTING REACTIONS

The reactions that take place during the hardening of amalgam are complex. The principal reactions for low- and high-copper alloys are summarized to illustrate the roles the various resulting reaction products—called *phases*—play in determining the properties of the amalgam and its behavior in the oral cavity.

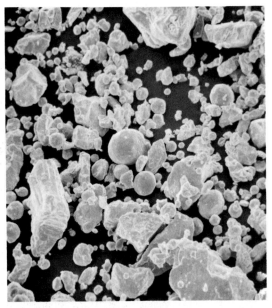

Figure 14–5. Typical admix (dispersion type) showing the lathe-cut particles and spheres.

Low-Copper Alloys

Although high-copper amalgam alloys have virtually replaced low-copper amalgams, a brief discussion of the setting reaction of the traditional alloys and the products of that reaction is necessary to explain the chemistry and behavior of the newer alloys.

The main component in the original alloy particle that reacts with the mercury during trituration is a combination of silver and tin (Ag_3Sn). This compound is referred to as the *gamma phase*.

During trituration, silver and tin on the surface of the gamma particles start to dissolve in mercury. The mercury then diffuses into the alloy particles, forming a plastic and workable mass. Because the dissolution of particles and the diffusion of mercury into the alloy particles reduce the total volume, an initial contraction occurs during the first hour. This contraction is shown in the graph in Figure 14–6, which depicts the contraction and expansion that occur during the first 24 hours in a low-copper alloy.

As the mercury becomes saturated with silver and tin, new compounds begin to precipitate. The silver-mercury compound that forms is Ag_2Hg_3, and the tin-mercury compound is Sn_8Hg. The silver-mercury compound is referred to as *gamma-1* and the tin-mercury compound, as *gamma-2*. Because the solubility of silver in mercury is lower than that of tin, gamma-1 starts to precipitate sooner than gamma-2. As the reaction continues, more and more crystals—particularly gamma-1—interlace and meet. They exert pressure against one another, resulting in an expansion similar to that described for plaster in Chapter 5. This phenomenon of crystal growth is responsible for the expansion of the alloy after about 1 hour, as shown in the dimensional change curve (see Fig. 14–6).

After 6 or 7 hours, this crystallization is completed. A second, very slight contraction occurs as any free mercury that remains is

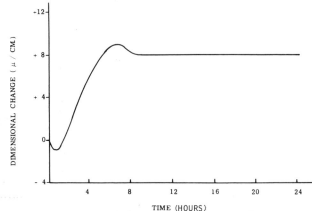

Figure 14-6. Dimensional change of an amalgam during the first 24-hour period after condensation.

taken up by the original particles of the alloy still present. Many factors can affect the dimensional change pattern of alloys during setting. These include alloy composition, setting time, and manipulative variables, such as the mercury-alloy ratio and trituration time.

The reaction that occurs between the low-copper alloy particles and the mercury is summarized in equation 14–1.

The hardened amalgam is a multiphase structure composed of unreacted particles of the original alloy surrounded and held together by a matrix of silver-mercury and tin-mercury compounds—the gamma-1 and gamma-2 phases, respectively.

The contribution each of the three phases makes to the properties of the amalgam and the clinical performance of the restoration is important. The strongest component is the original silver-tin phase (gamma). The weakest is the tin-mercury (gamma-2) phase. Gamma-2 also is more susceptible to corrosion than either the gamma or gamma-1 phase. Thus, the strength and corrosion resistance of the restoration depend on the rel-

ative percentages of each component. More specifically, the weak link is the tin–mercury phase.

High-Copper Alloys

Knowing the contribution of the various components of dental amalgam to clinical performance, one could assume that dental materials research set out to develop an amalgam that contained little, if any, of the gamma-2 phase. In fact, alloys that contain more than 6 per cent copper were originally developed for other reasons and only subsequently shown to have both improved clinical performance and an absence of the gamma-2 phase. This knowledge then led to changes in alloy formulations to eliminate or greatly reduce any gamma-2 phase formed. Empirically, high-copper alloys provide a mechanism to do this, accounting for their overwhelming popularity.

When a high-copper amalgam alloy is triturated with mercury, silver and tin dissolve in the mercury, and mercury diffuses into the particle, just as described for low-copper al-

Silver-tin alloy	+	mercury	→	silver-mercury	+	tin-mercury	+	silver-tin alloy	
Ag_3Sn	+	Hg	→	Ag_2Hg_3	+	Sn_xHg	+	Ag_3Sn	14–1
Gamma	+	mercury	→	gamma-1	+	gamma-2	+	gamma	

loys. The silver-mercury compound (gamma-1) is formed, and its crystals precipitate.

In these high-copper alloys copper becomes available to the reaction. Because tin has a greater affinity for the copper than for mercury, a copper-tin compound is formed instead of the tin-mercury compound. This copper-tin compound (Cu_6Sn_5) is referred to as the *eta phase*. Because the copper ties up the tin, little, if any, gamma-2 phase is formed. The exact amount of copper necessary to effectively suppress gamma-2 formation has not been defined but is believed to be around 12 per cent. *A good definition of a high-copper amalgam alloy is one that contains "enough" copper to suppress the formation of the gamma-2 phase.*

Although the exact setting reaction differs somewhat for admixed and single-composition alloys, equation 14–2 is representative of the basic reaction in both alloys.

Elimination of the gamma-2 phase results in improved corrosion resistance and strength.

Eutectic phase

PHYSICAL PROPERTIES OF AMALGAM

Clinical behavior of the restoration is based on the physical properties of the amalgam, which are the direct responsibility of both the dentist and the dental auxiliary. A proper understanding of these properties and their control is necessary to appreciate the importance of the manipulative factors discussed.

Dimensional Change

Because the hardening of amalgam is a solidification process, dimensional changes are to be expected. As noted, however, amalgam can exhibit either expansion or contraction, depending on whether the contraction resulting from dissolution of the original particles is greater or less than the expansion produced by crystal growth of the new phases. This depends on manipulation, composition, and the setting rate of the alloy.

Factors that favor the formation of gamma-1, such as higher mercury-alloy ratios, result in more expansion, because of greater crystal growth. On the other hand, anything that increases the solution of mercury into the alloy particles (such as increased trituration) increases the initial contraction that occurs, and thus reduces the net expansion. The final dimensional change in the amalgam thus is governed by various factors.

After the restoration has been placed into the prepared tooth cavity, dimensional change should be minimal. Excessive expansion can exert pressure on the pulp and result in postoperative sensitivity, protrusion of the restoration from the cavity, or even fracture of the surrounding tooth structure. Excessive contraction can cause the restoration to pull away from the cavity walls and permit gross leakage between the tooth and the restoration.

The ADA Specification no. 1 for amalgam alloy specifies that at the end of 24 hours, the dimensional change should be less than plus or minus 20 μm/cm (0.2 per cent). Considering that 1 μm is only 0.00004 inch, the allowed changes during the setting of amalgam are very small, and *minor* deviations from zero dimensional change apparently are not clinically significant. Because manipulation does influence the magnitude of the

Silver-tin	+	copper	+	mercury	$\rightarrow$	silver-mercury	+	copper-tin	+	silver-tin	
Ag_3Sn	+	Cu	+	Hg	$\rightarrow$	Ag_2Hg_3	+	Cu_6Sn_5	+	Ag_3Sn	14–2
Gamma	+	copper	+	mercury	$\rightarrow$	gamma-1	+	eta	+	gamma	

dimensional change that occurs, every precaution must be taken to prevent excessive expansion or contraction.

Strength

Sufficient strength to resist fracture is a primary requirement for any restorative material. Fracture—even of a small area—or chipping of exposed margins can lead to recurrent caries and clinical failure. Figure 14–7 shows an example of a gross fracture of an amalgam restoration. Amalgam must be handled in a manner that ensures maximum strength.

The strength of amalgam usually is measured under a compressive load. Table 14–1 lists some typical values for both high-copper and traditional amalgams. The 7-day compressive strengths of modern high-copper amalgams range from 431 MPa (62,600 psi) to more than 510 MPa (74,000 psi). As can be seen in the table, low-copper amalgams have lower compressive strengths than high-copper amalgams.

Although the principal stress involved during mastication may be compressive, other types of stress also are involved. Whenever those forces induce a tensile or bending stress, fracture is more likely to occur. As can be seen in Table 14–1, the tensile strength of amalgam is about one-eighth the compressive strength. An alloy that has a compressive strength of 431 MPa (62,600 psi) may have a tensile strength of only 48 MPa (7000 psi).

Compressive strength provides a convenient yardstick to assess the general strength characteristics of the material and is much easier to measure on a relatively brittle material like amalgam.

The compressive strength at 1 hour is used in the ADA Specification for dental amalgam as a measure of hardening rate. Typical values for early compressive strength are shown in Table 14–1.

The rate of hardening is of clinical interest. A patient may leave the operatory within 20 minutes after placement of an amalgam, when its strength is only 6 per cent of the value after 7 days. A vital question is whether the newly placed restoration is strong enough to support biting forces.

Amalgam does not gain its strength as rap-

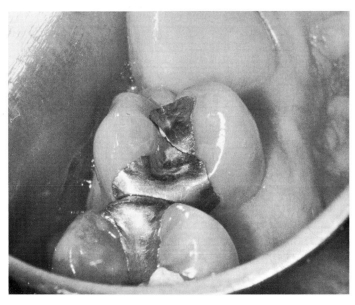

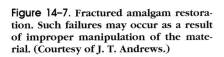
Figure 14–7. Fractured amalgam restoration. Such failures may occur as a result of improper manipulation of the material. (Courtesy of J. T. Andrews.)

TABLE 14–1. Physical Properties of Low- and High-Copper Dental Amalgams

Amalgam	Compressive Strength MPa (psi)		Tensile Strength MPA (psi)	Creep (%)
	1 Hour	7 Days	1 Hour	
Low-copper	145 (21,100)	343 (49,800)	60 (8700)	2.0
Admix, high-copper	137 (19,800)	431 (62,600)	48 (7000)	0.4
High-copper, single-composition	262 (38,000)	510 (73,900)	64 (9300)	0.13

idly as might be expected or desired. The strength during the first few hours is low. Many of the amalgam restorations that fracture probably do so in the first few hours, even though the break may not be apparent for several months. The patient should avoid biting on the restoration for the first 8 hours after leaving the dental office. (Certain high-copper alloys gain strength quite rapidly—this may be an advantage clinically.)

The manipulative variables that alter the compressive strength invariably seem to influence the tensile and shear strength of amalgam in the same manner. Undertrituration results in low strength, and within reasonable limits, longer trituration increases the strength.

The strength of amalgam is governed by two additional factors: the amount of residual mercury that remains after condensation (discussed in Chapter 15) and porosity. Internal voids always exist in the amalgam mass. As their number increases, strength decreases. For maximum strength, manipulation and placement must be designed to control the mercury content in the final restoration and to minimize porosity.

Creep

In Chapter 4, it is pointed out that a metal placed under a fixed stress may undergo continuing plastic deformation. This characteristic is called *creep*. Creep usually is a problem only for a metal used at tempera-

tures near its melting point. Because mercury is a liquid at room temperature, the phases in the set amalgam that contain mercury have relatively low melting points compared with mouth temperature. Hence, creep is a concern for dental amalgam.

Creep of amalgam is measured on a fully hardened specimen (7 days old) by placing it under a static compressive load for 3 hours. ADA Specification no. 1 permits a maximum creep of 3 per cent. The creep values for commercial amalgam alloys vary quite markedly, ranging from as high as 4 per cent to 0.10 per cent or less. As shown in Table 14–1, low-copper alloys have higher creep values than high-copper alloys. The creep of a high-copper alloy should be less than 1 per cent.

Manipulation also influences the creep of a given alloy. The high-copper alloys, as a group, seem to be less sensitive to some manipulative variables than low-copper alloys.

Creep appears to provide some indication of an amalgam's ability to withstand the rigors of the oral cavity. Amalgam restorations have been placed with alloys having different creep values, and their clinical behavior evaluated. Generally, the lower the creep of the amalgam, the better the marginal integrity of the restoration, as shown in Figure 14–8.

The tendency for reduced marginal fracture with reduced creep of the alloy applies only within certain limits. When creep is less

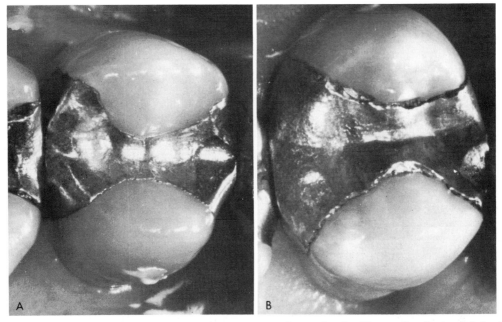

Figure 14–8. Four-year-old amalgam restorations. *A,* Amalgam placed with an alloy having minimal creep. *B,* Amalgam restoration of an alloy having a high creep value. (Courtesy of D. B. Mahler.)

than 1 per cent, little or no correlation appears between creep and marginal breakdown of high-copper amalgams. In other words, an amalgam with a creep value of 0.3 per cent may exhibit no more marginal breakdown than one with a creep value of 0.03 per cent.

Certain factors other than creep may be involved in the complex mechanism of marginal breakdown of the amalgam restoration. The differences in the restorations shown in Figure 14–8 might be related also to the corrosion resistance of the two alloys, differences in strength, or a combination of factors. At the moment, the creep test is a useful screening device for determining the clinical performance characteristics of amalgam alloys.

If satisfactory restorative dentistry is to be achieved, an appreciation of these properties is necessary. Failure to control them can result only in a clinical failure.

Selected Reading

Fairhurst, C. W.: Volume changes in the Ag-Sn-Hg reaction. IADR Program and Abstracts, No. M43, 1962.

Greener, E. H.: Amalgam—yesterday, today, and tomorrow. Oper. Dent. 4:24, 1979.

Innes, D. B. K., and Youdelis, W. V.: Dispersion strengthened amalgams. J. Can. Dent. Assoc. 29:487, 1963.

Mahler, D. B.: Behavior of three high-copper amalgams. J. Biomed. Mater. Res. 13:693, 1979.

Mahler, D. B., and Adey, J. D.: The influence of final mercury content on the characteristics of a high-copper amalgam. J. Biomed. Mater. Res. 13:467, 1979.

Mahler, D. B., Adey, J. D., and Marantz, R. L.: Creep versus microstructure of γ_2-containing amalgams. J. Dent. Res. 56:1493, 1977.

Mahler, D. B., Adey, J. D., and Van Eysden, J.: Quantitative microprobe analysis of amalgam. J. Dent. Res. 54:218, 1975.

Mahler, D. B., Terkla, L. G., Van Eysden, J., and Reisbick, M. H.: Marginal fracture versus mechanical properties of amalgam. J. Dent. Res. 49:1452, 1970.

Vrijhoef, M. M. A., Vermeersch, A. G., and Spanauf, A. J.: *Dental Amalgam.* Chicago, Quintessence Publishing Co., 1980.

Wing, G.: Dental amalgam. In von Fraunhofer, J. (Ed.): *Scientific Aspects of Dental Materials*. London, Butterworths, 1975.

Reviewing the Chapter

1. State the frequency of use of amalgam as a restorative material. When was it first used in dentistry?
2. Explain *amalgamation, trituration, condensation,* and *ditched* amalgam restoration.
3. Define *amalgam, gamma, gamma-1, gamma-2,* and *eta* phase.
4. What are the common types of failure seen clinically with amalgam restorations? List the probable causative factors involved in such failures.
5. Explain the statement "an amalgam restoration often is much better than it looks." How does that relate to the clinical performance of the material?
6. List the factors controlled by the manufacturer and those controlled by the dentist and auxiliary that influence the quality of the final restoration.
7. List the metals and their concentrations present in an amalgam alloy. Explain the effect of each.
8. What is the difference between *low-copper* and *high-copper* alloys in terms of composition, structure, properties, and clinical performance?
9. In what forms are the amalgam alloy particles supplied by the manufacturer? Do the physical properties and handling characteristics differ for amalgam made from these different types?
10. Describe the setting reaction that occurs between mercury and alloy particles of a low-copper alloy, making use of the chemical equation that depicts the reaction.
11. Illustrate by a graph the dimensional changes that occur during this hardening process.
12. What is the difference in the properties between the final phases that form? What effect does this have on clinical performance?
13. Explain how the setting reaction differs for a high-copper alloy. How does that affect behavior of the restoration in the oral cavity?
14. Explain the difference between an *admixed* and *single-composition* high-copper alloy.
15. List all the important physical properties of amalgam and the effect of manipulative variables on these properties.
16. Summarize the rationale behind the trend that has occurred in the formulation of high-copper alloys. What effect has this had on the improved clinical performance of amalgam restorations?

CHAPTER **15**

DENTAL AMALGAM: Manipulation

ALLOY SELECTION

PROPORTIONING THE ALLOY AND
MERCURY

THE FUNCTION OF MERCURY

TRITURATION
Mechanical Amalgamators
Consistency of Mix

CONDENSATION

EFFECT OF MOISTURE

FINISHING AND POLISHING

MARGINAL BREAKDOWN

SAFETY OF THE DENTAL AMALGAM

A good modern dental amalgam alloy can be manipulated so that the final restoration provides adequate clinical service. If the restoration is defective, the fault usually is with how it was prepared and not with the material. This chapter explains the manipulative procedures that assure optimum physical properties and the clinical success of the amalgam.

ALLOY SELECTION

Several factors enter into the selection of an alloy, and the weight given to each varies with the individual. First, the alloy must meet the requirements of the American Dental As-

sociation (ADA) Specification no. 1 or a similar specification.

Although some traditional low-copper alloys are still available, the high-copper alloys are preferred, as discussed in Chapter 14.

The manipulative characteristics, such as ease of amalgamation, rate of hardening, and smoothness of the finished surface, are extremely important and a matter of subjective preference. Coincident with this is the delivery system provided by the manufacturer and its convenience, expediency, and capability to reduce human variables. The physical properties discussed in Chapter 14 should be reviewed in light of claims made for superiority over competing products. Finally, documentation as to performance in well-controlled clinical studies should be requested and reviewed.

PROPORTIONING THE ALLOY AND MERCURY

The mercury used in dental amalgam must be chemically pure. Contaminants may influence the properties of the amalgam. Most mercury supplied by dental manufacturers is certified to meet ADA Specification no. 6 for mercury, which allows minimal amounts of impurities and no surface debris. Mercury should have a clean surface and pour cleanly from the dispenser, leaving no surface film on the walls of the container.

The amount of mercury in the dental amalgam mix may be specified as the alloy-mercury ratio—such as five parts alloy to six parts mercury by weight—or more simply as the percentage of mercury to be used in the mix. In this case, the mix would contain 54.5 per cent mercury. Consult the manufacturer's directions for the correct ratio to be used with a particular brand of alloy.

The ratio varies for different alloys and for the particular technique and handling characteristics used by the dentist. With the modern, small particle–size alloys, the alloy-mercury ratio has steadily decreased. The use of ratios equivalent to 50 per cent mercury is common, and as little as 40 per cent mercury may be used with some alloys. The use of these low alloy-mercury ratios is referred to as the *Eames* or *minimal mercury technique.*

Because the consistency of the amalgam and its properties are influenced by the amount of mercury in the original mix, using the correct alloy-mercury ratio is important.

Originally, mercury was purchased by the dentist in bulk containers that typically held 1 lb or more. The dentist was faced with the task of accurately measuring the correct amount of mercury and alloy powder needed for each amalgam mix.

Today, disposable mixing capsules, such as the one shown in Figure 15–1, have become popular. They contain preweighed alloy and mercury in separate compartments. In this particular capsule, mercury is released by twisting the cap before amalgamation is initiated. In other types, the motion of the amalgamator arms brings the mercury and alloy together.

The disposable, preproportioned mercury alloy capsule has few disadvantages other than the higher cost per mix of amalgam. The dentist has no opportunity to make minor adjustments in the alloy-mercury ratio for slightly wetter or dryer mixes, but this practice is not recommended with the low ratios used with modern high-copper alloys. On the other hand, the advantages are considerable.

- Using preproportioned capsules standardizes the amalgam technique—most products provide acceptable accuracy in the weights of alloy and mercury from one capsule to another.
- The capsules are convenient to use and save time by eliminating the step of proportioning the alloy and mercury.
- The use of bulk mercury is eliminated,

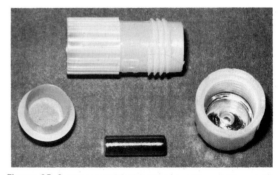

Figure 15–1. Disassembled, preproportioned disposable capsule. The preweighted mercury is in the top of the cap at right, and the alloy powder is in the compartment at left. When the cap containing the mercury is twisted, the mercury is released into the capsule with the alloy and pestle (*bottom center*). An assembled capsule is seen at right in Figure 14–3.

minimizing the chance for a major mercury spill.
- The dental team does not have to disinfect and clean capsules for reuse.

Accuracy is particularly important when the minimal mercury technique is used. At the very low alloy-mercury ratios used with modern alloys, a variation of as little as 0.5 per cent mercury may have a marked effect on the handling characteristics of the amalgam.

Some dentists prefer to use bulk mercury and dispense mercury and alloy into reusable capsules. In that case, one of the best methods of measuring the alloy and mercury is to use preweighed pellets of the alloy and to dispense the mercury from a volumetric dispenser that has been regulated to deliver the correct amount of mercury. Some typical mercury dispensers are shown in Figure 15–2.

If the amalgam alloy and the mercury dispenser are from different manufacturers, the pellet must be weighed on a pharmaceutical balance. The manufacturer of the dispenser usually does not supply the correct setting for a competitor's alloy. The amount of mercury required for the desired ratio can be calculated from the weight of the pellet. In-crements of mercury may then be dispensed and weighed on a pharmaceutical-type balance until the desired setting for the correct alloy-mercury ratio has been attained. Some mercury dispensers are not continuously adjustable, and the plunger in the dispenser must be changed to provide a different ratio.

If the weight of the alloy pellet were 0.310 g and if the desired alloy-mercury ratio were 52 per cent alloy and 48 per cent mercury, for example, the correct weight of mercury could be calculated as follows:

X = weight of mercury

Y = weight of alloy = 0.310 g

$$\frac{Y}{X} = \frac{52}{48} \qquad\qquad 15-1$$

$$\frac{0.310}{X} = \frac{52}{48} = 0.286 \text{ g mercury}$$

The dispenser should be adjusted to deliver 0.286 g of mercury.

Mercury dispensers that are adjusted correctly reliably deliver the correct amount of mercury for each mix if both the mercury and the dispenser are clean. The mercury should appear bright and shiny with no

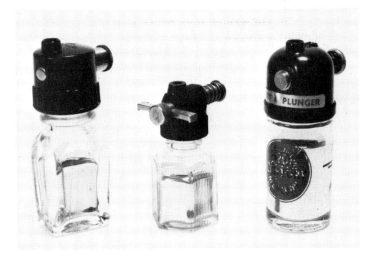

Figure 15–2. Three types of mercury dispensers that deliver a controlled weight of mercury.

scum present on its surface and should not wet the surface of the glass dispenser.

In any event, the correct amount of alloy and mercury must be proportioned before the start of trituration. Either excess mercury or insufficient mercury will have a deleterious effect on the properties of the restoration.

THE FUNCTION OF MERCURY

Mercury plays an important role in the clinical behavior of the individual restoration. An analysis of restorations shows a wide variation in mercury content. A well-placed modern amalgam characteristically contains 50 per cent or less mercury.

Note that the mercury concentration is invariably greatest in the marginal areas. This higher mercury content at the margins is important because it is these areas that are critical in terms of fracture and in which corrosion and secondary caries may occur.

Thorough amalgamation requires that each particle of alloy be wetted by the mercury. Mercury beyond this limit can result in a serious loss of strength. Conventional low-copper amalgams suffer a marked decline in compressive tensile and shear strength when the mercury content of the amalgam reaches 54 to 55 per cent. As can be seen in Figure 15-3, the compressive strength of high-copper alloys also is influenced by the mercury content. The admixed alloy lost strength when the mercury content exceeded 55 per cent, whereas the single-composition alloy underwent a reduction in strength at about the 50% per cent level. Undoubtedly, both tensile strength and shear strength of these amalgams also are reduced. In addition, both alloys undergo significant increases in creep when the mercury reaches these critical levels. Because of this effect on properties, clinical amalgam restorations that contain excess mercury show more marginal breakdown

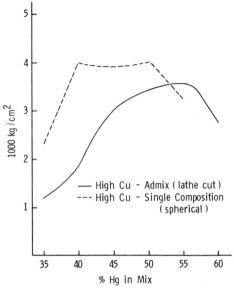

Figure 15-3. Effect of the alloy-mercury ratio on the compressive strength of high-copper amalgams.

than do restorations that contain mercury in the 50 per cent or lower range.

The curves in Figure 15-3 indicate that using too little mercury also can impair strength. This reduction may be due to several factors. First, there simply may not be sufficient matrix formation to bind together the unreacted alloy particles. Second, because such a mix is stiff, grainy, and difficult to condense, the restoration may contain voids that weaken it.

Manipulative variables that influence the amount of mercury that is present in the restoration include the following:

- The original alloy-mercury ratio
- The degree of trituration
- The technique used by the dentist in condensing the amalgam

The alloy-mercury ratio and trituration usually are the responsibility of the dental auxiliary.

TRITURATION

The object of trituration is to bring about an amalgamation of the mercury and alloy.

Each alloy particle is coated with a slight film of oxide that prevents penetration of mercury. During trituration, this film is abraded away, and the clean metal then is readily attacked by mercury. Combining the alloy and mercury correctly is essential. The composition of the final amalgam is largely determined at this stage, and this composition in turn determines the physical properties. The importance of correct trituration cannot be overemphasized.

Mechanical Amalgamators

The mixing of amalgam *(trituration)* usually is done with mechanical amalgamators, such as those shown in Figure 15–4. With a mechanical amalgamator, the mixing time is reduced to a few seconds and the procedure is readily standardized. Short amalgamation time becomes important in the restoration of large cavities, which require multiple mixes.

Many commercial brands of mechanical amalgamators are available. Capsules such as those shown in Figures 15–1 and 15–5 are inserted between the arms on top of the machine. A cylindrical metal or plastic piston in the capsule usually serves as a pestle.

Mercury and alloy are dispensed into the capsule. When the machine is activated, the arms holding the capsule oscillate at high speed, thus mixing the amalgam. Amalgamators have automatic timers for controlling the mixing time. Many of the newer amalgamators operate over a range of oscillation speeds and have a speed adjustment. Amalgamators should have hoods that cover the reciprocating arms that hold the capsule, as shown in Figure 15–4. The purpose of the hood is to confine mercury that might be sprayed if the capsule lid should not fit correctly. Capsules also occasionally rupture during trituration or may even be thrown from the arms of the amalgamator.

Reusable capsules are available with friction-fit and screw-type lids. With either type, the lid must fit the capsule tightly to prevent mercury from being sprayed from the capsule by the vigorous shaking action of the amalgamator. Loss of mercury alters the alloy-mercury ratio. More important, this fine mist of mercury droplets presents a potential for mercury inhalation. The fit of the lids deteriorates with time, so the lids should be checked periodically and defective ones discarded.

The piston or pestle should be considerably shorter and smaller in diameter than the

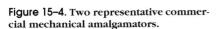
Figure 15–4. Two representative commercial mechanical amalgamators.

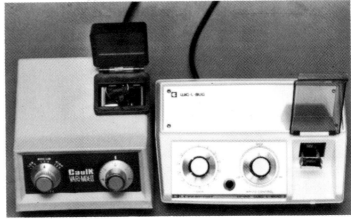

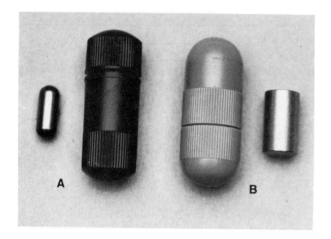

Figure 15–5. Capsule and pestle combinations, demonstrating a satisfactory size relation between the capsule and pestle (*A*) and an unsatisfactory pestle size (*B*).

inside dimensions of the capsule. The capsule shown in Figure 15–5*A* is satisfactory from this standpoint. If the piston is too large, such as that shown in Figure 15–5*B*, the mix may be unhomogeneous, particularly when the pellet form of the alloy is used. The pellet becomes wedged between the piston and the capsule and does not break up completely during trituration. With a few alloys, thorough amalgamation can be achieved without a pestle. To ensure correct trituration of the amalgam, the size of mix should never exceed two alloy pellets.

After trituration, the pestle can be removed, the capsule reinserted, and trituration continued without the pestle for 1 to 2 seconds. This procedure, referred to as *mulling*, is helpful in cleaning the capsule because the amalgam comes out in one piece. Small pieces of amalgam that are permitted to harden in the capsule contaminate future mixes. The use of preproportioned capsules eliminates this concern.

Consistency of Mix

The trituration time required to attain maximum properties and desired handling characteristics of the amalgam varies, depending on the brand of alloy, size of mix, alloy-mercury ratio, type of amalgamator, and speed setting. Most dental manufacturers suggest a trituration time and speed for specific types of mechanical amalgamators. Those directions, however, may not provide adequate trituration under the conditions present in an individual dental office.

The time recommended by the manufacturer should serve as a starting point to establish the optimum time with the particular equipment in the office. Trial mixes can be made, altering the time by a few seconds until mixes of optimum consistency are obtained. Because the size of the mix influences the time required, amalgamation time should be established for both single and double mixes.

Recognition of the appearance of the amalgam when it is correctly triturated is imperative. It serves as a guide for establishing mixing time for the particular equipment and technique used.

The grainy mix shown in Figure 15–6, for example, was undertriturated. Such a mix hardens too rapidly, and excess mercury is left in the restoration. The increase in mercury content leads to a marked loss in strength. The amalgam restoration made from this mix is weak, and the rough surface left after the granular amalgam has been carved leads to greater danger of corrosion, as explained in Chapter 13. Carefully con-

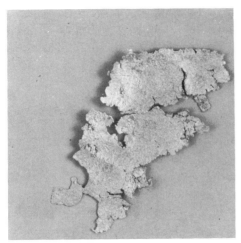

Figure 15–6. Undertriturated mix of amalgam. Such a mix has low strength and poor resistance to corrosion.

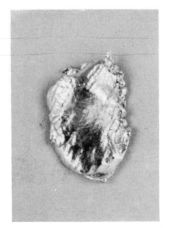

Figure 15–7. Correctly triturated amalgam having maximum properties.

trolled clinical studies have demonstrated that a marked increase in marginal fracture results when such a mix is used.

If trituration is carried to a point at which the consistency of the mass has the general appearance shown in Figure 15–7, the handling characteristics are optimal, the strength higher, and the smoother surface less susceptible to corrosion. At this point, the amalgam has a smooth, velvety consistency.

Continuing trituration beyond this stage is undesirable. Because of the excessive heat generated, the mix sets unduly fast, resulting in insufficient working time.

Amalgam alloys differ in their sensitivity to trituration variables. Figure 15–8 shows the hardening rate for two alloys mixed at low-, medium-, and high-speed settings. Alloy A is sensitive to mixing speed, whereas alloy B is generally unaffected.

Most amalgam alloys that are predispensed in self-activating capsules require amalgamators that are capable of operating at higher speeds than those needed for older alloys. As a result, many of the older, single-speed amalgamators will not reliably activate these capsules. The replacement of older amalgamators with modern, multiple-speed

units is recommended. Dental restorative materials other than amalgam are being sold increasingly in a precapsulated form to be mixed in an amalgamator. These materials also require higher mixing speeds than the older amalgamators can produce.

CONDENSATION

Once the mix is made, amalgam should not be permitted to stand before its conden-

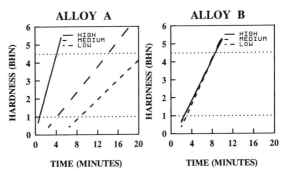

Figure 15–8. Hardening rates of two amalgam alloys mixed at low, medium, and high settings of the amalgamator. The horizontal broken lines at 1.0 and 4.5 represent consistencies at the end of condensation and the beginning of carving, respectively. (Brackett, W. W.: Master's thesis. Indiana University School of Dentistry, 1986.)

sation into the prepared cavity. The longer the time lapse between trituration and condensation, the weaker the amalgam. The crystals that are forming are fractured during condensation. Also, more mercury may be retained in the restoration. Using an amalgam mix that is 5 minutes old, for example, can result in a 40 per cent decrease in compressive strength. Consequently, each mix of amalgam should be triturated immediately before the condensation begins. Condensation should be as rapid as possible. A fresh mix of amalgam should be used if condensation requires more than 3 minutes.

Condensation is carried out by the use of hand instruments or by mechanical devices that make use of an impact or vibratory action. Either procedure is satisfactory in terms of the ultimate properties, although mechanical condensers aid in standardizing the technique and reduce fatigue to the operator. In either case, the goal is to bond the increments into a homogeneous mass that has minimal porosity and residual mercury.

The pressure needed for optimal condensation depends upon the type of amalgam alloy used. Spherical-particle alloys require lower condensation pressure than lathe-cut alloys. Because pressure is equal to the force divided by the area over which it is applied, lower forces and larger condenser tips are used with spherical alloys. Application of too high a condensation pressure punches holes in the amalgam mass instead of condensing it.

Because residual mercury plays such a vital role in the behavior of the restoration, the factors that influence the final mercury content should be summarized again:

- The original alloy-mercury ratio of the mix
- The amount of trituration
- The pressure and technique of condensation
- The time that has elapsed during the process.

EFFECT OF MOISTURE

Excessive expansion caused by the incorporation of moisture during the manipulation and insertion of the amalgam is a definite clinical problem. Such contamination may result from moisture on the condensing instruments, from perspiration on the hands or fingers while the material is being handled, or from saliva being incorporated into the amalgam during its placement into the cavity preparation.

If the amalgam alloy contains an appreciable amount of zinc, any water incorporated reacts with the zinc, and hydrogen gas is liberated. The gas, trapped within the mass of the amalgam, exerts pressure, and a delayed expansion starts about 1 week after the restoration has been inserted. By the end of 6 months, the expansion may be 0.5 mm or more. The resulting protruding restoration, as shown in Figure 15–9, can lead to secondary caries at the overhanging margins, corrosion, and, possibly, postoperative pain from pressure exerted by the amalgam

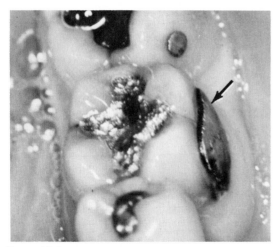

Figure 15–9. Amalgam failure (*arrow*) caused by moisture contamination. Reaction between the zinc in the alloy and moisture has produced the severe expansion. Caries then developed around the protruding restoration. (Courtesy of J. Osborne.)

against the pulp. Also, the amalgam undergoes a significant loss of strength.

Moisture contamination during amalgam placement must be avoided. The amalgam mix should never be touched with bare hands. The increments of amalgam should be carried into the cavity preparation with suitable instruments, *not* the fingers.

Many alloys today are zinc-free, thus eliminating the problem of delayed expansion. In instances in which moisture in the oral cavity cannot be controlled, such as in the child patient in whom maintenance of a dry field is difficult, the use of this type of alloy is recommended. Some non-zinc spherical alloys contaminated by moisture suffer a loss of strength, however. Amalgam should not be contaminated with perspiration or saliva, regardless of whether the alloy does or does not contain zinc.

FINISHING AND POLISHING

After the amalgam is placed into the prepared cavity, the restoration is carved to reproduce the correct anatomy. At that time, the surface and margins may be smoothed by *burnishing* the amalgam with a ball burnisher, using light pressure. Final smoothing and debris removal can be done with a moist cotton pellet or by lightly going over the surface with a polishing cup and paste.

It is essential to avoid the generation of heat. This requirement applies to any step associated with finishing and polishing. Any temperature above 60° C (140° F) results in release of mercury, and the mercury-rich amalgam is more susceptible to breakdown.

The amalgam restoration finally is carefully polished, not less than 24 hours after insertion. Premature polishing disturbs the structure of the hardening amalgam and reduces the effectiveness of the procedure. If desired, polishing may even be done a considerable time after placement of the restoration.

Amalgams should be polished for aesthetic reasons and to produce the most homogeneous surface possible. Polishing reduces surface roughness and, as discussed in Chapter 13, provides a surface more resistant to corrosion. In particular, it smooths out pits left after carving, thus eliminating defects that can result in concentration cell–type corrosion, such as those shown in Figure 13–2. The difference in surface texture and in general appearance between amalgam restorations before and after polishing can be seen in Figure 15–10.

During prophylaxis, the dentist or dental hygienist should take special care to polish all amalgam restorations thoroughly, thereby increasing their length of service by preventing tarnish and corrosion. A wet powder or paste is used. Dry polishing powders and disks should not be used because they increase the surface temperature. The polishing must be done in a manner to avoid generating heat. An incorrectly polished restoration is inferior to one that is finished correctly but not polished.

MARGINAL BREAKDOWN

A commonly observed type of amalgam failure is the restoration in which the marginal areas have become markedly chipped and frayed. Figure 15–11 shows an example of such a condition, often referred to as the *ditched* amalgam, as noted in Chapter 14. This condition, with time, develops in most amalgam restorations.

Although the exact mechanisms that produce this breakdown of the amalgam and/or the adjoining tooth structure are not as yet established, a number of causative factors are recognized.

The condition often is attributed to contraction of the amalgam during hardening. This is probably not the cause. The deterioration more likely is precipitated by the na-

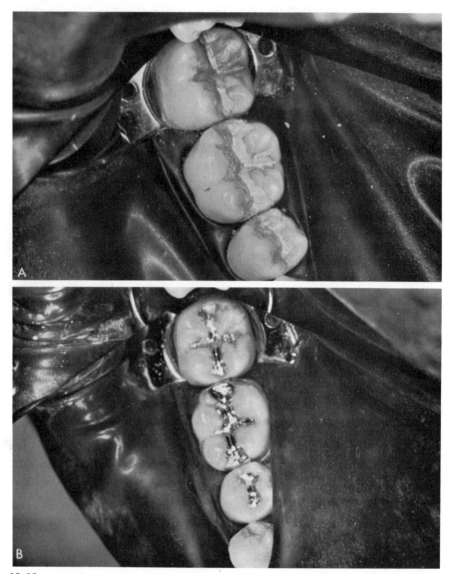

Figure 15–10. *A,* Amalgam restorations as they appear after carving. *B,* The same restorations after polishing. (From Gilmore HW and Lund MR: *Operative Dentistry,* 2nd ed. St. Louis, C. V. Mosby, 1975, p. 306.)

ture of the alloy used and the manipulation and technique of finishing rather than by dimensional changes during setting.

The higher the creep value of the alloy, apparently the greater the tendency for marginal breakdown (see Fig. 14–8). If the manipulative technique results in a high mercury content at the marginal areas, the strength is lower and the susceptibility to fracture is greater.

Incorrect finishing of the restoration by the dentist may result in a thin ledge of amalgam being left extending slightly over the enamel at the margins. These thin edges of

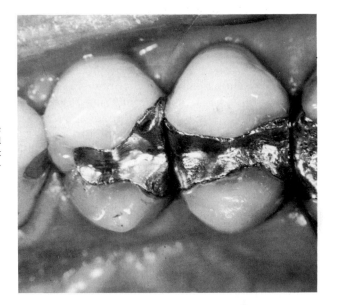

Figure 15-11. *Ditched* amalgam restoration. The severe marginal breakdown may be associated either with improper manipulation or incorrect placement of the material or with inherent properties of the alloy used. (Courtesy of M. Cochran.)

such a brittle material cannot support the forces of mastication. In time, they fracture, leaving an opening at the margins.

This chapter and Chapter 14 have continually referred to the role corrosion plays in reducing the aesthetics of the restoration and contributing to marginal breakdown. The theory is that the tin-mercury phase of the amalgam along the tooth-restoration interface undergoes corrosion. The margins of the restoration are thereby weakened and susceptible to fracture. On the basis of that theory, then, one should select high-copper alloys that are formulated to eliminate the gamma-2 phase.

Even with the best of techniques, minute marginal discrepancies occur as the restoration ages. Such deterioration can be minimized if all steps involved in selecting the alloy, preparing it, and placing it are carefully controlled.

The end result of the standardized amalgam technique is restorations such as are shown in Figure 15-10*B*. The clinical success of the amalgam restoration depends on meticulous attention to detail.

SAFETY OF THE DENTAL AMALGAM

The amalgam restoration is possible only because of the unique characteristics of mercury. This liquid metal provides the plastic mass that can be inserted into the tooth and contoured. It then hardens to a structure that resists the rigors of the oral environment surprisingly well. Mercury is also the metal that causes the concerns previously mentioned about the safety of the amalgam restoration.

Controversy regarding the safety of the dental amalgam restoration has existed since the material was introduced to the profession more than 150 years ago. Between 1988 and 1991, this controversy surfaced in the press and other news media and became a matter for public as well as professional debate. A popular television program in the United States devoted its weekly hour to this issue. As a result, the dentist and auxiliaries in an office that places dental amalgam can expect patients to raise questions and, possibly, request replacement of intact amalgam restorations with other materials. Amalgam, however, is still the most commonly used material for restoring the carious lesion. Although other restorative materials, such as composite resins, are seeing increased usage, dental amalgam's popularity will continue until the longevity of composite resins and their suitability as general amalgam replacements in the permanent dentition can be determined.

From the earliest use of amalgam, it has been asked whether mercury can produce local or systemic toxic effects in humans. It occasionally is conjectured that mercury toxicity from dental restorations is the cause for certain undiagnosed illnesses.

Mercury is one of the more toxic materials found in the dental office. A potential hazard does exist for the dentist or dental auxiliary when mercury vapor is inhaled during mixing, thus producing an accumulative toxic effect. Reading the Materials Safety Data Sheet for mercury is a sobering experience. By law the manufacturer of dental materials must supply this information.

Undoubtedly, mercury penetrates from the restoration into tooth structure. An analysis of dentin underlying amalgam restorations reveals the presence of mercury, which in part may account for a subsequent discoloration of the tooth.

The possibility of toxic reactions to the patient from these traces of mercury penetrating the tooth or sensitization from mercury dissolving from the surface of the amalgam is remote. The danger has been evaluated in numerous studies. The patient's encounter with mercury vapor during insertion of the restoration is too brief, and the total amount of mercury vapor is too small to be injurious. Furthermore, any mercury leached from the amalgam apparently is excreted by the body and not converted to the lethal forms of methyl or ethyl mercury.

In August 1991, a symposium was held by the National Institutes of Health to examine the evidence for risk of the dental restorative materials to the patient. It was concluded that except for the very small fraction of the population with a true allergic reaction to mercury or other constituents of amalgam, the dental amalgam restoration remains a safe and effective treatment. No evidence was found that related the presence of amalgam restorations to disorders such as arthritis, multiple sclerosis, or the other diseases with which amalgam has been implicated. The symposium also noted that no restorative material is completely risk-free and that patients should be informed of the relative risks associated with treatment alternatives.

As mentioned at the beginning of this section, the amalgam controversy has entered the public domain. The practitioner who uses amalgam must be prepared to answer questions about its safety. The question about the replacement of existing serviceable amalgams with other materials remains one of professional judgment. Patients who believe that they have medical problems related to the presence of any dental restorative material should be referred to a physician for diagnosis and treatment recommendations.

What about dental office personnel? Dentists and their auxiliaries are exposed daily to the risk of mercury intoxication. Although metallic mercury can be absorbed through the skin or by ingestion, the primary risk to dental personnel is from inhalation.

The maximum level of exposure considered safe for occupational exposure is 50 μg of mercury per cubic meter of air. This is an average value to be calculated when instantaneous exposures are averaged over a standard workday. Mercury is volatile at room temperature and has a vapor pressure almost 400 times the maximum level considered acceptable. Mercury vapor has no color, odor, or taste. It cannot be readily detected by simple means at levels near the maximum safe exposure. Because liquid mercury is almost 14 times denser than water, a small spill can be significant. An eyedropper-sized drop of mercury contains enough mercury to saturate the air in a typical operatory.

The ADA has estimated that one dental office in 10 exceeds the maximum safe-exposure level for mercury. Health screening of dental personnel indicates that they have a higher average blood mercury level than the general population. However, only a few cases of serious mercury intoxication caused by dental exposure have been reported. The potential hazard can be greatly reduced, if not eliminated, by attention to a few simple precautions.

The operatory should be well ventilated. All excess mercury, including waste and amalgam removed during condensation, should be collected and stored in well-sealed containers. If spilled, mercury must be cleaned up as soon as possible. It is extremely difficult to remove mercury from carpeting. Ordinary vacuum cleaners merely disperse the mercury farther through their exhaust. Mercury suppressant powders are helpful but should be considered temporary measures. If mercury comes into contact with the skin, the skin should be washed with soap and water.

If mercury dispensers and bulk mercury are used, particular care must be exercised in filling and handling the dispensers. A typical mercury dispenser holds as much as 250 g of mercury. A spill of this magnitude is a major spill. Pediatric patients should never be left unattended with mercury dispensers within their reach. The attraction of this silvery liquid metal may be irresistible.

The capsule used with a mechanical amalgamator should have a tightly fitting cap to avoid mercury leakage. As noted earlier, the use of preproportioned capsules reduces the risk of mercury exposure. When cutting amalgam, a water spray and high-speed evacuation should be used. More detailed recommendations can be obtained from the *Regulatory Compliance Manual* published by the ADA.

An important part of a hygiene program for handling toxic materials is periodic monitoring of actual exposure levels. Recommendations suggest that this procedure be conducted at least annually. Several techniques are available. Instruments can be brought in to sample the air in the operatory and yield a time-weighted average for mercury exposure. Film badges similar to radiation-exposure badges are available and can be worn by office personnel. Biological determinations can be performed on office staff to measure mercury levels in blood or urine.

The risk from mercury exposure to dental personnel cannot be ignored. Close adherence to simple hygiene procedures, however, will help to ensure a safe working environment.

Another precaution related to handling mercury and mercury-containing materials should be noted. Waste materials that contain amalgam or mercury should be disposed of responsibly in accordance with Environmental Protection Agency regulations in the area in which a dentist works. These materials should not be incinerated or subjected to heat sterilization. Biologically contaminated wastes that contain mercury should be sterilized with a cold chemical agent before disposal.

In the past, amalgam scrap often was collected and sold to companies that specialized in silver recovery. The dentist should be aware that a generator of hazardous waste is ultimately responsible for its proper disposal. Selling amalgam scrap to a recovery firm or even paying a company to dispose of it does not limit the dentist's liability. Caution should be exercised to make certain that any company that disposes of such waste is licensed and does so in accordance with the law.

Ironically, the most significant threat to the continued use of dental amalgam may be from regulations on environmental waste discharge. In certain areas in Japan, the use of amalgam has been discontinued because it is not economically feasible for a dental office using amalgam to meet local restrictions on mercury discharge into sanitary sewers. Amalgam-mercury separators on waste water discharge lines are now required in several countries in Europe.

One final precaution about handling mercury and mercury-containing materials should be noted. Mercury rapidly amalgamates with most precious metals, especially gold. Watches, rings, and other jewelry should be removed before mercury or dental amalgam is handled. Contact with mercury may seriously damage the jewelry.

Selected Reading

Anusavice, K. J.: *Quality Evaluation of Dental Restorations: Criteria for Placement and Replacement.* Chicago, Quintessence Publishing Co., 1989.

Barbakow, F., Gaberthuel, T., Lutz, F., and Schuepbach, P.: Maintenance of amalgam restorations. Quintessence Int. 19:861, 1988. Federation Dentaire Internationale, Technical Report 33: Safety of dental amalgam. Int. Dent. J. 39:217, 1989.

Council on Dental Materials, Instruments and Equipment, Council on Dental Therapeutics. Safety of dental amalgam. J. Am. Dent. Assoc. 106:519, 1983.

Frykholm, K. O.: On mercury from dental amalgam. Its toxic and allergic effects and some comments on occupational hygiene. Acta Odontol. Scand. 15:7, 1957.

Greener, E. H.: Amalgam: Yesterday, today and tomorrow. Oper. Dent. 4:24, 1979.

Jorgensen, K. D.: The mechanism of marginal fracture of amalgam fillings. Acta Odontol. Scand. 23:347, 1965.

Klausner, L. H., Green, T. G., and Charbeneau, G. T.: Placement and replacement of amalgam restorations: A challenge for the profession. Oper. Dent. 12:105, 1987.

Leinfelder, K. F.: Clinical performance of amalgams with high content of copper. Oper. Dent. 5:125, 1980.

Letzel, H., van't Hof, M. A., Vrijhoef, M. M. A., et al.: A controlled clinical study of amalgam restorations: Survival, failures, and cause of failure. Dent. Mater. 5:115, 1989.

Letzel, H., and Vrijhoef, M. M. A.: The influence of polishing on the marginal integrity of amalgam restorations. J. Oral. Rehabil. 11:89, 1984.

Mahler, D. B.: Research on dental amalgam: 1982–1986. Adv. Dent. Res. 2:71, 1988.

Mahler, D. B., and Adey, J. D.: The influence of mercury content on the characteristics of a high-copper amalgam. J. Biomed. Mater. Res. 13:467, 1979.

Marshall, G. W., Jackson, B., and Marshall, S.: Copper-rich and conventional amalgam restorations after clinical use. J. Am. Dent. Assoc. 100:43, 1980.

Marshall, G. W., Marshall, S. J., and Letzel, H.: Mercury content of amalgam restorations. Gen. Dent. Nov.-Dec., 1989, p. 473.

Mjor, I. A.: The safe and effective use of dental amalgam. Int. Dent. J. 37:147, 1987.

Rogers, K. D.: Status of scrap (recyclable) dental amalgams as environmental health hazards or toxic substances. J. Am. Dent. Assoc. 119:159, 1989.

Sutow, E. J., Letzel, D. W., and Hall, G. C.: Correlation of dental amalgam crevice corrosion with clinical ratings. J. Dent. Res. 68:82, 1989.

Reviewing the Chapter

1. List all the factors that enter into the selection of a commercial amalgam alloy.
2. What criteria are used in ensuring purity of dental mercury?
3. Explain what is meant by the alloy-mercury ratio and describe how it is determined.
4. Give the reasons that support the use of only high-copper amalgam alloys.
5. Describe the factors and precautions associated with proportioning the alloy and mercury. What are the advantages and disadvantages of preweighed disposable capsules?
6. Discuss in detail the potential toxic effect of mercury to (1) the patient and (2) the dentist and auxiliary. List the precautions to be taken to reduce the danger of mercury inhalation in the dental office. What is the limit for occupational exposure to mercury vapor?
7. Describe the effect of excess mercury on the properties and clinical behavior of the amalgam restoration. Be specific.
8. What factors control the final mercury content in the restoration?
9. Describe the appearance of an undertriturated and thoroughly triturated mix of amalgam. Explain the differences in the

properties and the clinical behavior of amalgam as related to trituration time.

10. Explain the components of a mechanical amalgamator and how it operates. How does one establish the correct trituration time with such a device? What is the function of the speed control on some units?

11. What precautions are exercised in selecting the correct capsule and pestle and in their use?

12. Describe the amalgam condensation procedure and the factors to be ob-

served in ensuring a successful restoration. What is burnishing?

13. What happens if a zinc-containing amalgam is contaminated with moisture? What is the difference, if any, between zinc-free and zinc-containing alloys?

14. Describe the polishing procedure and the various factors that must be controlled for optimum results.

15. Discuss all possible mechanisms associated with marginal breakdown of amalgam restorations.

CHAPTER 16

ALLOYS FOR DENTAL CASTINGS

CONVENTIONAL GOLD CASTING ALLOYS
Gold Content and Fineness
COMPOSITION OF NOBLE METAL ALLOYS
COMPOSITION OF BASE METAL ALLOYS

CLASSIFICATION OF CASTING ALLOYS
Metal-Ceramic Alloys
BASE METAL ALLOYS
ALTERNATIVE CASTING ALLOYS
CASTING SHRINKAGE
RECYCLING CASTING ALLOYS

In contrast to the direct filling restorative materials discussed in previous chapters, many metallic restorations are fabricated outside the mouth to fit casts, dies, and other replicas of oral tissues obtained from an impression taken by the dentist. Although this may be done in the dental office, it usually is done in a dental laboratory. At one time, most of these restorations were fabricated from gold-based casting alloys. Alternative casting alloys that contain either much smaller amounts of gold or no gold at all have recently been used.

The casting process is described in detail in Chapter 19. Briefly, the following steps are involved:

1. A pattern of the missing tooth structure or the dental prosthesis is constructed in wax.

2. The pattern is embedded in *investment*, a mixture of a binder, such as gypsum, and silica.

3. The investment is mixed and poured over the pattern.

4. After the investment has hardened, the wax is removed, forming the *investment mold.*

5. Molten metal is forced (cast) into the space left by the wax.

The resulting casting is an accurate duplicate of the wax pattern. This casting process is used for small structures, such as inlays or crowns, to replace part of a single tooth and for larger structures, called *bridges*, which replace one or more missing teeth. These prostheses are cemented to existing tooth structure and are referred to as *fixed restorations*. Examples are shown in Figure 16–1.

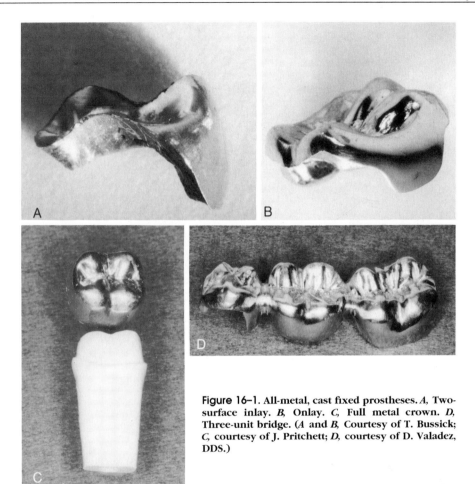

Figure 16–1. All-metal, cast fixed prostheses. *A,* Two-surface inlay. *B,* Onlay. *C,* Full metal crown. *D,* Three-unit bridge. (*A* and *B,* Courtesy of T. Bussick; *C,* courtesy of J. Pritchett; *D,* courtesy of D. Valadez, DDS.)

Larger castings also are made to construct appliances that can be removed from the mouth by the patient. The removable partial denture shown in Figure 16–2 is an example of such a *removable* appliance.

The role played by the dental assistant or hygienist in the construction of these castings usually is limited. The assistant helps in the impression-taking process and may pour the cast or die. The assistant also plays an important role in cementing the fixed restoration, discussed in Chapter 22. The hygienist cleans and polishes fixed restorations

when the natural teeth are cleaned. Hygienists may also clean as well as advise patients on cleaning removable prostheses.

As the average age of the dental population increases and people retain their natural teeth longer, the need for restorative dentistry involving castings is expected to increase. Constructing a successful cast appliance is an involved and expensive process, as demonstrated by this and the next three chapters.

Dental auxiliaries need to be familiar with the process to be able to answer patient

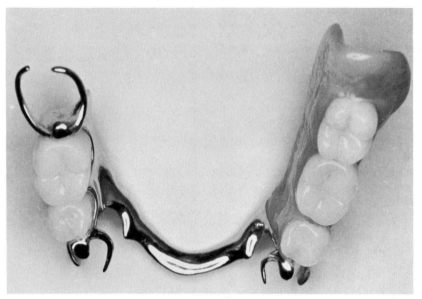

Figure 16–2. Finished removable partial denture appliance cast with a chromium-based alloy. An acrylic resin "ridge" and artificial teeth have been attached.

questions, to help ensure that the restoration is fabricated and placed in a satisfactory manner, and to ensure that it will provide service for its expected lifetime. The recent development of a large number of alloys that differ in composition from the traditional gold alloys requires that the auxiliary understand how the behaviors of these materials differ to handle them appropriately.

CONVENTIONAL GOLD CASTING ALLOYS

As noted in Chapter 13, gold is the most corrosion-resistant of all pure metals and, hence, was a natural choice for use in dental restorations. Pure gold is too soft and weak for most dental applications. The art of alloying gold with other metals to obtain improved properties is an ancient one. Numerous gold alloys had been developed for casting jewelry long before the technique was introduced to dentistry. The dental profession quickly adopted these alloys, which became the starting point for the development of modern dental gold casting alloys.

Gold Content and Fineness

Jewelry gold alloys usually are designated according to their *karat*. The same designation originally was used for dental gold alloys. The karat of an alloy is the number of the parts of pure gold in 24 parts of the alloy—24-karat gold would be pure gold; 18-karat gold is an alloy of which 18 parts are pure gold and the remaining 6 parts are other metals (75 per cent gold).

If dental gold alloy is rated for gold content today, the *fineness* of the alloy is used. The fineness of a gold alloy is the parts per thousand of pure gold. A 750-*fine* alloy would contain 750 parts of gold per 1000 parts of alloy (75 per cent gold).

The karat or fineness of dental gold alloys is important primarily to the intrinsic or resale value of the alloy. With the possible exception of corrosion resistance, it usually is of secondary importance as an estimate of the physical properties of the alloys.

Gold, silver, platinum, palladium, and other members of the platinum group of metals are referred to as *precious metals* because they have intrinsic value associated with the international monetary system. Sometimes the conventional gold-based casting alloys are referred to as *precious metal alloys.*

More important from a dental point of view, the precious metals are *noble metals,* as described in Chapter 13. Except for silver, these metals are inherently resistant to corrosion in the oral environment. This is the reason they were used in traditional dental casting alloys.

Instability in the price of precious metals was a significant driving force in the development of alternative alloys. Many contained significantly lower amounts of noble metals than the conventional alloys, and the term "semiprecious alloy" was coined. This term has no accepted definition in terms of composition and should not be used.

Alloys that do not depend on noble metal content for corrosion resistance are called *base metals.* As noted in Chapter 13, their corrosion resistance depends on the presence of metals that *passivate.* Although they have been referred to as "nonprecious," the preferred designation is *base metal alloys.*

The precious metal content of a dental casting alloy is no longer the definitive predictor of clinical acceptability. Many lower gold content alloys can provide excellent service when used appropriately. Some base metal alloys are even the materials of choice for certain dental applications.

COMPOSITION OF NOBLE METAL ALLOYS

The basic composition of dental gold alloys is gold and copper. Gold provides the corrosion resistance and copper strengthens the gold. Modern alloys are much more complex than this binary-type alloy. Silver usually is added, along with platinum, palladium, or both, to make the strongest and hardest alloys. About 1 per cent of zinc also is present in most alloys.

As described in Chapter 12, each metal has a special contribution to the alloy:

- If sufficient *copper* is added to the gold, the alloy can be subjected to heat treatment to change its properties.
- Copper reddens the alloy, and *silver* is used to counteract this redness.
- Silver can lead to tarnish problems unless the copper-silver ratio is controlled and sufficient *palladium* is added to the alloy.
- Addition of significant amounts of *platinum* or *palladium* raises the melting point and whitens the alloy.
- *Zinc* is added as a deoxidizer to keep the alloy clean during the melting and casting process.

COMPOSITION OF BASE METAL ALLOYS

Base metal alloys have been used since the 1930s for the construction of removable partial denture frameworks. Today, they are accepted as the materials of choice for this application. Their use for fixed prostheses is more recent, but their acceptance is growing.

Most base metal alloys depend on *chromium* for passivation and, hence, their corrosion resistance. Chromium is a reactive metal that rapidly forms a tough, stable oxide coating when exposed to air or water. Most common base metal alloys are either nickel- or cobalt-based alloys and contain adequate amounts of chromium to ensure passivation.

Iron-based alloys (stainless steels) are

used as wrought metals but not commonly used as casting alloys in dentistry.

Aluminum is another metal that passivates readily. Sometimes its alloys are used for construction of bases for complete dentures.

The newest of the base metal alloys systems are *titanium-based*. This metal and its alloys are extensively used in dental implants and as wrought metals in orthodontics and have recently been investigated as casting alloys. The extreme reactivity of titanium with oxygen results in rapid passivation, and it is considered one of the most biologically compatible of dental materials. Its reactivity, however, also complicates the casting process, and successful applications of titanium casting alloys are still under development.

CLASSIFICATION OF CASTING ALLOYS

Several classification systems have been developed to encompass the wide array of casting alloys available today. No single composition of alloy meets the varied requirements for all types of dental restorations. The demands placed on a three-quarter crown that is to serve as a bridge abutment are entirely different from those placed on a small, one-surface inlay. Therefore, different properties are needed in the alloy, depending on the purpose for which it is intended.

The classification presented in Table 16–1 is according to the American Dental Association (ADA) Specification no. 5 for the traditional gold-based casting alloys. As indicated, alloys are placed into four classes. The composition limits on the precious metals contents were restricted to ensure tarnish resistance. In general, the hardness and strength increase from the first to the fourth type as the platinum group metals are added.

Although this classification system originally applied only to gold alloys with high noble metal content, it has come to be used as a general classification to identify the clinical application of a given alloy. A Type IV casting alloy, for example, refers to an alloy suitable for Type IV applications, whether or not the alloy meets the compositional requirements in ADA Specification no. 5.

- *Type I.* Type I alloys are used for small inlays that are not subject to stress, such as the restorations of gingival cavities. They seldom are used today because several types of direct filling materials serve the same purposes. Although these alloys are quite ductile, they exhibit a rather low proportional limit. They cannot be hardened by heat treatment, and they have relatively high melting points.
- *Type II.* Type II alloys are used chiefly for inlay restorations that are not subject to high stresses. These alloys are harder than the Type I alloys. Type II alloys also are not used extensively today.
- *Type III.* These alloys are harder than the other two types and have largely replaced Type I and Type II alloys. They

TABLE 16–1. Classification of Dental Casting Gold Alloys (ADA Specification No. 5)

Type	Minimum Percentage Content of Gold and Platinum Group Metals	VHN (softened)	
		Minimum	*Maximum*
I	83	50	90
II	78	90	120
III	78	120	150
IV	75	150	—

VHN, Vickers Hardness Number.

are indicated for crowns and bridge abutments, which are subject to considerable stress during mastication. They also are used for casting inlays and onlays. The gold-based Type III alloys usually are amenable to hardening heat treatment—a marked decrease in ductility may result, although the other tensile properties are significantly increased.

- *Type IV.* These alloys must be especially strong because they are used for large castings, such as long span bridges, partial dentures, clasps, and bars. They are the strongest and hardest of all the types.

Types III and IV alloys often are referred to as *crown and bridge* alloys because this describes their principle clinical applications.

Metal-Ceramic Alloys

Although not part of the ADA specification for gold-based casting alloys, a fifth type, based on clinical application, commonly is recognized. These alloys are intended for use in metal-ceramic restorations. Their clinical application is described in more detail in Chapter 20.

These casting alloys are used to make metal substructures over which dental porcelain is fused to construct tooth-colored fixed restorations. An example is shown in Figure 16–3. All or, in some cases, only part of the exterior surface of the metal casting is covered with porcelain. As the demand for aesthetic dentistry has grown, these restorations have become common and today constitute the majority of anterior fixed prostheses.

Development of these metal-ceramic alloys required considerable modification from Types I through IV to be suitable for this application.

- They must have higher melting points to withstand porcelain fusing temperatures.

- Their thermal coefficient of expansion must be reduced to be compatible with the porcelain used.
- They must provide a mechanism for chemically bonding to the porcelain but must not discolor the porcelain.

The first metal-ceramic alloys were composed of gold-platinum-palladium with more than 90 per cent noble metal content. The balance consisted of base metals such as tin, iron, and indium used to provide a bond to the porcelain. Not only were these alloys expensive, but they had relatively poor mechanical properties because they lacked the copper and silver that effectively harden the other gold alloys.

A large number of alternative alloy systems have been developed for this clinical application with goals of reduced cost and improved properties.

BASE METAL ALLOYS

From a clinical application point of view, this section on base metal casting alloys could be titled *removable partial denture alloys.* Long successful use of base metals led to their acceptance as alloys of choice for this application and resulted in the development of ADA Specification no. 14 for alloys intended for this clinical application. The specification requires a composition of not less than 85 per cent of nickel, cobalt, and chromium, along with appropriate physical properties.

Base metal alloys are also used for metal-ceramic applications and have been widely accepted by dental laboratories. The nickel-based alloys commonly are used for metal-ceramic restorations. The following characteristics of base metal alloys are important in dental applications:

- Base metal alloys have about twice the elastic modulus of the gold-based alloys. This results in the ability to construct thinner, lighter restorations.

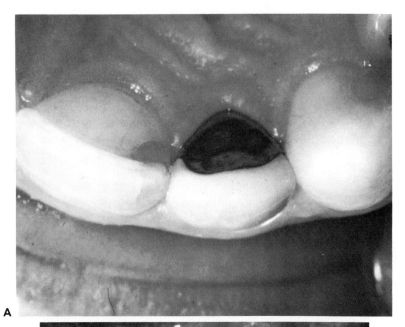

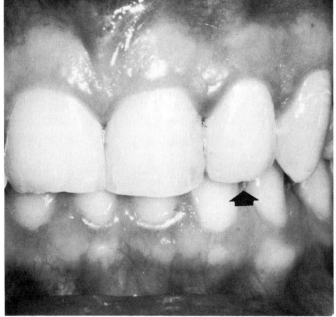

Figure 16–3. *A*, Lingual view of a metal-ceramic showing the metal coping partially covered by porcelain. *B*, Cemented restoration, as shown by arrow. (Courtesy of C. Goodacre.)

- Base metal alloys have higher melting points, which is advantageous for metal-ceramic use but makes casting somewhat more difficult.
- They are much harder than gold alloys and, thus, are difficult to cut and finish.
- Base metal alloys also have low ''as in cast'' ductility and work harden rapidly. Patients should be cautioned about bending the clasps on partial denture frameworks because their brittleness can lead to fracture.
- Unlike noble metal alloys, base metal alloys depend on the formation of an oxide film to protect them from corrosion. Base metals formulated for dental applications should have stable oxides in the oral environment. Their corrosion resistance depends more on their environment than does the corrosion resistance of most noble metals.
- Chlorine is known to cause rapid corrosion attack on some chromium-containing base metals, particularly those with high nickel content. As a result, base metal appliances should not be immersed in chlorine-containing substances, such as hypochlorite bleaches.

An estimated 8 to 10 per cent of the female population exhibits an allergic reaction to nickel. The incidence in males is about one tenth as high. Although oral manifestations of this allergy are not common, extraoral responses may be incited in a previously sensitized person. The ADA recommends against the use of nickel alloys in patients who are known to have nickel sensitivity. The ADA requires labeling of such alloys by manufacturers and labeling of appliances constructed of nickel alloy by dental laboratories. These labels must indicate that the alloys contain nickel and may cause allergic reactions.

ALTERNATIVE CASTING ALLOYS

A useful approach to simplify the large number of casting alloy types marketed is to consider them as alternatives for various clinical applications. Within each application, the alternatives can be grouped by composition. Then what is known about the properties and performance of each group can be compared and a choice made among the different alternatives. Viewed in this manner, the traditional high noble metal content alloys often are just one alternative for a given restorative function. For most applications, they serve as benchmarks for comparison because the longest term clinical data are available for these traditional alloys.

In summary, modern casting alloys can be described as follows:

- Yellow gold alloys that meet ADA Specification no. 5 with respect to both properties and composition for Types I and II applications
- Yellow gold alloys that meet Specification no. 5 for Types III and IV applications
- Low-gold alloys (40 to 60 per cent gold) that have properties comparable to the traditional ADA specification golds for Types III and IV applications
- Silver-palladium (white) alloys that have properties comparable to Types III and IV gold alloys
- Yellow gold alloys (gold-platinum-palladium) for metal-ceramic restorations
- White gold alloys (gold-palladium with or without silver) for metal-ceramic applications
- Palladium-silver alloys for metal-ceramic applications
- Palladium-based metal-ceramic alloys with significant amounts of metals other than silver (e.g., gold, copper, cobalt)
- Base metal alloys (nickel-chromium, cobalt-chromium) for metal-ceramic applications
- Base metal alloys for removable partial denture frameworks (nickel-chromium, cobalt-chromium, cobalt-nickel-chromium)

When comparing these various alternative

alloys, the physical properties are reasonably similar in most cases. For some of the tests used—for example, those for measuring the metal-ceramic bond strength—the data are somewhat controversial and the results are not in good agreement. The final evaluation, as always, is the clinical performance in the mouth. The traditional ADA Specification no. 5 alloys have clinical records dating back 30 to 40 years. The metal-ceramic alloys with high noble metal content (gold-platinum-palladium) were developed in the early 1960s. Most of the other alloy systems date only to the late 1960s or even more recently. Thus, the clinical data available are not as long-term as for the former systems.

CASTING SHRINKAGE

With water an important exception, most crystalline substances contract when they change from the liquid to the solid state. Casting alloys are no exception. Another shrinkage that occurs is the thermal shrinkage as the solid alloy cools to room temperature. The total shrinkage inherent in the casting process from all sources is known as the *casting shrinkage.*

As described at the beginning of this chapter, the casting procedure consists of forming a mold around a wax pattern that is a reproduction of the casting to be obtained. The wax is then eliminated, and a molten alloy is forced into the mold. As the metal solidifies, it takes the place of the wax. If the wax pattern is an accurate reproduction of the missing part, it follows that as the alloy shrinks during solidification and cooling, the casting will be too small by the total amount of this shrinkage. Consequently, the amount of this shrinkage becomes important. As shown in Chapter 18, the mold must be enlarged by the same amount as the shrinkage so that the casting will be accurate.

This casting shrinkage ranges from 1.2 to

2.3 per cent when measured in a linear direction. It depends on the composition of the alloy and, to a certain extent, the shape of the casting. A value of about 1.4 per cent is typical for the traditional gold-based dental alloys. Other alloys with higher solidification temperatures, such as base metal and metal-ceramic alloys, exhibit higher casting shrinkages.

RECYCLING CASTING ALLOYS

A surplus of alloy always remains after the casting has been prepared for cementation in the mouth. If the alloy has significant precious metal content, care should be taken to sort out this excess gold alloy according to its type and composition.

Under no circumstances should the excess metal from different types or brands of alloys be mixed. The mixture might result in the formation of an alloy that has low corrosion resistance and ductility. The resulting properties tend to be unpredictable.

A gold alloy can be remelted and recycled two or three times without harm if an equal amount of new alloy is added to compensate for the loss of some of the zinc. Noble metal–ceramic alloys can be recast similarly if new metal is added.

Any gold alloy that cannot be reused should be stored by itself as scrap gold and sent to a metal refiner. Most companies that sell gold casting alloys purchase gold alloy scrap from the dental office. Again, it should be emphasized that unidentified scrap gold should never be used for dental casting purposes.

Under no circumstances should two alloys of different compositions be mixed and melted together for subsequent use in the mouth.

Contamination of gold alloys must be avoided. As little as 0.05 per cent of certain base metals may make the alloy so brittle that it is unusable. The alloy should not be stored in a drawer that contains metal dies.

Mercury is particularly injurious because it diffuses rapidly into gold. Cast gold restorations should not be placed on a bracket table or on top of a laboratory bench where amalgam scrap is present.

The manufacturer's recommendations for the reuse of scrap metal from base metal or low gold alloys should be followed. In general, the intrinsic value of the alloy is so low as to make such a practice questionable. The cost of remakes and refinishing may well offset any savings.

Selected Reading

American Dental Association Report: Classification system for cast alloys. J. Am. Dent. Assoc. 109:838, 1984.

Asgar, K., and Peyton, F. A.: Effect of microstructure on the physical properties of cobalt-base alloys. J. Dent. Res. 40:63, 1961.

Bertolotii, R. L.: Selection of alloys for today's crown and fixed partial denture restorations. J. Am. Dent. Assoc. 108:959, 1984.

Burse, A. B., Swartz, M. L., Phillips, R. W., and Dykema, R. W.: Comparison of the in vitro and in vivo tarnish of three gold alloys. J. Biomed. Mater. Res. 6:267, 1972.

Council on Dental Materials, Instruments and Equipment.: Report on base-metal alloys for crown and bridge applications: Benefits and risks. J. Am. Dent. Assoc. 111:479, 1985.

Covington, J. S., McBride, M. A., Slagle, W. F., and Disney, A. L.: Quantization of nickel and beryllium leakage from base metal casting alloys. J. Prosthet. Dent. 54:127, 1985.

Hollenback, G. M., and Skinner, E. W.: Shrinkage during casting of gold and gold alloys. J. Am. Dent. Assoc. 33:1391, 1946.

McLean, J. W.: *The Science and Art of Dental Ceramics*. Vols. 1 and 2. Chicago, Quintessence Publ. Co., 1979 and 1980.

McLean, J. W.: The metal-ceramic restoration. Dent. Clin. North Am. 27(4):747, 1983.

Moffa, J. P.: Alternative dental casting alloys. Dent. Clin. North Am. 27(4):733, 1983.

Moffa, J. P., Guckes, A. D., Okawa, M. A., and Lilly, G. E.: An evaluation of nonprecious alloys for use with porcelain veneers. Pt. II. Industrial safety and biocompatibility. J. Prosthet. Dent. 30:432, 1973.

Moffa, J. P., Jenkins, W. A., Ellison, J. A., and Hamilton, J. C.: A clinical evaluation of two base-metal alloys and a gold alloy for use in fixed prosthodontics: A five-year study. J. Prosthet. Dent. 52:491, 1984.

Moffa, J. P., Lugassy, A. A., Guckes, A. D., and Gettleman, L.: An evaluation of nonprecious alloys for use with porcelain veneers. Pt. I. Physical properties. J. Prosthet. Dent. 30:424, 1973.

Morris, H. F.: Veterans Administration Cooperative Studies Project No. 147, Pt. I: A multidisciplinary, multicenter experimental design for the evaluation of alternative metal-ceramic alloys. J. Prothet. Dent. 56:402, 1986.

Morris, H. F.: Veterans Administration Cooperative Studies Project No. 147, Pt. IV: Biocompatibility of base metal alloys. J. Prosthet. Dent. 58:1, 1987.

Morris, H. F.: Veterans Administration Cooperative Studies Project No. 147, Pt. VII: Comparison of the mechanical properties of different metal-ceramic alloys in the as cast condition and after simulated porcelain firing cycles. J. Prosthet. Dent. 61:160, 1989.

Nielsen, J. P., and Tuccillo, J. J.: Grain size in cast gold alloys. J. Am. Dent. Assoc. 45:964, 1966.

Nitkin, D. A., and Asgar, K.: Evaluation of alternative alloys to Type III gold for use in fixed prosthodontics. J. Am. Dent. Assoc. 93:622, 1979.

Prystowsky, S. D., Allen, A. M., Smith, R. W., et al.: Allergic contact hypersensitivity to nickel, neomycin, ethylenediamine and benzocaine. Arch. Dermatol. 115:959, 1979.

Reviewing the Chapter

1. Outline the general steps involved in fabricating a cast restoration.
2. What metals provide resistance to tarnish in a gold-based alloy? In a base metal alloy?
3. Define *noble metal, karat, fineness,* and *base metal.*
4. List the constituents present in a dental gold alloy and explain the effect of each one.
5. Which gold alloys can be subjected to heat treatment for hardening or softening?
6. Classify conventional gold alloys according to the ADA Specification and explain the use of each type. Do manufacturers market only one alloy of each type?

7. Why were alternate alloy systems developed to replace the traditional gold alloy?

8. Classify the alternate alloys as related to composition and usage.

9. Is the precious metal content of a dental alloy a satisfactory method of classification? Explain your answer.

10. Describe a metal-ceramic restoration. Discuss the various types of alloys used for that application and the requirements of such an alloy.

11. What is the composition of the base metal alloys used in fabricating a metal-ceramic restoration? How do the properties differ from a gold-based alloy? Is there a biological consideration in the use of such an alloy? Explain.

12. Give the composition of the various base metal alloys used in the construction of a removable partial denture. How do the properties of these alloys differ from noble metal alloys?

13. Describe the modern casting alloys and compare them in terms of properties and performance.

14. What is meant by *casting shrinkage?* What is its magnitude, and how does one compensate for it?

15. Which alloys can be economically recycled? What precautions should be followed?

CHAPTER 17

DENTAL CASTING WAXES AND OTHER PATTERN MATERIALS

THE WAX PATTERN	**WAX DISTORTION**
THE DIE	**Causes of Distortion**
COMPOSITION	**OBTAINING THE PATTERN**
FLOW	**OTHER DENTAL WAXES**
DESIRABLE PROPERTIES	

Many kinds of waxes are used in dentistry. The dental auxiliary most frequently comes in contact with those used in the fabrication of cast restorations. Thus, the major part of this chapter focuses on casting waxes. Many characteristics of this wax are common to those used for other dental procedures.

Of all dental restorations, the cast restoration is the one that is most likely to be prepared entirely outside the patient's mouth. The fabrication of this restoration might be the responsibility of the dental assistant or hygienist, if either is serving in the capacity of a dental technician.

The accuracy of the inlay, crown, or more complex appliances, such as bridges and partial dentures, depends on the physical properties of the dental materials involved.

Of equal importance are the intelligence and skill of the people who manipulate the materials and tools to produce the finished restoration. The technique is not difficult, but knowledge of the materials and strict attention to detail are essential to success.

The weakness in a fixed cast restoration is the layer of cement present at the margins after the casting has been cemented in place. Many dental cements are somewhat soluble in oral fluids, as discussed in Chapters 21 and 22. In some areas of the mouth, detecting marginal discrepancies is difficult. Openings as large as 100 μm may pass unnoticed in the gingival areas that are not visible. Thus, layers of cement are exposed even though the restoration may appear to be clinically acceptable. Accuracy greater than that which can be detected by eye or routine clinical methods of evaluation is required.

THE WAX PATTERN

As summarized in Chapter 16, the essential steps in the casting procedure are as follows:

1. An accurate pattern that duplicates the missing tooth structure is constructed, using inlay wax.

2. The wax pattern is then surrounded by a gypsum product, known as *investment*, which is allowed to harden.

3. The wax is removed or *eliminated* from the investment. The mold remaining should be an accurate reproduction of the wax pattern.

4. The casting alloy is melted and forced into this mold.

If all principles have been followed, the resulting casting should fit the original cavity preparation accurately.

If the wax pattern is not precise, the casting will not fit. The accuracy of the mold depends on the accuracy of the pattern. On solidification, the alloy reproduces the mold space, which in turn has reproduced the shape of the pattern.

The fit of the casting depends initially on the accuracy of the wax pattern.

The pattern can be prepared directly on the tooth by the dentist—the *direct technique*. More commonly, a die reproducing the tooth and the prepared cavity obtained from an impression is used. The wax pattern is formed on the die outside the mouth—the *indirect technique*.

THE DIE

The die is constructed from an impression obtained by the dentist. An impression material with good accuracy and detail reproduction should be used, either a rubber impression material or reversible hydrocolloid. Most dies are constructed with a Type IV (Class II) dental stone. Resin die materials also are available. Because of the polymerization shrinkage of the resin, such a die may be somewhat undersized in contrast to stone, which expands as it hardens. This factor must be taken into consideration and the technique adjusted accordingly. In comparison to stone, pouring resin into the impression without trapping voids is more difficult.

The disadvantage of the stone die is the tendency to abrade the stone surface while carving the wax pattern. With careful handling, however, Type IV die stone provides an adequate cast for the construction of the wax pattern.

COMPOSITION

The American Dental Association (ADA) Specification no. 4 divides dental inlay casting waxes into two types:

- Type I is a medium wax used in the direct technique.
- Type II is a soft wax designed for the indirect technique.

These waxes differ chiefly in their softening or melting ranges. A Type I wax must melt at a higher temperature than a Type II wax because the former is used in the mouth. *Under no circumstances should these two types be used interchangeably.*

To meet the specification requirements, the waxes must be carefully compounded by the manufacturer. The primary component wax is paraffin, usually in a concentration of 40 to 60 per cent.

Obtained from petroleum, *paraffin wax* is a complex mixture of organic compounds of varying molecular weights. The components with lower weights melt at lower temperatures than those with higher weights. Thus, paraffin can be obtained with almost any desired melting point. The paraffin used for Type I waxes has a higher melting point than the paraffin used for Type II waxes.

Other modifying waxes are added to provide desirable properties of the wax, such as smoothness, firmness, carvability, and toughness. An important additive is *carnauba wax*. It increases the melting range and reduces the flow at mouth temperature. *Synthetic waxes* often are used to replace, in part, the carnauba wax. The synthetic waxes are quite pure and assist the manufacturers in standardizing the batch-to-batch production, as compared with the natural carnauba wax, which comes from the leaves of a tree. The same problem is inherent in other natural waxes, such as *gum dammar*, which is added to paraffin to increase toughness and enhance surface smoothness.

FLOW

Inlay waxes do not solidify with a definite space lattice as does a metal. Instead, the structure is more likely to be a combination of crystalline and amorphous materials, displaying limited ordering of the molecules. The wax lacks rigidity and flows under stress at room temperature.

Flow or plasticity of the wax is necessary when it is heated to its softening temperature because the cavity in the die often is filled by pressing the softened wax into position. In Type I wax, the softening temperature must be above mouth temperature but still low enough to be tolerated by the patient.

Because Type II wax is used at room temperature, its softening point can be lower than a Type I wax but must not be so low that the wax flows significantly at room temperature.

After the wax pattern has been formed on the die, the pattern must be withdrawn from the die. If the wax flows during the removal of the pattern, the pattern is distorted. It is important that the flow of the wax be as low as possible while the pattern is being removed from the die and during subsequent handling. The composition of the wax is regulated to achieve this objective.

The flow of the wax at various temperatures is specified in ADA Specification no. 4, as shown in Table 17–1. The maximum flow permitted for Type I waxes at 37° C (98° F) is 1 per cent. This low flow permits carving and removal of the pattern from the prepared tooth at oral temperatures without distortion.

Both Type I and Type II waxes must have a minimum flow of 70 per cent at 45° C (113° F). At about this temperature, the wax is inserted into the prepared cavity. If the wax does not have sufficient plasticity, it will not flow into the preparation and reproduce the necessary detail.

DESIRABLE PROPERTIES

The following properties are desired in an inlay wax:

- When softened, the wax should be homogeneous. It should be compounded with ingredients that blend with one another so that there will be no graininess or hard spots.
- Its color should contrast with the die material (or tooth). The wax margins must be carved close to the die, and a well-defined contrast in color facilitates proper finishing of the margins.

TABLE 17–1. Flow Requirements for a Dental Casting Wax

	30° C (Max)	37°C (Max)	40° C Min.	40° C Max.	45° C Min.	45° C Max.
Type I	—	1.0	—	20	70	90
Type II	1.0	—	50	—	70	90

- There should be no flakiness or surface roughening when the wax is bent and molded after softening. Such flakiness is present in pure paraffin wax. This is one of the reasons modifiers are added.
- After the wax pattern has solidified, it must be carved to the exterior contours of the restoration. The wax must be carved so the pattern conforms exactly to the surface of the die at the margins. This may require carving the wax to a very thin layer. If the wax pulls or chips with the carving, such precision cannot be attained.
- After the investment has hardened, the wax must be eliminated from the mold space. This is accomplished by heating the mold and burning the wax. The wax must burn cleanly, leaving no residue or coating on the mold walls.
- The wax pattern should be rigid and dimensionally stable until eliminated. Unless handled carefully, the wax pattern actually flows and is subject to stress relaxation—a factor that must be taken into consideration in its manipulation.

WAX DISTORTION

The first opportunity for distortion of the wax pattern occurs during its removal from the die. During subsequent manipulations, the pattern may be further distorted by handling. With proper care, such distortions can be kept to a minimum.

The chief cause of distortion is the relaxation of stresses induced during manipulation. The phenomenon of relaxation was discussed in Chapter 4. Such distortion can easily be demonstrated. A piece of inlay wax can easily be softened, bent into the shape of a horseshoe, and chilled in this position in cold water. It then is floated in a pan of water at room temperature, as in Figure 17–1A. After remaining in this position for several hours, the wax horseshoe opens. Figure 17–1B shows its appearance after 24 hours. The stick of wax has tried to return to its original shape.

The reason for this change in shape is relaxation of stresses induced when bending the wax. As can be noted (see Fig. 17–1A), the wax was stretched on the outer part of

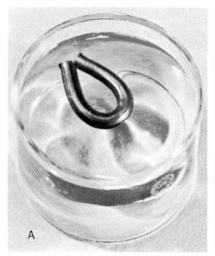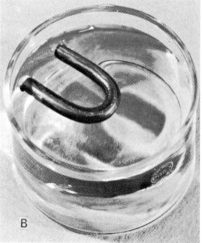

Figure 17–1. *A,* A piece of inlay wax is bent into the shape of a horseshoe and floated on water at room temperature. *B,* After 24 hours, the same wax appears as shown.

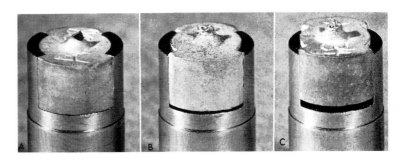

Figure 17–2. Effect of storage of the wax pattern on the fit of the casting. *A,* Casting made from a pattern invested immediately. *B,* Casting made from a pattern stored for 2 hours before investing. *C,* Casting made from a pattern stored for 12 hours before investing.

the horseshoe and compressed on the inner arch. This results in trapped stresses in the wax horseshoe. According to the theory of relaxation, in time the stresses will be released. Because the molecules of the upper arch are too far apart, they tend to move together, whereas the molecules on the lower arch tend to move apart. As a result, the wax tends to straighten out.

The stresses relax more rapidly when the temperature is increased. If the water in the bath is heated, relaxation may take place within a matter of minutes.

Such stresses are inadvertently introduced when the wax is softened, molded to the form of the cavity, and then carved. Given sufficient time, the pattern is likely to distort for the same reason as the stick of inlay wax in Figure 17–1.

Causes of Distortion

A number of factors may cause distortion. Although partially under the control of the operator, they cannot be entirely eliminated. If the wax is not at a uniform temperature when it is adapted to the cavity, for example, some parts of the wax pattern will contract more than others as it cools, and stresses are introduced. If the wax is not held under uniform pressure during cooling, some molecules will be compressed more than others. If wax has to be melted and added to the pattern, the added wax will introduce stresses during cooling. During the carving operation, some of the molecules of the wax

will undoubtedly be disturbed, and a stress will result.

Any change in the state of internal stress in the wax results in an accompanying change in strain and, thus, in distortion of the pattern.

A technique that minimizes the amount of carving and change in temperature as well as similar factors results in less subsequent relaxation and distortion of the pattern.

Most important is the rule to invest the pattern as soon as possible after it is finished. Once the pattern is surrounded by the hardened investment, no further distortion can occur. Remember that stress relaxation depends on time and temperature.

The possible effect of storing a wax pattern is shown in Figure 17–2. Note that the casting fits best when the pattern is invested immediately after it has been completed.

Wax distortion may appear to be relatively unimportant if the indirect technique is used and the pattern is stored on the die. The die confines the pattern and aids in preventing distortion. Relaxation of stress may still take place, however, in directions away from the die, such as the marginal areas or a surface that is not enclosed by the die. The margins of the wax pattern should be checked and adjusted as needed just before the pattern is removed from the die.

OBTAINING THE PATTERN

The wax should always be softened with dry heat and never in water. The lower melting constituents of the wax can dissolve or leach out and change its properties. The wax may become brittle and unmanageable.

If the wax is softened over a flame, this should be done with care. The safest method is to hold a stick of wax at some distance above the flame and then to rotate it rapidly until it softens. If the surface becomes shiny, the wax is too hot, and the outer layers are beginning to melt. It should not be placed directly in the flame because this procedure may volatilize some of the wax constituents.

After softening, the wax is kneaded with the fingers and pressed into the prepared cavity in the die and held under pressure, if possible, until it has hardened.

The die should be lubricated in some manner so that the wax does not stick to the stone. A number of commercial lubricating agents that provide ready release of the pattern are available. The film thickness of the agent should be a minimum; excess prevents adaptation of the wax to the die.

Melted wax may then be added in layers with a wax spatula or painted on with a camel's hair brush. If the die is for a full crown restoration, it may be dipped repeatedly into molten wax.

The prepared cavity should be overfilled, and the wax carved to the correct contour. When carving is done along the margin with the stone die, care should be taken not to abrade the surface of the die.

OTHER DENTAL WAXES

Other types of dental waxes are used for different purposes than the casting waxes described. The composition of each is adjusted for the particular clinical application. One of the most common is *baseplate* wax. Baseplate wax is used principally to establish the initial arch form in the construction of complete dentures. Supplied in 1- to 2-mm-thick red or pink sheets, the wax is

about 75 per cent paraffin or *ceresin*, with additions of *beeswax* and other resins or waxes.

ADA Specification no. 24 includes Types I, II, and III—designated as soft, medium, and hard. The differentiation from one to another is by the percentage of flow at room temperature, at mouth temperature, and at 45° C (113° F). The harder the wax, the less the flow at a given temperature. The difference in flow of the three types is advantageous in the particular usage.

As with casting wax patterns, residual stress is present within denture base wax from contouring and manipulating the wax. The finished denture pattern should be invested as soon as possible after completion.

Other waxes include the *sticky* waxes, which are tacky when melted but firm and brittle when cooled. These waxes are used to join and stabilize temporarily the components of a bridge before soldering or the pieces of a broken denture before the repair. The auxiliary is likely to use *boxing* wax for enclosing an impression before the plaster or stone cast is poured.

Selected Reading

Craig, R. G., Eick, J. D., and Peyton, F. A.: Strength properties of waxes at various temperatures and their practical application. J. Dent. Res. 46:300, 1967.

Baum, L., Phillips, R. W., and Lund, M. R.: Textbook of Operative Dentistry, 2nd ed. Philadelphia, W. B. Saunders Co., 1985.

McCrorie, J. W.: Some physical properties of dental modelling waxes and of their main constituents. J. Oral Rehabil. 1:29, 1974.

Steinbock, A. F.: An overview of dental waxes. Dental Lab News July, 1989, p. 50.

Reviewing the Chapter

1. What is the weak link in the cemented cast restoration?
2. Summarize the steps involved in the casting procedure.

3. Explain the difference between *direct* and *indirect* techniques.
4. List the materials used in the construction of a die. What are the advantages and disadvantages of each?
5. How are inlay waxes classified by the ADA Specification? How do they differ?
6. Discuss the components present in inlay waxes and the effect of each.
7. How does the flow of a Type I wax differ from that of a Type II wax at various temperatures? Explain the significance.
8. List the properties desired in an inlay wax.
9. Discuss the factors that influence distortion of the wax pattern and how these can be controlled. How does the phenomenon of *relaxation* enter into the matter?
10. Explain the technique of constructing the wax pattern and discuss cautionary factors to be exercised.
11. List other types of waxes used in dental procedures and how they are used.

CHAPTER 18

CASTING INVESTMENTS

GYPSUM-BONDED INVESTMENTS	**Thermal Expansion**
Composition	**Strength**
Purpose of the Investment	**Porosity**
Setting Time	**Care of Dental Investments**
Normal Setting Expansion	**OTHER TYPES OF INVESTMENTS**
Hygroscopic Setting Expansion	

After the wax pattern has been formed, a *sprue former* or *sprue pin* is attached. A sprue pin is a short metal, wax, or plastic rod that is attached to the pattern by melting the wax at the point of attachment. The pattern and sprue pin are then surrounded with the *casting investment*, which is mixed in the same manner as plaster or stone. After the investment hardens, the sprue former is removed and the wax eliminated. The molten metal is forced through an opening called the *sprue* or *ingate*—left when the sprue pin was removed—into the mold space left by the wax. These procedures are described in detail in Chapter 19.

Two types of dental casting investment—*gypsum-bonded* and *phosphate-bonded*—are used, depending on the alloy's melting range and individual preference. The gypsum-containing materials traditionally are used for conventional noble metal alloys. The phos-phate-bonded investments frequently are used with noble metal alloys but originally were designed for metal-ceramic restorations alloys.

Silica-bonded investment, a third type, is used principally in the casting of base metal alloys for large castings, primarily partial dentures. Because this type is used only in dental laboratories, it is not discussed further.

GYPSUM-BONDED INVESTMENTS

Investments can be viewed as composite structures composed of a matrix material called the *binder* and a filler called the *refractory*. Gypsum-bonded investments use gypsum as the binder. Many considerations presented are common to other investment types as well.

Composition

The essential ingredients are calcium sulfate hemihydrate (see Chapter 5) and silica. The hemihydrate constitutes about 30 to 45 per cent of the total content. The remainder of the investment consists mainly of silica (SiO_2) with small amounts of modifiers, such as accelerators, retarders, reducing agents, and thermal expansion regulators.

When the investment is mixed with water, the hemihydrate reacts as described in Chapter 5 to form dihydrate crystals, which bind the silica particles into a solid material.

Purpose of the Investment

An investment's primary function is to form the mold into which the molten metal is poured to make a casting. Silica strengthens the investment during elimination of the wax pattern as the investment is heated above the temperature at which the dihydrate reverts to the hemihydrate.

Silica also is included to enlarge the mold space into which the alloy is cast. Casting shrinkage of a noble metal alloy is discussed in Chapter 16. Before the metal is cast, the mold must be enlarged by an amount equal to the casting shrinkage of the alloy. Otherwise, the casting will be too small.

The casting investment is so compounded that the mold can be enlarged by normal setting expansion, by hygroscopic setting expansion, by thermal expansion, or by all three methods at once. The total expansion of the investment must be carefully controlled to obtain an accurately fitting cast restoration.

Setting Time

After the investment is mixed with water, sufficient time must be available for investing the wax pattern before the investment sets—usually in 9 to 18 minutes. The setting of investments, like other gypsum products, is accelerated by longer and/or more vigorous mixing. Increasing the water-powder (W/P) ratio slows the set.

Normal Setting Expansion

The setting expansion of a gypsum investment is caused by the outward thrust of the growing gypsum crystals. As each crystal grows, it pushes on the silica crystals, thereby multiplying the expansion. The mass tends to gain its strength slowly, so the outward thrust of the growing gypsum crystals meets less resistance, prolonging growth. The setting expansion of a mixture of silica and calcium sulfate hemihydrate, therefore, is greater than the setting of hemihydrate alone. Increasing the W/P ratio reduces the setting expansion.

Because the setting expansion of the investment aids in enlargement of the mold space, it should be accurately controlled. Its magnitude usually is between 0.3 and 0.6 per cent. Small adjustments in the W/P ratio commonly are used to adjust the setting expansion.

Hygroscopic Setting Expansion

If the investment is allowed to set in contact with additional water, the setting expansion is greatly increased, as shown in Figure 18–1. Curve A indicates the setting expansion obtained when the investment was allowed to set on wax paper. In curve B, the same investment was allowed to set on the wax paper under water. The setting expansion in curve A was 0.3 per cent, whereas it was 1.8 per cent when the investment set under water. The metal casting ring, used to contain the investment, tends to restrict the setting expansion. For this reason, the ring is lined with a cushion of cellulose or ceramic paper, which helps to offset the restriction from the ring.

To distinguish between the two setting expansions, the expansion obtained when the

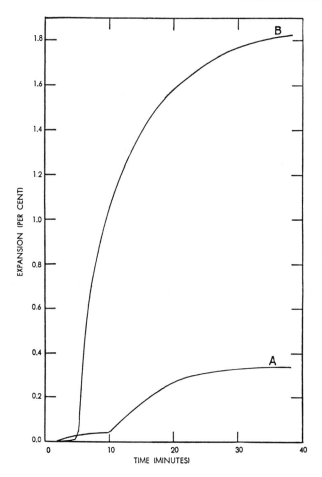

Figure 18-1. Curve *A*, normal setting expansion; curve *B*, hygroscopic setting expansion for the same investment.

investment sets without contact with water other than that used in the mix is called the *normal setting expansion*. The expansion obtained when the investment sets while exposed to additional water is designated the *hygroscopic setting expansion*.

The higher the silica content of the investment or the lower the W/P ratio, the greater is the hygroscopic expansion. Hygroscopic setting expansion can expand the mold sufficiently to compensate almost entirely for the casting shrinkage of a noble metal alloy.

Thermal Expansion

Thermal expansion of the investment also contributes to expansion of the mold space.

If gypsum alone is used for an investment, its contraction on heating is so great that it causes warpage and cracking. This adds to the casting shrinkage of the casting alloy rather than compensating for it. When the proper type of silica is added in a sufficient amount to the gypsum hemihydrate, however, the investment can be made to expand on heating.

Two types of silica are used, *quartz* and *cristobalite*. Both are the same chemical compound, silicon dioxide (SiO_2), but they have different space lattices. Both expand thermally but do so at different rates.

- When quartz is heated to 575° C (1070° F), its space lattice changes form and a marked expansion takes place.

- When cristobalite is heated, the change occurs between 200° and 270° C (390° and 518° F), and the expansion is greater than for quartz.

If either quartz or cristobalite is added to gypsum hemihydrate in the correct amount, the thermal shrinkage of the gypsum is compensated and a net thermal expansion results.

Dental investments often are classified as *quartz investments* or *cristobalite investments*. The more quartz or cristobalite in the investment, the greater is the thermal expansion. The W/P ratio also affects the thermal expansion: the lower the W/P ratio, the greater the thermal expansion.

The W/P ratio of the investment must be measured carefully. Although the water is measured by volume, the investment powder must be weighed—or preweighed packages used—to obtain the correct ratio.

Strength

The strength of an investment is important. The investment should be sufficiently strong that the mold will not be damaged when the molten alloy is forced into the mold.

The strength of an investment usually is measured under compressive stress. The compressive strength of an investment is increased according to the amount and type of gypsum present in the hardened product.

As with other gypsum products, the greater the W/P ratio, the lower the compressive strength. The investment may be heated as high as 700° C (1290° F) without greatly decreasing its compressive strength. The quartz or cristobalite acts as a *refractory*, which gives the investment strength at high temperatures. After the investment has cooled to room temperature, its strength is considerably reduced, presumably because of fine cracks that occur during cooling. For this reason, once the mold has been heated,

it should not be allowed to cool before casting.

Porosity

The molten alloy is forced into the mold through the sprue. To provide entry of the molten metal into the mold, the investment must be sufficiently porous for the air in the mold space to be forced out ahead of the metal. If the air is not eliminated, pressure builds up in the investment and prevents the molten metal from completely filling the mold space. An incomplete casting results. The greater the number of gypsum crystals present in the set investment, the lower the porosity. Therefore, the lower the hemihydrate content and/or the higher the W/P ratio used to make the mix, the more porous the investment.

Care of Dental Investments

Dental investments should be given the same care as a dental stone or plaster. If the investment is stored under conditions of high relative humidity, not only is the setting time altered, but also the setting expansion and hygroscopic expansion are affected. The investment should always be stored in airtight, moistureproof containers. During use, the container should be opened for as short a period as possible.

The ingredients in the investment may settle out according to their specific gravity under the normal vibration present in a dental laboratory. The container periodically should be shaken to maintain a homogeneous distribution of the various components.

OTHER TYPES OF INVESTMENTS

Gypsum investments cannot be used to cast alloys whose high melting range would result in fracture or surface breakdown of the investment. An example is the metal–ceramic restoration (see Fig. 16–3). Other types of investments are used in such cases. The most common of these, the phosphate-bonded investment, is composed of *refractory fillers* and a *binder*. The filler is silica, which provides high temperature strength and thermal expansion. The binder consists of magnesium oxide and a phosphate.

Phosphate investments may be mixed with water or a special liquid that contains silica suspensions (hydrocolloid sols), which increases both the setting and the thermal expansion. A mixture of water with the special liquid also can be used to "fine-tune" the total investment expansion.

Because the metal-ceramic and base metal alloys have higher melting temperatures than traditional noble metal alloys, their solidification contraction is greater, as mentioned in Chapter 16. This requires a greater total expansion in the investment. Phosphate-bonded investments are considerably stronger than gypsum-bonded materials, making it more difficult to remove the casting from the investment. The same principles involved in manipulation of gypsum-bonded investments, such as control of the liquid-powder ratio, also apply to these investments.

Phosphate investments are satisfactory for use with conventional noble metal alloys. Their chief disadvantage is the difficulty in recovering the casting from the investment. Chemical investment removers that are safe and effective are available for gypsum-bonded investments. These are not effective with phosphate investments. Phosphate investments can be dissolved only with hydrofluoric acid solutions. Use of these solutions is *not* advisable because of the risk of serious personal injury.

Selected Reading

Cooney, J. P., and Caputo, A. A.: Type III gold alloy complete crowns cast in a phosphate-bonded investment. J. Prosthet. Dent. 46:414, 1981.

Earnshaw, R.: The effect of casting ring liners on the potential expansion of a gypsum-bonded investment. J. Dent. Res. 67(11):1366, 1988.

Earnshaw, R.: The effects of additives on the thermal behavior of gypsum-bonded casting investments. Pt. 1. Aust. Dent. J. 20:27, 1975.

Finger, W., Jørgensen, K. D., and Ono, T.: Strength properties of some gypsum-bonded casting investments. Scand. J. Dent. Res. 88:155, 1980.

Jenkins, C. B. G., and Phillips, R. W.: An evaluation of five inlay investing techniques employed with different types of wax patterns. J. Prosthet. Dent. 25:211, 1971.

Jørgensen, K. D., and Okamoto, A.: Restraining factors affecting setting expansion of phosphate-bonded investments. Scand. J. Dent. Res. 94:178, 1986.

Junner, R. E., and Stevens, L.: Anisotropic setting expansion of phosphate-bonded investment. Aust. Dent. J. 31(6):434, 1986.

Mahler, D. B., and Ady, A. B.: An explanation for the hygroscopic setting expansion of dental gypsum products. J. Dent. Res. 39:578, 1960.

Mahler, D. B., and Ady, A. B.: The influence of various factors on the effective setting expansion of casting investments. J. Prosthet. Dent. 13:365, 1963.

Matsuya, S., and Yamane, M.: Decomposition of gypsum-bonded investments. J. Dent. Res. 60:1418, 1981.

Neiman, R., and Sarma, A. C.: Setting and thermal reactions of phosphate investments. J. Dent. Res. 9:1478, 1980.

Santos, J. F., and Ballester, R. Y.: Delayed hygroscopic expansion of phosphate-bonded investments. Dent. Mater. 3(4):165, 1987.

Verrett, R. G., and Duke, E. S.: The effect of sprue attachment design on castability and porosity. J. Prosthet. Dent. 61:418, 1989.

Reviewing the Chapter

1. Define *sprue, sprue former, ingate, investment, mold, inversion,* and *refractory.*
2. Describe the process of sprue attachment to the wax pattern.
3. What types of investments are used in dentistry? What is the purpose of an investment?
4. Give the compositions of a *gypsum-bonded investment* and a *phosphate-bonded investment.*
5. Explain the importance of a proper setting time of an investment. What factors influence it?

6. Describe what occurs to produce setting expansion of an investment.

7. What is the *magnitude of setting expansion*?

8. What is meant by *hygroscopic expansion*? How is that different from *normal setting expansion*?

9. Explain the purpose of the *ring liner*. What materials are used for ring liners?

10. Discuss the thermal expansion of a gypsum-bonded investment and the difference between a *quartz*- and a *cristobalite*-containing investment.

11. List the factors that influence (1) setting expansion, (2) hygroscopic expansion, and (3) thermal expansion.

12. What is the significance of having a high strength in an investment? List the factors that control the strength.

13. Discuss the role played by porosities in an investment as related to the casting process.

14. What precautions should be exercised in caring for an investment in terms of storage and dispensing?

15. What are the principal uses for phosphate- and silica-bonded investments?

16. What function does the "special liquid" play in the use of phosphate investments? How does it influence the properties of the investment?

CASTING THE INLAY OR CROWN

The fundamentals associated with the casting procedure are common to all types of dental investments and vary only slightly according to the type of alloy used. Although the following discussion focuses on gypsum investments and the traditional noble metal alloys, most of it is relevant to other types of investments and alloys.

PREPARATION FOR INVESTING

The Pattern

A typical *inlay casting ring*, shown in Figure 19–1, is a short length of metal or polymer tube. Its dimensions vary according to the size of the casting but average about 29 mm (1⅛ in) in diameter and 38 mm (1½ in) in height. Metal rings must be constructed of a material that will not be attacked by the investment. If the rings are to be left around the investment during burnout, they also must be constructed of a material that is not appreciably oxidized during heating. Polymer rings are removed before burnout.

The ring is lined with a layer of ceramic fiber or cellulose called the *ring liner*. The liner should be trimmed so that it ends 3.2 mm (⅛ in) short of each end of the ring, as can be seen in Figure 19–1. A more accurate casting is obtained when the casting ring is not completely lined.

The liner cushions the investment expansion, which is essential to offset the shrinkage that occurs as a molten alloy solidifies.

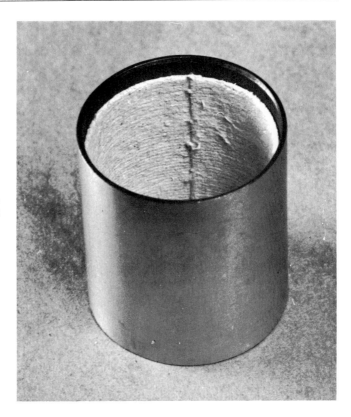

Figure 19-1. Typical casting ring with liner inserted. Note that the liner does not extend to the ends of the ring.

Thicker ring liners offer less restriction to expansion in the direction of the casting ring. Expandable or split casting rings, which do not require the use of a ring liner, have become popular. A better name for this flexible polymeric tube is *investing ring* because it must be removed from the investment before burnout.

The Sprue Former

The *sprue former* or *sprue pin* provides an exit way for the molten wax pattern and then, in turn, an access channel for the molten alloy to enter the mold after the wax has been eliminated. It usually is formed from wax or low-melting plastic, although sprue pins originally were metal and were removed before burnout.

A sprue former with a larger diameter is preferred to one with a smaller diameter. Premature solidification of the molten alloy before the mold is completely filled is less likely with the larger diameter. The sprue must be small enough, however, to be easily attached to the wax pattern without altering pattern details, such as margins or occlusal anatomy. The sprue former is attached to the pattern with a small drop of sticky wax heated only enough to ensure firm attachment.

The position of the sprue former attachment to the pattern usually is a matter of individual judgment coming from experience. The general rule is to attach the sprue former in a position in which the molten metal will reach all the mold areas farthest from the point of attachment of the sprue former simultaneously. In Figure 19–2, for example, the pattern is sprued on the proxi-

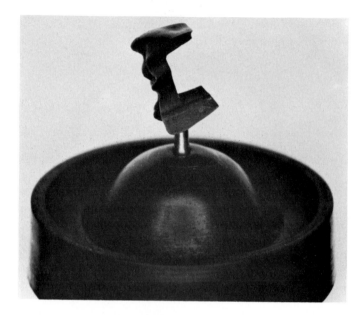

Figure 19-2. Sprue former attached to wax pattern and crucible former.

mal area so that the molten metal fills the mold beginning in the gingival area. The sprue should be attached also to the thickest section of the pattern, provided that this thickness does not exceed the sprue diameter.

The pattern is carefully lifted from the die by means of the sprue former. As shown in Figure 19-2, the free end of the sprue former is inserted in a *crucible former* or *sprue base*. The crucible former can be made of metal, rubber, or some type of plastic.

The distance from the extreme end of the pattern to the sprue base should be adjusted according to the length of the casting ring. When the casting ring is in position on the crucible former, the pattern should be about 6.4 mm (¼ in) below the top or open end of the ring (top of Fig. 19-2).

INVESTING

As noted in Chapter 18, the investment and water must be accurately proportioned, and the same precautions should be used in mixing the investment as described for mix-

ing plaster or stone. A variation of only 1 ml of water can alter the setting expansion significantly. Likewise, the manipulation of the investment and the smoothness of the surface of the casting are affected. Elimination of air from the mix is of even greater importance than when mixing dental stone or plaster. Air bubbles cling to the wax pattern, creating round nodules of metal on the surface of the casting.

Although investment may be hand-mixed, motor-driven mechanical mixers typically are used. The use of a machine that mixes the investment under vacuum is strongly encouraged. Devices also are available for both mixing and investing the pattern in a vacuum. After the investment is spatulated by hand or with a mechanical mixer, it is painted with a brush onto the pattern, the ring is placed over the crucible former, and the investment is flowed into the ring under vibration. A wetting agent can be applied to the pattern before investing to help prevent air bubbles on the surface. The wetting agent decreases the surface tension of the wax, causing the investment mix to spread smoothly over the wax surface. If such an agent is used, it should be applied thinly and dried before investing. The wetting agents also are referred to as *wax pattern cleaners.*

Vacuum Investing

Several types of vacuum investing equipment that both mix the investment and invest the pattern in a vacuum are available. One such device, shown in Figure 5–11, is being used for the mechanical mixing of plaster or stone under vacuum. This apparatus is also used for vacuum investing.

With this equipment, the following steps are used to invest the pattern automatically without the use of a brush:

1. Water is measured and placed in the mixing bowl supplied with the unit.
2. Investment powder is added to the water and spatulated by hand just enough to wet the powder.
3. Air is evacuated through a vacuum tube attached to the top of the mixing unit.
4. The casting ring assembly is attached to the top of the mixing unit with the open end of the ring opening into the mixing bowl.
5. During mixing, additional air is evacuated, reducing the possibility of bubble formation.
6. While still under vacuum, the investment is vibrated into the casting ring and over the wax pattern.

Although equally good results can be obtained with hand investing, the use of vacuum investing is more likely to ensure consistently smooth castings that are free of nodules from trapped air bubbles.

After investing is completed, subsequent treatment of the invested pattern depends on the casting technique to be used.

BURNOUT

After the investment has hardened, the crucible former is removed and the ring

placed in an electric furnace to eliminate the wax and thermally expand the mold space. The ring and invested pattern are heated slowly and uniformly to the temperature at which required thermal expansion of the investment is obtained, usually 650° C (1200° F). This temperature depends on the type of investment and whether a hygroscopic expansion technique is used.

Wax Elimination

As the temperature in the mold is increased, the wax melts, boils, and, finally, burns. When the temperature reaches 650° C (1200° F), the wax is entirely eliminated and the casting should be completed immediately, as described in a subsequent section. The total elapsed time for complete wax elimination should be about 1 hour. If a low-temperature burnout is used with a hygroscopic technique, the total burnout period may need to be extended to ensure complete wax elimination.

CASTING

Casting Machines

A casting machine forces the molten alloy into the mold under pressure. Almost any type of pressure can be used—air pressure, for example. In Figure 19–3, the casting ring is positioned with the crucible end up. The piston through which air pressure is applied is above the ring. The following process takes place in this type of casting machine:

1. The alloy is placed into the crucible and melted.
2. The piston is pushed downward into contact with the top of the ring, enclosing the molten alloy.
3. Air pressure is applied automatically, forcing the molten metal into the mold.
4. Optionally, a vacuum may be applied

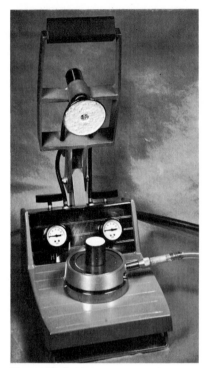

Figure 19–3. Air pressure casting machine.

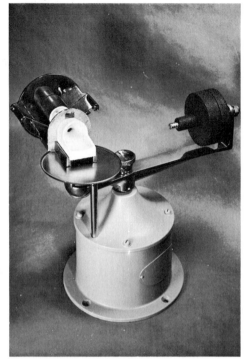

Figure 19–4. Centrifugal casting machine.

through the base beneath the casting ring, drawing the molten alloy into the mold.

5. A combination of air pressure and vacuum may also be used.

A more popular type of casting machine is shown in Figure 19–4. A strong spring is encased in the base of the casting machine that can be wound into tension by rotating the arms with the weights at one end and the casting ring at the other. The casting ring is in the cradle on the left arm. Just in front of the ring is a separate crucible in which the gold alloy is melted. When the spring is released, the two arms rotate rapidly, forcing the molten metal into the mold by centrifugal force.

Either type of casting machine produces clinically acceptable castings if the correct technique is used. If an air pressure machine is used, a minimum air pressure of 15 psi is

necessary. With a centrifugal machine, the arm must be wound a minimum of three or four turns, depending on the type of machine. The machine should rotate for 15 seconds—or until the metal has solidified.

The size of the sprue former varies with different machines. A sprue former larger than 1.7 mm, for example, should not be used for castings made by air pressure or by any other method in which the alloy is melted directly in the investment crucible. If too large a sprue pin is used, the molten alloy flows into the ingate under the force of gravity and solidifies prematurely while the metal in the crucible is still molten.

Centrifugal casting machines do not function as effectively with some of the low-density alternative casting alloys. The force with which the molten metal is driven into the mold is directly proportional to the weight of the molten metal. A metal with a density of 8.5 g/cm³ has only one half the casting force of a similar volume of traditional gold alloy with a density of 17.0 g/cm³.

Other types of casting machines melt the alloy automatically in an electrically heated furnace inside the casting machine, as opposed to manual heating with a torch.

Melting the Alloy

The alloy usually is supplied as small square sheets of metal. In most cases, the manufacturer's trade name and the type of alloy are stamped on the face of the metal squares. Two or three of these squares, or *ingots,* are placed in the crucible to one side of the sprue or ingate. When a crucible separate from the casting ring is used, the ingots may be leaned against the side of the crucible.

A flame fed by gas and compressed air usually is used. Accurate proportioning of the gas and air is important in obtaining the correct flame temperature and casting atmosphere. Exact details of such adjustment vary with the type of gas to be used. In general, the correct mixture produces a blue, nonluminous flame.

Depending on the intended use as well as base metal content, some dental casting alloys melt at temperatures beyond those attainable with a gas and air flame. A gas–oxygen mixture or an electrically heated casting machine is required. Metal-ceramic alloys must have melting temperatures well above the fusion temperature of the ceramic veneer and cannot be melted with a gas-air torch. The alloys commonly used for removable partial denture frameworks are base metal alloys with casting temperatures far beyond the limits of the gas-air torch.

Proper care must be given during the heating and eventual liquefying of a dental alloy before casting. An incorrectly adjusted torch can cause oxidation of the alloy during melting, volatilize necessary constituents of the alloy, or fail to completely liquefy the melt. Any error leads to an unacceptable casting.

After casting, the mold is removed from the casting machine. An excess of alloy, known as the *button,* is seen at the entrance to the mold.

The investment and casting within retain considerable heat. The rate at which cooling occurs can have a dramatic effect on the physical properties of the casting. Quenching in water should be avoided until the red glow disappears from the button.

Casting Time

Casting should be completed within 1 minute of the time the casting ring is removed from the furnace. Once the casting ring is removed from the furnace, it begins to cool, and the mold contracts thermally. The effect of the time lapse between the time the ring is removed from the furnace and the completion of the casting is shown in Figure 19–5. As can be noted, the fit of the casting is adequate only if the casting is completed within a time lapse of 1 minute.

Flux for Casting Procedure

Just before casting, *flux* usually is added to the molten metal to remove any oxides on the surface of the molten alloy. If the surface becomes dull through inadvertent misuse of the flame, it can be cleared easily by the use of a reducing flux. The flame then should be readjusted or repositioned immediately to prevent a recurrence of dulling.

Flux also tends to increase the fluidity of the molten alloy and should be used routinely regardless of whether used or new alloy is melted. The type of flux used depends on the alloy being cast. With metal-ceramic alloys, fluxes usually are not used.

Under no circumstances should the flux

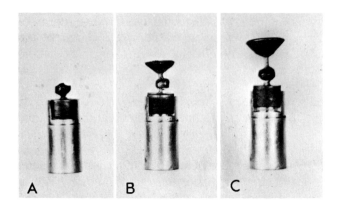

Figure 19–5. Experimental castings made after certain elapsed times after removal from the furnace. *A,* Casting completed in 1 minute. *B,* Casting completed in 2 minutes. *C,* Casting completed in 3 minutes. The castings were made with small diameter ingates, and the use of a reservoir was necessary, as shown. Note in *A* that the sprue parted from the casting because of the porosity between the reservoir and the button.

be used in excess. It may be carried into the mold with the molten metal and, thus, cause defects in the casting.

DEVESTING THE CASTING

If the hot casting ring is quenched in water, the violent reaction between gypsum and water may remove a considerable amount of investment from the casting. Quenching is not as effective with phosphate investments, which usually must be removed mechanically.

Sometimes a reducing agent is added to dental investments to produce a reducing atmosphere in the mold during casting. As a result, the casting may come out clean and bright; otherwise, its surface may be blackened by oxides.

Pickling

The casting is cleaned with a *pickling solution,* which can be made with a 50 per cent hydrochloric acid–water solution or sulfuric acid and water in the same proportion. Hydrochloric acid readily cleans remnants of investment from the casting. Its fumes, however, can corrode laboratory furnishings. If the acid solution is made in the laboratory, care should be taken to pour the concen-

trated acid into the water. Either acid must be handled with great care to avoid personal injury. Commercial pickling solutions also are available.

The cleaning procedure, known as *pickling,* involves the following steps:

1. The casting is placed in a porcelain dish or test tube.
2. Acid is poured over the casting.
3. The acid is heated to boiling, and the casting becomes bright and clean.
4. The acid then is poured off.
5. The casting—still in the pickling container—is washed in running water.

At no time should the casting be touched with bare metal tweezers or otherwise allowed to come into contact with a foreign metal while it is covered with acid because of the possible effect of electrolytic corrosion. Tweezers with rubber-insulated ends as well as plastic tweezers are available if the casting must be handled in acid.

Heating the casting and quenching it in the pickling acid, as sometimes is practiced, is not a desirable method. This can lead to warpage or melt a delicate margin.

The casting is then washed thoroughly and examined with a magnifying lens so that small nodules or irregularities may be detected and removed. If they are not removed, the casting probably will fail to seat in the cavity preparation.

DEFECTIVE DENTAL CASTINGS

With an understanding of the technical considerations and some practice, extremely accurate castings can be routinely obtained for dental use.

The most common causes for defective castings are included below.

- *Surface roughness.* Only a smooth wax pattern can produce a smooth casting and only if the investment is able to intimately surround the pattern. The use of a wetting agent on the wax pattern surface is recommended, but an excess can increase surface roughness. Without a wetting agent, the investment may trap air bubbles on the surface of the pattern. The air bubbles then are cast into spherical metal surface nodules, as shown in Figure 19–6.
- *Fins.* As shown in Figure 19–7, fins on the internal or external surface of a casting indicate that the investment has cracked before the casting was made.

Thermal shock is the most likely cause of investment cracking. Too rapid burnout or allowing the investment to completely dry out before burnout also can cause finning.
- *Porosity.* Visibly evident voids in a casting are probably due to *shrinkage porosity*. Improper sprue placement or inadequate diameter of the sprue results in solidification occurring in the sprue before the casting is solidified. If the ingate is blocked with frozen metal, solidification shrinkage cannot be compensated by flow of additional molten alloy. This results in porosity in the areas of the casting that solidify last. Turbulence as the molten metal flows into the mold also can result in a porous casting. Fragments of investment broken loose as the melt enters the mold cause solitary irregular casting voids.
- *Incomplete casting.* Incomplete elimination of the pattern during burnout results in a carbon residue–contaminated mold that does not fill completely. An incomplete casting with

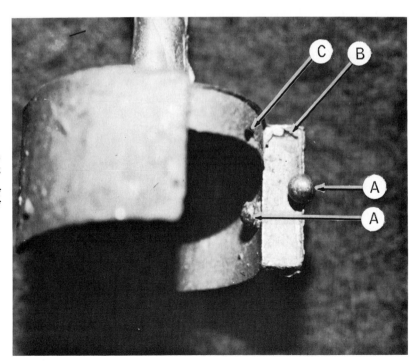

Figure 19–6. Surface roughness on an experimental casting caused by air bubbles *(A)*, water film *(B)*, and inclusion of foreign body *(C)*. (Courtesy of D. Vieira.)

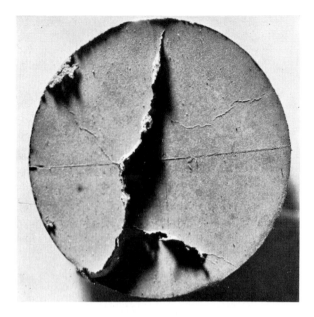

Figure 19-7. Fins caused by too rapid heating of the investment.

rounded, shiny edges as shown in Figure 19–8 usually indicates incomplete wax burnout. Underheating of the alloy also produces an incomplete casting. In the case of underheating, edges are rounded but not shiny. The button of an underheated alloy melt also shows a rounded base with rolled edges.

• *Warpage.* If a wax pattern is distorted before investing, there is no hope for clinical success. As described in Chapter 17, time- and temperature-dependent dimensional change of the wax pattern occurs after it is removed from the die. Completed patterns should be quickly and carefully invested to minimize distortion.

• *Overheating of investment.* When overheated, gypsum-bonded investments break down, releasing sulfur compounds. Sulfur contamination of a precious metal dental casting results in a restoration from which black surface deposits cannot be removed (Fig. 19–9).

The clinical life of a dental casting can be measured in decades if the preceding principles are carefully applied. Injudicious instrumentation of delicate margins or proximal contact areas can quickly transform a successful restoration into a clinical failure.

Removing, repairing, and reseating a damaged cemented restoration is virtually impossible. Occlusal wear or endodontic therapy may leave an opening that can be restored using gold foil, but other efforts at repair seldom produce long-term clinical success.

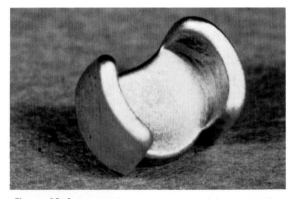

Figure 19-8. Incomplete casting caused by incomplete wax elimination. Note shiny appearance of margins.

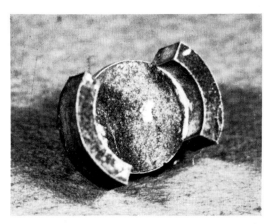

Figure 19-9. Roughness caused by overheating either the investment or the alloy. Also, the alloy may have been oxidized during melting.

Selected Reading

Baum L., Phillips, R. W., and Lund, M. R.: *Textbook of Operative Dentistry.* Philadelphia, W. B. Saunders Co., 1981, ch. 17.

Dootz, E. R., and Asgar, D.: Solidification patterns of single crowns and three-unit bridge castings. Quintessence Dent. Technol. 10:299, 1986.

Leinfelder, K. F., Fairhurst, C. W., and Ryge, G.: Porosities in dental castings. II. Effects of mold temperature, sprue size and dimension of wax pattern. J. Am. Dent. Assoc. 67:816, 1963.

Macasaet, A. A., and Dickson, G.: Some factors affecting the dimensional changes of gold-alloy investments. National Bureau of Standards Report 7574. Washington, D.C., U.S. Government Printing Office, June 30, 1962.

Naylor, W. P.: Spruing, investing, and casting techniques. Section 4. Non-gold base dental casting alloys: Vol. II. Porcelain-fused to metal alloys. USAF-SAM-TR-5, 1986, pp. 75-99.

Naylor, W. P., Moore, B. K., and Phillips, R. W.: A topographical assessment of casting ring liners using scanning electron microscopy (SEM). Quintessence Dent. Technol. 11:413, 1987.

Nelson, J. P., and Ollerman, R.: Suck-back porosity. Quintessence Dent. Technol. 1:61, 1976.

O'Brien, W. J., and Nielsen, J. P.: Decomposition of gypsum investments in the presence of carbon. J. Dent. Res. 28:541, 1959.

Phillips, R. W.: *Skinner's Science of Dental Materials,* 9th ed. Philadelphia, W. B. Saunders Co., 1991, ch. 23.

Skinner, E. W.: Casting technics for small castings. Dent. Clin. North Am. March 1965, pp. 225-239.

Tombasco, T., and Reilly, R. P.: A comparison of burn-out temperatures and their effects on elimination of plastic sprues. Trends and Techniques 4:36, 1987.

Vaidyanathan, T. K., Schulman, A., Nielsen, J. P., and Shalita, S.: Correlation between macroscopic porosity location and liquid metal pressure in centrifugal casting technique. J. Dent. Res. 60:59, 1981.

Reviewing the Chapter

1. What is meant by *shrinkage compensation*? What three methods are used?
2. Explain the difference between the *thermal expansion* and *hygroscopic expansion* techniques. How does one select the technique preferred?
3. Describe the purpose and correct use of the *liner* for the inlay ring.
4. Define *sprue former, crucible former,* and *reservoir button.*
5. What precautions should be exercised in the selection and use of the sprue former?
6. Sketch a cross section through an inlay ring containing an invested wax pattern and identify the various components.
7. Describe the hand investing of a wax pattern. What are the advantages of vacuum investing?
8. List and describe the use of different types of casting machines.
9. What is an effective technique for removing gypsum investment from a casting (*devesting* the casting)?
10. What is the composition and purpose of the flux?
11. Explain the *pickling* procedure.

DENTAL CERAMICS

As noted in Chapter 2, dental materials can be classified as either metals, polymers, or ceramics. This chapter presents the basic principles of ceramic materials and briefly discusses the dental materials that can be considered ceramics.

One of the first solid materials—if not the very first—that humans learned to use was a ceramic, natural stone. It was suitable for various uses because of the characteristic properties of a ceramic: hardness, strength, and resistance to thermal and chemical attack.

By definition, a *ceramic* is a material composed of a metal chemically bonded to a nonmetal. The chemical bond usually is an ionic bond, although some ceramics have covalent bonds. Ceramics owe many of their physical and chemical properties to the strength of the ionic bond. Solid ceramics usually are crystalline materials. The exception is the important group of materials known as glasses that are amorphous solids considered to be supercooled liquids.

Because ceramics, by definition, are composed of at least two chemical elements, the mechanism that provides for easy plastic deformation of metals—*dislocation motion*—does not occur readily in most ceramics at low temperatures. Although ceramics typically have high compressive strengths, they have very low ductility: they are brittle. They also have much lower tensile and bending strengths than their compressive strengths. As a result, their use in load-bearing structures must be carefully planned.

The use of ceramic materials in dentistry is not new. Porcelains, the type of ceramic most commonly used in dentistry, have a long history of use. The demand for aesthetic, tooth-colored restorative materials has led to increased use of the traditional porcelain materials as well as the development of new dental ceramic systems.

The inorganic component of natural tooth structure is a ceramic composed of the metal calcium bonded to the nonmetal phosphate and hydroxyl groups, forming crystalline calcium hydroxyapatite.

DENTAL PORCELAIN

There are two types of dental porcelain: one is used in the construction of artificial teeth and the second, in certain kinds of restorations. These latter restorations may be one of the following:

- An inlay made of porcelain
- A restoration that covers the entire crown of the tooth—referred to as a *jacket crown* (Fig. 20–1)
- A metal cast restoration on which a layer or veneer of porcelain is placed (see Fig. 16–3)
- A thin layer of porcelain covering only the facial surface of the tooth—called a *laminate veneer.*

Most porcelain restorations are fabricated by the dental technician. Because the manipulation of porcelain is a highly skilled art, the following discussion is confined to a summary of the general procedures used.

The basic principles of composition, chemistry, and technique are the same for all these porcelains. This discussion focuses on the type used in fabricating jacket crowns or veneers. As discussed in Chapter 16, the porcelain veneer is fused directly to the casting. Such a restoration is called a *metal-ceramic crown.* Basically, the technique involves the following steps:

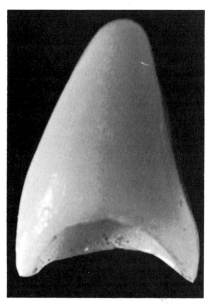

Figure 20–1. Porcelain jacket crown.

1. A finely powdered ceramic is mixed with water to form a paste.

2. The paste is formed into the desired shape and heated, or *fired,* at a high temperature.

3. The grains of powder fuse to form a ceramic material.

If the material is correctly compounded by the manufacturer and carefully handled during construction, the porcelain restoration will possess excellent aesthetics in the mouth.

Composition of Restorative Porcelain

Dental porcelains used for crowns and bridges are classified according to their *fusion temperature,* that is, the temperature to which the powder must be heated to form the ceramic restoration. The three varieties of porcelain recognized and the temperatures required for firing are as follows:

High-fusing   1300°–1370° C (2360°–2500° F)
Medium-fusing 1090°–1260° C (2000°–2300° F)
Low-fusing   870°–1065° C (1600°–1950° F)

The use of high-fusing porcelains normally is limited to the manufacture of denture teeth. Medium-fusing materials are used in all ceramic restorations. Low-fusing porcelains used in metal-ceramic restorations minimize the chance of damage to the cast metal substructure during porcelain firing.

Dental porcelains are essentially mixtures of feldspar and quartz. The feldspar melts first to provide a glassy matrix for the quartz, which is held in suspension within the matrix. The quartz thus acts as a filler to provide strength in this ceramic-ceramic composite. Part of the quartz may be replaced by alumina (Al_2O_3), resulting in what is referred to as *aluminous porcelain*. The alumina particles are much stronger than quartz and have a higher modulus of elasticity. The fracture of porcelain is caused by propagation of cracks through the structure; the alumina crystals obstruct the path of the cracks. The use of aluminous porcelain has markedly reduced the frequency of fracture in porcelain jackets.

Opaque porcelain is fused to a metal coping in a metal-ceramic restoration and is used as an initial layer to mask the color of the dentin or the color of the metal. The opaquing agent usually is zirconium oxide. This opaque layer then is covered with other layers of porcelains to simulate the color and translucency of different portions of the tooth, such as the gingival and incisal areas. Metallic oxide pigments are used for tinting and staining.

In the manufacturing of dental porcelains, the pure powdered components are fired together to form a fused mass called a *frit*. The frit is then ground to a fine powder for use in fabricating the crown.

Manipulation and Condensation

The general technique for constructing a porcelain jacket crown includes the following steps:

1. An impression of the prepared tooth is obtained, and a die is made.
2. A thin sheet of platinum, called the *matrix*, is adapted onto the die.
3. The porcelain powder is mixed with distilled water to form a thick paste.
4. Small portions of the paste are applied to the matrix until the desired shape of the crown has been built up.
5. Excess water is removed by blotting with some absorbent material in a process called *condensation*.
6. Different shades of porcelain are used to produce shades to match the natural teeth.

Firing

After condensation, the formed crown is placed in a porcelain furnace and fired. There are various stages in the firing. The temperature for each firing stage depends on the type of porcelain used.

The porosity in the porcelain jacket may be reduced by firing the porcelain in a vacuum rather than in air. The denser structure results in a more translucent material having a greater impact and compressive strength.

The surface of the restoration should be smooth when the restoration is placed in the mouth. Otherwise, food and other debris may adhere to it and lead to stain and discoloration. Soft tissue irritation also can result if the restoration contacts gingival tissue. After final adjustments are made in the mouth, a crown is fired to *glaze* its surface. At this stage, an extremely smooth translucent surface is formed, similar to tooth enamel in appearance.

If this glaze is removed, a rough and somewhat porous surface of porcelain is exposed. For this reason, care should be taken to protect the glaze. Porcelain restorations may be almost indistinguishable from natural teeth. During prophylaxis, care should be taken not to confuse the margins of a porcelain crown with calculus because the brittle margins of the crown can be damaged readily with a sharp instrument, such as a scaler.

Dental ceramics are resistant to chemical attack by most agents in the mouth. An exception is an acid solution that contains fluoride ion. Acidulated fluoride prophylaxis agents will etch dental ceramics in the time required for the treatment. If a patient has any ceramic restorations, the restorations must be protected with a coating of an agent such as petroleum jelly or cocoa butter during an acidulated fluoride treatment. A safer procedure is to not use this type of fluoride agent in these cases. The student also should remember that a ceramic filler is a major component of composite resin restorations. The dental restorative cements discussed in Chapter 21 are also ceramic materials. Either of these dental materials can be attacked by an acid fluoride treatment.

General Properties

The porcelain restoration possesses excellent aesthetic qualities. It is completely insoluble in mouth fluids and dimensionally stable after it has been fired. Porcelain is compatible with the soft tissues and resistant to abrasion.

The principal reason for the choice of porcelain as a restorative material is its aesthetic qualities in matching the adjacent tooth structure in translucence, color, and intensity. Color and the terminology associated with it are discussed in Chapter 4. Those matters are of primary importance to the dentist and technician in achieving the optimal cosmetic result. In addition to the differences in light reflection and refraction between the enamel and dentin, there may also be some dispersion, giving a color shade that varies in different teeth. The appearance of the teeth, therefore, may vary according to whether they are viewed in direct sunlight, reflected daylight, or fluorescent light (the phenomenon of *metamerism*).

Completely duplicating the optical properties of the natural dentition is impossible. The manufacturer, dentist, and technician, however, can approach the aesthetic characteristics sufficiently that the difference is apparent only to the trained eye. In the last analysis, the coloring of a porcelain restoration is an art more than an exact science. This dental material provides the best choice today for an aesthetic, long-lived restoration.

The tensile and shear strength of the fired porcelain is very low. The low tensile strength is partially the result of surface irregularities, such as microscopic cracks and porosities. Stress concentrates around these imperfections. When the restoration is placed in tension, the accumulated stress can easily exceed the stress required to cause cracks and other defects to grow until brittle fracture occurs.

Although dental porcelain probably has adequate compressive strength to resist masticatory forces, it readily fractures under the tensile stress that may be induced in the restoration. The dentist must design the porcelain restoration in such a manner that this shortcoming is minimized.

THE METAL-CERAMIC RESTORATION

The most serious limitation to the use of porcelain as a restorative material is its low tensile strength. This disadvantage is minimized if the porcelain is fused directly to a metal casting that fits the prepared tooth. With proper design, the porcelain is reinforced so that brittle fracture is avoided.

The metal-ceramic restoration is shown in Chapter 16. The special types of alloys used in its construction and the factors related to attaining an adequate bond of the porcelain to the metal are discussed. The reader is referred to that chapter for details.

The metal-ceramic restoration is a relatively recent addition to prosthodontics, even though the ancient Egyptians fused porcelain to metal. As early as 1887, restorations of dental porcelain bonded to metal were constructed. These original veneered dental restorations and prostheses were failures because of lack of proper fit, brittleness of the porcelain, and poor bonding of the porcelain to the metal. The materials and techniques have been so perfected that this type of restoration now is extremely popular. Its use far exceeds that of the all-porcelain jacket crown.

Applications of the Metal-Ceramic Restoration

Single metal-ceramic units are the most commonly used anterior restoration for full coverage. The alloy systems used have adequate strength for the construction of multiunit bridges, which are also common. The use of porcelain to cover the occlusal surface of posterior teeth is more controversial. Dental porcelains can result in accelerated wear of the opposing natural dentition. Some practitioners use porcelain to cover only the buccal surfaces of posterior teeth, leaving the occlusals in metal.

Despite its high degree of acceptance, the metal-ceramic restoration has a number of drawbacks.

- Its construction is time-consuming and expensive, involving the casting of a precision metal coping followed by porcelain buildup and contouring.
- Its aesthetics are limited by the total opacity of the metal core.
- The necessity for a minimum thickness of metal covered by enough porcelain to mask the metal outline may require excessive tooth reduction. This is particularly a problem in the younger patient who has relatively large pulp chambers and a minimal thickness of dentin.

The traditional all-ceramic jacket crown also has numerous liabilities.

- Its construction is even more technique-sensitive than the metal-ceramic crown.
- The adaptation of the jacket crown to the tooth often is poor.
- The lack of tensile and bending strength may compromise the longevity of these restorations.

Numerous attempts have been made to develop a ceramic material with improved strength and easier fabrication. The high-alumina-content porcelains resulted in much improved strengths for jacket crowns. Other recent advances in ceramic technology have led to even higher-strength dental porcelains. Some of these materials are considered comparable to the properties of a metal-ceramic restoration.

CASTABLE DENTAL CERAMICS

The lost wax casting technique used for fabricating metal restorations, as described in Chapter 19, has also been adapted to fabricating ceramic restorations.

In the system originally introduced, ceramic cores or copings were formed over which veneering porcelain was applied in a technique similar to the metal-ceramic crown. This resulted in a much stronger porcelain material with a somewhat more complicated technique than the metal-ceramic process. The technique involved the following steps:

1. A gypsum investment mold was formed, using the lost wax process.
2. The ceramic powder was injection-molded into that mold.
3. The "green" molded porcelain was retrieved from the mold and subjected to a complex, high-temperature firing cycle.

The resulting core material was opaque, and the system did not make a significant impact on the use of metal-ceramic crowns.

More recently, *castable ceramic materials* have been marketed. These are liquefied at very high temperatures and cast directly into an investment mold using equipment similar to that used to cast dental alloys. The material that has gained the most commercial acceptance, Dicor, is technically a *glass-crystalline ceramic composite*. Developed by Corning Glass Works, Dicor is chemically similar to the material used in Corning pyroceram cooking ware.

The material retrieved from the investment mold is a transparent glass with low strength and very brittle behavior (Fig. 20–2). This glass is "cerammed" at temperatures around 800° C, which results in the precipitation of a crystalline component. The resultant structure is acceptably translucent for dental use and has reasonable strength and fracture resistance. In this system, a complete crown is formed, not just a coping.

The final stage of processing involves the application of a thin layer of low fusing porcelain to color-match and characterize the restoration.

An example of a Dicor crown is shown in Figure 20–2. The resulting aesthetics are excellent and rival those of a conventional porcelain jacket crown. The crown usually is etched and silanated on its internal surface and then cemented with a dual-cured resin cement, as described in Chapter 22. The castable glass-ceramic material has received good acceptance for use in anterior restorations and finds some use for posterior crowns. The tensile and shear strengths of the material normally limit its use to single units.

CERAMIC VENEERS, INLAYS, AND ONLAYS

The preceding discussion focused on the use of ceramics for full-coverage crowns, either as single units or in bridges. The discovery that dental ceramics could be etched with an appropriate acid to form micromechanical retention has led to the acid-etched, resin-bonded ceramic restoration. These use the acid-etched retention to enamel used with the composite resin restorations, as dis-

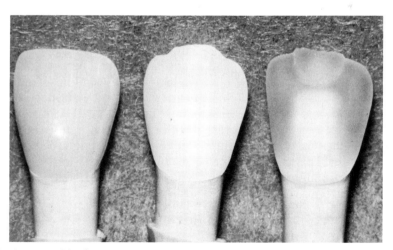

Figure 20–2. Dicor castable glass-ceramic restoration at three stages of preparation. *Right,* As removed from the casting investment, the material is entirely a glass and transparent. *Center,* After ceramming to form the glass-ceramic. *Left,* Finished restoration with stain and glaze porcelain applied. (From Phillips RW: *Skinner's Science of Dental Materials,* 9th ed. Philadelphia, WB Saunders Co., 1991.)

cussed in Chapter 10. Dentin bonding agents are used, particularly when any margins are in dentin.

This technique forms thin veneers, which are laminated over the facial surfaces of teeth—usually to mask discolored or malformed tooth structure. These ceramic laminate veneers have proved popular and are a more durable alternative to the direct placement composite or composite resin veneer.

Improved ceramic materials and techniques, such as the castable glass-ceramic, have also encouraged the use of resin-bonded ceramics for aesthetic inlays and onlays. These are more durable than posterior composites and have better aesthetics than dental amalgam but are considerably more difficult and expensive to fabricate and place. The concern previously mentioned about the wear on dentition opposing a porcelain occlusal surface is also a limitation.

COMPUTER-AIDED DESIGN AND MANUFACTURING—CAD-CAM

Although computer-aided design and manufacturing (CAD-CAM) is a manufacturing technology that is not limited to a specific dental material, its use has been particularly suggested for constructing ceramic restorations.

Briefly, this technology involves four steps.

1. The prepared tooth surfaces to which the restoration will be cemented are reproduced as a three-dimensional digitized image stored in a computer. This may be done directly by an optical scanning process in the mouth or mechanically from a stone die constructed from a dental impression.

2. The dentist or technician uses computer graphics to define the margins of the restoration and construct a three-dimensional image of the external surfaces of the restoration. Libraries containing data for den-

tal anatomy and computer images of the opposing dentition may be utilized to assist in this process. The end result is a digitized, computer image of the total restoration.

3. This image is used to control a multiaxis milling machine that uses conventional rotating dental abrasive tools (Chapter 25) to machine a block of material into a finished restoration.

4. Some hand machining and polishing are required to make final adjustments, and the restoration is colored and stained to match the adjacent dentition. It then is cemented in the mouth.

In principle, this procedure can be accomplished in a relatively short period of time—chairside construction of the restoration is possible with delivery in a single patient appointment. The manpower and skill required are considerably less than those required for a metal-ceramic or cast ceramic crown. The materials used can be any dental material that is reasonably machinable, including metals, machinable ceramics, and composite resins. The latter two are the most attractive because they can be used for aesthetic restorations.

Although commercial systems are available (Fig. 20–3), this technology is still under development and has not been widely used in dentistry. Existing hardware is expensive, and there are limits to the precision with which the restorations can be machined and the types of restoration that can be formed.

CAD-CAM in dentistry is a developing technology with considerable potential. The development of new dental materials specifically formulated for computer-controlled machining will probably result as CAD-CAM matures in its dental application. The applications of other types of machining, such as laser cutting, are also likely to occur. The 21st century will see increasing demands for aesthetic dental restorations with a concurrent demand for faster, more economical technology for delivery of this service.

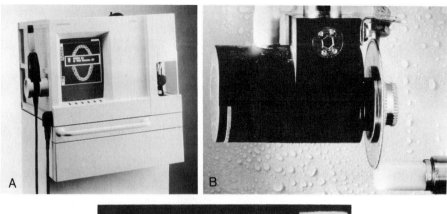

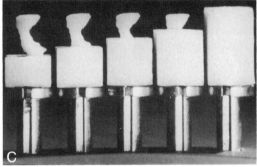

Figure 20-3. CEREC CAD-CAM system (Siemens Dental Products Division). *A,* The complete CEREC console—the intraoral scanner is on the left, computer monitor on the front, and automated milling machine on the right. *B,* Closeup of the computer-controlled milling machine using a water-cooled diamond disk to shape a block of ceramic into a three-surface inlay. *C,* Ceramic block at various stages of machining from start to finish.

Selected Reading

Brown, D. T., Munoz, C. A., Moore, B. K., and Goodacre, C. J.: Topical fluoride effect upon cerapearl and dicor castable ceramics. IADR Abs. 813, J. Dent. Res. (special issue) 67:214, 1988.

Dorsch, P.: Thermal compatibility of materials for porcelain-fused-to-metal (PFM) restorations. Ceramic Forum International/Ber. Dt. Keram. Ges. 59:1, 1982.

Duret F., Blouin, J. L., and Duret, B.: CAD-CAM in Dentistry. J. Am. Dent. Assoc. 117:715, 1988.

Fairhurst, C. S., Anusavice, K. J., Hashinger, D. T., et al.: Thermal expansion of dental alloys and porcelains. J. Biomed. Mater. Res. 14:435, 1980.

Jones, D. E.: Effects of topical fluoride preparations on glazed porcelain surfaces. J. Prosthet. Dent. 53:483, 1985.

Mörmann, W. H.: Chairside computer-generated ceramic restorations: The cerec third generation im-provements. Pract. Periodontics Aesthet. Dent. 4(7):9–16, 1992.

McLean, J. W.: *The Science and Art of Dental Ceramics,* Vol 1. Chicago, Quintessence Publ. Co., 1979.

McLean, J. W.: *The Science and Art of Dental Ceramics,* Vol. 2. Chicago, Quintessence Publ. Co., 1980.

McLean, J. W.: The metal-ceramic restoration. Dent. Clin. North Am. 27(4):747, 1983.

McLean, J. W., and Hughes, T. H.: The reinforcement of dental porcelain with ceramic oxides. Br. Dent. J. 119:251, 1965.

Phillips, R. W.: *Science of Dental Materials,* 9th ed. Philadelphia, W. B. Saunders Co., 1991, chs. 20, 26.

Preston, J. D. (Ed.): Perspectives in dental ceramics. Proc. 4th Int. Symposium on Ceramics. Chicago, Quintessence Publ. Co., 1988, p. 53.

Rekow, D.: Dental CAD-CAM systems, What is the state of the art? J. Am. Dent. Assoc. 122:42–48, 1991.

Wunderlich, R., and Yaman, P.: In vitro effect of topical

fluoride on dental porcelain. J. Prosthet. Dent. 55:385, 1986.

Reviewing the Chapter

1. What is a *ceramic material*?
2. Describe the mechanical properties of ceramic materials. Why is the ductility of these materials usually very low?
3. Name a natural ceramic dental material.
4. What are the man-made dental ceramics usually called?
5. Classify three types of dental porcelains by their firing temperatures and explain the dental applications of each type.
6. What are the basic chemical components of dental porcelain, and what is the function of each one?
7. What is a *jacket crown*? A *metal-ceramic crown*?
8. Briefly describe the construction of the jacket crown and the metal-ceramic crown.
9. List the clinical advantages and disadvantages of the jacket crown and the metal-ceramic crown.
10. Why are porcelain restorations *glazed* as part of the finishing procedure? How is this done? What precautions should be taken to protect the glaze?
11. How can a fluoride prophylaxis treatment pose a risk to a ceramic restoration? What other types of restoration can this procedure harm? How can these restorations be protected?
12. What is a *castable ceramic*? Name one commercial product.
13. Describe the construction of a glass-ceramic crown.
14. What are the clinical advantages and disadvantages of a castable glass-ceramic restoration?
15. What is CAD-CAM? Why is this topic included in this chapter?
16. Describe the technique for constructing a dental restoration using CAD-CAM with a ceramic material.
17. What are the advantages of CAD-CAM compared with the techniques for construction of conventional jacket crowns, metal-ceramic crowns, and castable glass-ceramic crowns?
18. Describe the properties of the casting alloys used for metal-ceramic restorations (Chapter 16).

DENTAL CEMENTS: Restorative Materials

Dental cements are relatively low-strength materials that are used extensively in dentistry when strength is not the prime consideration. With a few exceptions, they do not actually form adhesive bonds to enamel or dentin. Except for the resin cements, they dissolve and erode in oral fluids with time. Such defects are likely to reduce their permanency.

Despite these shortcomings, they possess

many desirable characteristics and are used in 40 to 60 per cent of all restorative procedures.

Dental cements are used in the following ways:

- As permanent, intermediate, and temporary restorations
- As luting cements for indirect restorations and orthodontic bands
- As thermal insulators under metallic restorations (bases)
- As pulp-capping agents and cavity liners
- As root canal sealants
- As periodontal packing or bandages

Because the chemical and physical properties of these materials leave much to be desired, correct manipulation is essential for optimal clinical performance.

CLASSIFICATION OF DENTAL CEMENTS

Dental cements are classified according to composition, as presented in Table 21–1.

Except for calcium hydroxide and resin materials, the setting reactions are typical acid–base reactions that form a more or less insoluble salt. The liquid component acts as the acid and the powder, as the base. When mixed together, the acid and base react to form salts, forming the matrix that bonds the mass together as the cement hardens.

Overview of Dental Cements

Table 21–1 shows that many cements are designed to perform multiple tasks. In these instances, the basic formulations are modified to provide handling characteristics and properties appropriate for the particular use. For this reason, the American Dental Association (ADA) Specifications for the various cements further classify certain cements as Type I, Type II, Type III, and so on based on their properties and, hence, their intended use. A Type I *zinc phosphate cement* is a fine-grain cement recommended for ce-

TABLE 21–1. Classification and Uses of Dental Cements

Cement	Principal Uses	Secondary Uses
Zinc phosphate	Luting agent for restorations and orthodontic appliances	Intermediate restorations; thermal insulating bases
Zinc oxide–eugenol	Temporary and intermediate restorations; temporary and permanent luting agent for restorations; thermal insulating bases; cavity liner; pulp capping	Root canal restorations; periodontic bandage
Polycarboxylate	Luting agent for restorations; thermal insulating bases	Luting agent for orthodontic appliances; intermediate restorations
Silicate	Anterior restorations	
Silicophosphate	Luting agent for restorations	Intermediate restorations; luting agent for orthodontic appliances
Glass ionomer	Anterior restorations; luting agent for restorations and orthodontic appliances; cavity liners	Pit and fissure sealant; thermal insulating bases
Metal-modified glass ionomers	Conservative posterior restorations; core buildups	
Resin	Luting agent for restorations and orthodontic appliances	Temporary restorations
Calcium hydroxide	Pulp-capping agent; thermal insulating bases	

mentation of precision castings. Type II cements are for all other uses—for example, thermal-insulating bases and cementation of orthodontic bands. The requirements for Type I and Type II cements differ: Type I cements must be able to form a thinner film.

Historically, zinc phosphate cement has been the permanent luting cement of choice. It was used almost universally until the development of polycarboxylate, glass ionomer, and improved resin cements.

As discussed in Chapter 2, when the thickness of remaining dentin on the floor of the prepared cavity approaches the pulp, a layer of cement—called a *cement base*—is used to replace the lost dentin and to protect the pulp against mechanical and thermal trauma. Zinc phosphate cement is an excellent thermal insulator with a thermal conductivity in the same range as dentin. The cement base functions as a dentin replacement material in this application.

Different types of *zinc silicophosphate* cement also are available, including a translucent cement used for cast restorations. Its optical properties make it particularly useful for cementing porcelain jacket crowns.

Zinc oxide–eugenol cements are popular as base materials and liners and for temporary and intermediate restorations. Their most outstanding feature is their palliative effect on the pulp. They also are good thermal insulators.

Polycarboxylate cements develop chemical adhesion to tooth structure. Such cements are used primarily as luting agents for cast restorations. Because their biological characteristics are comparable to zinc oxide–eugenol cement, they also are used frequently as a base material.

Resin cements are used extensively for direct attachment of orthodontic brackets and in the acid-etch resin bonded-bridge technique. They also are used in luting aesthetic veneers to anterior teeth and cementing ceramic restorations and composite resin inlays.

Silicate is a translucent cement that for many years was used for the direct restorations of anterior teeth. The cement, however, is a pulpal irritant and gradually deteriorates in the oral environment. In time, silicate restorations stain, craze, and erode. Composite resins and glass ionomer cements have replaced silicate for aesthetic restorations.

The newest cement system is the *glass ionomer*, a translucent cement. Glass ionomer cements are designated as Types I, II, and III.

- Type I glass ionomer cement is a luting cement for metal and ceramic restorations.
- Type II glass ionomer cement is used in the restoration of anterior teeth. It is similar to polycarboxylate cement in its potential to bond chemically to tooth structure. Because of its adhesive properties, glass ionomer cement is well suited for restoration of gingival erosion lesions without the need of a retentive cavity preparation.
- Type III is designated for uses such as liners and dentin bonding agents.

A group of cements in Table 21–1 is described as *metal-modified glass ionomers*. These materials were developed in an effort to upgrade the mechanical properties of the glass ionomer cement to permit it to serve in stress-bearing locations.

Calcium hydroxide materials are used for pulp capping, liners, and bases. They are not used for restorations or as luting cements.

With most cements, the manipulation of the material is critical. When the powder and liquid are mixed, the manufacturing process is continued by the person who mixes the cement. The correct procedure must be followed for optimum properties to be achieved.

CEMENTS FOR RESTORATIONS

Silicate Cement

Although *silicate cement* is not in general use today, discussion of the material is warranted because this material has demonstrated a unique anticariogenic action, with a well-explained mechanism. Glass ionomer cement also is based, to a certain extent, on the silicate cement.

Composition and Chemistry

Silicate cement is a powder–liquid system. The powder is a finely ground ceramic (glass) that is acid-soluble. It is composed of silica (SiO_2), alumina (Al_2O_3), lime (CaO), and fluoride salts, such as cryolite (Na_3AlF_6) or calcium fluoride (CaF_2). The ingredients are melted together at high temperature to form the glass. The fluoride component is called a *flux* because it melts first and dissolves the other components. The fluoride content of the cement powder usually ranges from 12 to 15 per cent.

The liquid is a solution of phosphoric acid in water. When the powder and liquid are mixed together, the following process takes place:

- The phosphoric acid attacks the surface of the glass particles.
- This forms reaction products that serve as a matrix to bind the remaining particles.
- The cement sets.

The major constituent of the matrix is aluminum phosphate with small amounts of other phosphates. Fluoride salts are dispersed in the matrix but are not part of its structure. In an aqueous environment, the fluoride leaches from the cement.

The major weaknesses of silicate cement are its vulnerability to degradation in the oral environment and its irritating effect on the pulp. Compared with other cements, silicate cement is ranked as a severe pulpal irritant. Its most advantageous feature is its anticariogenic activity.

Anticariogenic Action

The incidence of secondary (recurrent) caries around silicate restorations was mark-

edly less than that around other restorative materials in use. A silicate restoration may undergo marginal leakage and even partially disintegrate, but secondary caries adjacent to the restoration seldom was seen.

This unique anticariogenic property seems to be related to the presence of fluoride. Fluoride in small amounts is slowly dissolved or leached from the silicate cement. The amount of fluoride leached from a silicate cement over a 30-day period is plotted in the graph in Figure 21–1. The fluoride released from the cement apparently reacts with the surrounding tooth structure and decreases its acid solubility.

This reaction is shown in Table 21–2 where the effects on adjacent enamel of fluoride-free and fluoride-containing silicate restorations are compared. There is a marked increase in the fluoride content and a subsequent decrease in the solubility of enamel in contact with the fluoride-containing silicate. There was no increase in the fluoride content of enamel in contact with

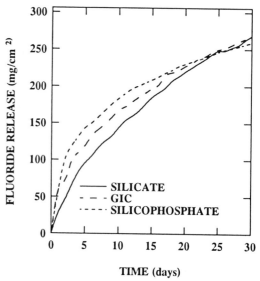

Figure 21–1. Fluoride release from three dental cements.

TABLE 21-2. Changes in F⁻ Content and Acid Solubility of Tooth Enamel Adjacent to Cement Restorations

Cement	Percentage of Change in F⁻ Content	Percentage of Change in Acid Solubility
Silicate (without F)	0	+20
Silicate (with F)	3500	−40
Zinc silicophosphate	5000	−50
Glass ionomer	3000	−30

the fluoride-free cement and no decrease in its solubility.

In essence, the silicate restoration provides a continuous topical application of fluoride to the cavity walls and to the surrounding tooth structure. The decrease in the solubility of the enamel increases its resistance to acid attack in the caries process.

A second effect of the fluoride appears to be that the small amount of fluoride continually released at the surface of the restoration and the cement-tooth interface serves as an enzyme inhibitor, preventing bacterial metabolism of the constituents of plaque. It thereby aids in reducing microbial activity, acid production, and caries.

The question arises as to the length of time the fluoride in these cements is available. Research has shown that after 1 year, measurable amounts of fluoride still are being released from cement. It seems likely that this leaching of the fluoride persists throughout the life of the restoration, thus affording a continuous protection from caries.

Identification of the anticariogenic action of silicate cement has led to attempts to incorporate fluorides into other restorative materials, such as amalgam, resins, and other cements. This research sought to incorporate anticariogenic activity through a slow and continuous release of fluoride without degradation of the physical and mechanical properties of the materials. With the exception of glass ionomer cements, these efforts have not met with great success.

Research continues—particularly in the area of composite resin—to seek a means of incorporating effective anticariogenic action.

Glass Ionomer Cement—Type II

Glass ionomer is the generic name for this cement because the setting mechanism and the adhesive bond to the tooth structure involve ionic bonds. The cement, often abbreviated GIC, also is referred to as *polyalkenoate cement.*

Many advances have recently been made in dental materials, including composite resins, bonding techniques, and casting alloys. None has had a greater impact on restorative dentistry than the glass ionomer system.

The basic formulation of glass ionomer cement has been modified to provide characteristics suitable for a variety of uses. The discussion in this chapter focuses on the Type II glass ionomers intended for use in dental restorations. Examples of two commercial Type II glass ionomer cements are shown in Figure 21-2.

The Type II glass ionomer cement is used for aesthetic restorations in anterior teeth. It is recommended for restoring Class III and Class V cavities. Its ability to chemically bond to both enamel and dentin makes it particularly applicable for these restorations as well as for restoring erosion lesions in the gingival area. The retention provided by the adhesive property eliminates or minimizes the need for mechanical retention and cavity preparation other than the removal of caries. As discussed in Chapter 10, treatment of lesions with composite resins relies on acid etching of enamel margins and the use of dentin bonding agents when margins are located in dentin or cementum. Glass ionomer cement is *not* recommended for restoration of the incisal portion of the tooth (Class IV) or for Class II cavities in posterior teeth or other high stress-bearing areas.

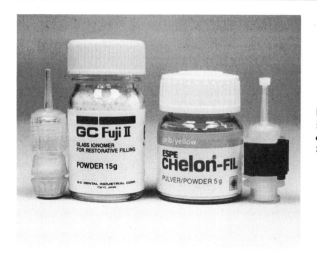

Figure 21-2. Representative Type II restorative glass ionomer cements. (From Phillips RW: *Skinner's Science of Dental Materials,* 9th ed. Philadelphia, WB Saunders Co, 1991.)

Composition and Chemistry

Glass ionomer cement powder is an acid-soluble calcium fluoroaluminosilicate glass that is similar in composition to silicate cement powder.

Most glass ionomer cement liquids are aqueous solutions of polyacrylic acid and copolymers with other polyalkenoic acids such as maleic and itaconic. The liquid also contains tartaric acid, which regulates working and setting time. The water content of the liquid is important to the reaction, so the liquids must be protected from water loss or gain.

Some manufacturers freeze-dry the poly-acid copolymer and combine that powder with the glass powder component. In this case, the liquid is water or a water solution of tartaric acid. When the cement powder is mixed with water, the polyacid dissolves to form a liquid acid, and the setting reaction proceeds by the same chemistry as powder–liquid acid systems. These cements often are referred to as "water-settable" cements.

When the glass powder is mixed with the polyacid liquid, the surface of the glass particles is attacked. Calcium and aluminum ions are freed to react to form calcium and aluminum polysalts. The new salts form a matrix surrounding the unattacked glass. The residual glass powder particles in the polysalt matrix are visible in the micrograph of a set glass ionomer cement (Fig. 21–3).

The setting reaction occurs in two steps. The calcium salts form first and are responsible for the initial hardening of the cement. The aluminum salts form slowly over a number of hours and give the cement its ultimate properties and final set. Although the material appears to be set shortly after insertion in the cavity, maximal properties and resistance to the oral environment are not developed for 24 hours or longer.

When the acid attacks the glass, fluorides also are freed from the surface of the particles, along with calcium and aluminum. Just as with silicate cement, fluoride products are dispersed throughout the matrix. These are *not* part of the structural matrix that holds the set cement together.

Light-activated glass ionomer formulations were first introduced for use as Type III liners, but Type II versions are appearing on the market. These contain copolymers of resin groups like those described in Chapters 9 and 10 with polyacrylic-type acids. The goal is to capture the best qualities of both

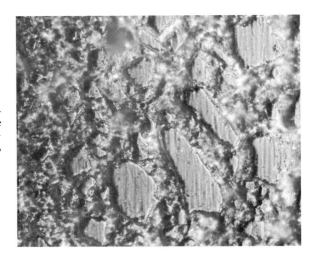

Figure 21–3. Micrograph of a set glass ionomer cement showing powder particles surrounded by the matrix. (From Phillips RW: *Skinner's Science of Dental Materials,* 9th ed. Philadelphia, WB Saunders Co, 1991.)

materials. The basic composition and chemistry of these light-activated glass ionomers is discussed with the liner materials.

Mechanism of Adhesion

Adhesion of glass ionomer cement to tooth structure results primarily from an ionic reaction between the polyacid and the calcium in the tooth structure with the formation of calcium polysalts. The adhesion mechanism is further described in the section on polycarboxylate cement in Chapter 22. The bond to enamel is stronger than the bond to dentin. This is not surprising because enamel has a higher inorganic content (more calcium) and its surface is not interrupted by dentinal tubules.

Properties

The properties of typical Type II glass ionomer cements are listed in Table 21–3. The compressive strength and hardness are somewhat lower than those of a silicate cement. The compressive strength of glass ionomer cement is about one third that of posterior composite resin. The fracture

TABLE 21–3. Properties of Cement Restorative Materials

	Silicate	Glass Ionomer (Type II)	Metal-Modified Glass Ionomer (Cermet)
Compressive strength (24 h)			
MPa	180	150	150
psi	26,000	22,000	22,000
Diametral tensile strength (24 h)			
MPa	3.5	6.6	6.7
psi	500	960	970
Hardness (KHN)	70	48	39
Pulp response	Severe	Mild	Mild
Anticariogenic	Yes	Yes	Yes
Solubility (ADA test)	0.7	0.4	—

toughness is only 25 to 30 per cent of that of composite resin and 10 to 25 per cent of that of amalgam.

This low fracture toughness characterizes glass ionomer cement as a brittle material. The cement is extremely vulnerable to occlusal wear by opposing teeth. This is shown in Table 21–4, which presents the results of laboratory tests conducted to determine the amounts of various materials that were worn away by rotating them against a cylinder of synthetic enamel (hydroxyapatite). Under this test, the volume of glass ionomer cement worn away is 15 times that of a composite resin and 30 times that of amalgam. This is why glass ionomer cement is not recommended for restorations that are subjected to high stress or wear by opposing teeth.

Glass ionomer cement's 24-hour solubility in distilled water is in the same range as that of silicate. As discussed in Chapter 22, the high initial solubility is probably due to the slow setting reaction because the rate of dissolution decreases markedly with time. Tests conducted in the oral cavity indicate that glass ionomer luting cements rank high in resistance to degradation compared with most other cements.

Anticariogenic and Biological Properties

Considerable evidence indicates that glass ionomer cements possess the same anticar-iogenic properties as silicates. As shown in Figure 21–1, the amount of fluoride released from a typical Type II glass ionomer cement is comparable to that released from a silicate cement. Likewise, the enamel adjacent to the restoration (see Table 21–2) exhibits a comparable uptake of fluoride and an increase in resistance to acid attack.

On the basis of years of experience with silicate cement, it can be assumed that glass ionomer cements would inhibit caries. A survey of 1700 glass ionomer restorations in service for 2 to 7 years reports only one instance of secondary caries associated with those restorations. In Class V studies of eroded-lesion restorations, recurrent caries seldom are reported with glass ionomer cement, even in cases where the restorations have been partially lost.

Histological studies indicate that Type II glass ionomer cements are "relatively" biocompatible. They produce slightly more pulp reaction than zinc oxide–eugenol but less than that produced by zinc phosphate cements. As a safety precaution, a small amount of calcium hydroxide preparation should be placed in deep areas of the cavity before restoration with glass ionomer cement.

Manipulation

As with most materials, manipulation of the glass ionomer cement governs, to a large degree, its properties and, ultimately, its clinical performance.

SURFACE TREATMENT. As noted in Chapter 10, clean surfaces are essential to encourage adhesion. The presence of a smear layer on the cut tooth surface after cavity preparation was also discussed. This layer of debris acts as a barrier, preventing contact between the tooth structure and the potential adhesive. Thus, in the Type III or Type V cavity, the smear layer should be removed from the cut dentin to achieve the strongest adhesive bond.

TABLE 21–4. Material Loss of Restorative Materials in Simulated Occlusal Wear

Material	Volume Loss (mm³)*
Amalgam	0.2
Composite resin	0.4
Glass Ionomer	6.0
Cermet glass ionomer	0.3

*Material lost in sliding wear against a synthetic hydroxyapatite cylinder.

The aim in smear layer removal is to remove the debris from the tooth structure while leaving the dentinal tubules occluded by collagen plugs so that they can act as a barrier to fluid transfer into or out of the dentin.

An efficient cleansing method is to apply a 10 per cent solution of polyacrylic to the cut dentin surface for 10 to 15 seconds, followed by a 30-second rinse with water. A cut dentin surface with intact smear layer and one after a 10-second treatment with 10 per cent polyacrylic acid is shown in Figure 21–4. The smear layer is removed from the dentin, but the tubules remain plugged. Deep areas in the preparation should be protected by calcium hydroxide before treatment by the polyacrylic acid. Erosion lesions

are cleaned with pumice followed by a 5-second treatment with polyacrylic acid.

After the cavity preparation has been conditioned (treated with the polyacrylic acid) and rinsed, it is dried but not desiccated. There should be no contamination of the conditioned surface with blood or saliva.

DELIVERY SYSTEMS. As shown in Figure 21–2, the cements are supplied by manufacturers in bulk form, bottles of powder and liquid, or in preproportioned capsules. The latter are similar to the preproportioned amalgam capsules described in Chapter 14 and contain both the cement powder and the liquid.

When the bulk form of the cement is used, it should be dispensed in accordance with the manufacturer's recommended powder-

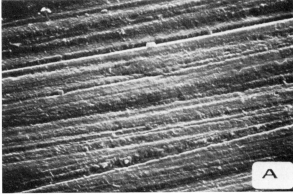

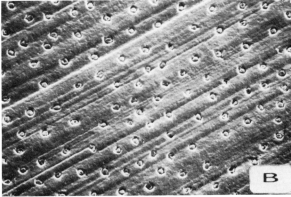

Figure 21–4. *A,* **Cut dentin surface showing presence of the smear layer.** *B,* **After cleansing with poly-acrylic acid, the smear layer is removed, yet tubules remain plugged. (From Phillips RW:** *Skinner's Science of Dental Materials,* **9th ed. Philadelphia, WB Saunders Co, 1991.)**

liquid ratio. This is in the range of 3:1 by weight. A reduction in the amount of powder in the mix reduces the properties of the cement and increases its acidity so that it is more likely to be an irritant.

MIXING. Reducing the temperature of the mixing slab slows the setting reaction. This enables the optimum amount of powder to be incorporated while the mix retains its plasticity. The mix must be plastic for good adaptation and adhesion to the walls of the cavity.

Although disposable, nonabsorbent paper pads are convenient for mixing, a glass slab is preferred. It is easier to cool and remains cold for a longer period. The glass slab may be chilled under cool water or in a refrigerator, but the surface should be dried before use. The slab should not be cooled below the temperature at which moisture condenses on the surface.

If the liquid contains polyacid, the bottle should not be stored in a refrigerator—the liquid will become very viscous.

The following steps are required to hand-mix the cement:

1. The liquid is dispensed onto the slab *just before* the mix is to be started. Prolonged exposure to the air alters the acid-water ratio of the liquid.

2. The powder is dispensed onto the slab and divided into two or three parts.

3. A stiff spatula is used to rapidly incorporate each into the mix. The total mixing time should not exceed 45 seconds.

4. The cement must be immediately inserted into the cavity.

At the time of its insertion, the cement must have a glossy appearance. A shiny surface indicates the presence of free polyacid not yet consumed by the setting reaction. This free acid reacts with the calcium in the tooth to form the adhesive bond.

If mixing is prolonged, a dull surface develops, indicating that little free polyacid re-

mains to bond with the calcium of the tooth. This precaution applies to all polyacid cements. The correct appearance of a polycarboxylate mix is shown in Chapter 22 (see Fig. 22–10).

Preproportioned capsules are mixed in an amalgamator. In making the mix mechanically, the amalgamator must be operated at high speed. Note in Figure 21–2 that the capsules have nozzles for direct injection of the mix into the cavity.

Capsulated mechanical mixing has several advantages:

- The mixing time is reduced.
- The delivery system is convenient.
- The dentist has more consistent control of the powder-liquid ratio and the degree of mixing.

Disadvantages are that the size of the mix cannot be adjusted to provide the amount needed for a specific task and that cement color cannot be matched by mixing powders of different shades.

PLACEMENT. The mixed cement is either "packed" by means of a plastic instrument or injected into the cavity. Immediately after placement, the dentist applies a preshaped matrix. The matrix provides optimal contour, so that minimal finishing is required.

The most important function of the matrix is to protect the setting cement from the environment during the initial set. Glass ionomer cements are extremely vulnerable to loss of water by exposure to air and to gain of water when exposed to moisture before the setting reaction has been completed. The matrix provides protection from both. The matrix is left in place for at least 5 minutes—or for the time suggested for the particular product.

On removal of the matrix, the surface *immediately* must be protected while the excess material is trimmed from the margins. The varnish supplied by the manufacturer can be used or an unfilled, light-activated resin bond agent can be applied.

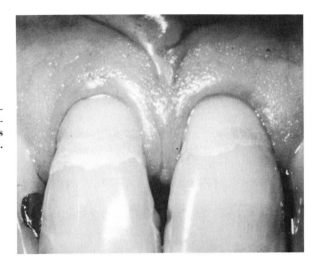

Figure 21-5. Crazed and chalky surface on glass ionomer restoration resulting from inadequate protection of the cement during maturation. (From Phillips RW: *Skinner's Science of Dental Materials*, 9th ed. Philadelphia, WB Saunders Co, 1991.)

If further finishing is needed, it is delayed for at least 24 hours. With some of the faster-setting cements, finishing times of as little as 10 minutes are suggested.

Before dismissing the patient, the restoration must again be coated with a protective agent. Finishing exposes the cement, which then is vulnerable to the environment until it reaches full maturity.

If the correct procedures are not followed, a chalky or crazed surface, as shown in Figure 21–5, results.

If the correct manipulative procedures are followed, glass ionomer cement can provide a durable and aesthetic restoration as illustrated by the restorations shown in Figure 21–6.

SUMMARY. Type II glass ionomer cements have now been in use for more than 20 years. Clinical studies of eroded-area glass ionomer cement restorations report retention rates of about 90 per cent over 2- to 6-year periods. Glass ionomer restorations probably are vulnerable, to some degree, to dehydration throughout their lifetime. Therefore, it is prudent to protect existing glass ionomer restorations with a coat of varnish or light-activated resin when other dental procedures are carried out.

Three cardinal requirements for successful placement of glass ionomer restorations are as follows:

1. Conditioning of the tooth surface with dilute polyacrylic acid
2. Correct manipulation of the cement
3. Protection of the cement during setting

Metal-Modified Glass Ionomer Cements

Metal filler particles have been added to glass ionomer cements to improve strength, fracture toughness, and wear resistance to enable the cements to be used in stress-bearing applications, such as restoration of posterior teeth.

Two methods of incorporating the metal fillers have been used.

- In the first method, a spherical-particle amalgam alloy is mixed with a Type II glass ionomer cement—referred to as a *silver alloy admix*.
- In the second system, silver powder is fused to the surface of the glass powder particles at a high temperature. Such a material is called a *cermet* (ceramic-metal composite), and glass ionomer cements of this type are referred to as *cermet cements*. Examples

of representative commercial products are shown in Figure 21–7.

Properties

The properties of a cermet glass ionomer are compared to those of a conventional Type II glass ionomer cement in Table 21–3. Neither the strength nor the fracture toughness of the cermet is improved over the conventional Type II cement. As can be seen in Table 21–4, however, cermet has appreciably better resistance to occlusal wear than conventional cement. Fluoride is leached from both types of metal-modified cement in significant amounts, and the cements bond to tooth structure.

A major shortcoming of both metal-modified cements is poor aesthetics. The restorations look like metallic restorations.

With their increased wear resistance and the anticariogenic potential, metal-modified cements have been suggested for limited use as an alternative to amalgam. Remember, however, that these cements are relatively weak and brittle compared with amalgam and composite resin. For this reason, their use is restricted to *conservative* Class I restorations. They appear to perform relatively well in this situation, particularly in young patients prone to caries.

Sometimes metal-modified glass ionomers are used for a core buildup on severely damaged teeth that are to be restored with cast crowns. Because they are brittle and have low fracture toughness, this use is recommended *only if* they constitute no more than 40 per cent of the total core structure.

Zinc Oxide–Eugenol Cement

The zinc oxide–eugenol cements (ZOE) usually are dispensed in the form of a powder and liquid or as two pastes. The compo-

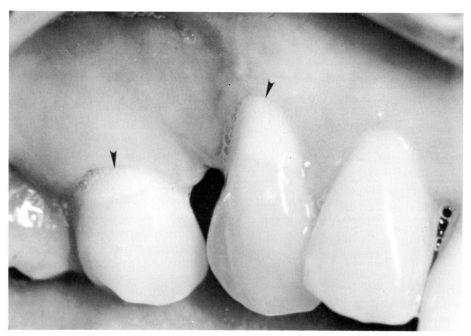

Figure 21–6. Six-year-old glass ionomer restorations restoring erosion lesions. The restorations were protected during maturation of the cement and remained free of crazing and cracks. (From Phillips RW: *Skinner's Science of Dental Materials,* 9th ed. Philadelphia, WB Saunders Co, 1991.)

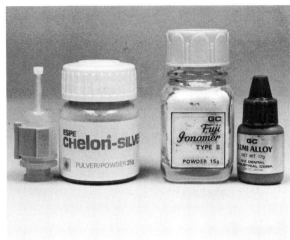

Figure 21–7. Representative commercial metal-modi-fied glass ionomer cements. Cermet material at left. At right is an admix of amalgam added to Type II ionomer cement (Miracle Mix). (From Phillips RW: *Skinner's Science of Dental Materials,* 9th ed. Phila-delphia, WB Saunders Co, 1991.)

nents are combined by mixing on a slab with a spatula. As indicated in Table 22–1, a wide variety of zinc oxide–eugenol formulations are available for use as temporary and inter-mediate restorations, cavity liners, thermal insulating bases, and temporary and perma-nent cements. The pH is about 7.0 at the time they are inserted into the tooth. They are one of the least irritating of all dental materials.

The various formulations and uses are re-flected in ADA Specification no. 30 for zinc oxide–eugenol restorative materials, which lists four types.

- Type I preparations are designed for tem-porary cementation.
- Type II formulations are designed for per-manent cementation of restorations or appliances fabricated outside the mouth.
- Type III cement is used for temporary fill-ings and thermal insulating bases.
- Type IV is used as a cavity liner—a thin coating is applied on the pulpal wall to provide protection from chemical in-sult.

In this chapter, the zinc oxide–eugenol ce-ments used for temporary and intermediate restorations, bases, and liners are discussed.

Those used for cementation are discussed in Chapter 22.

Composition and Chemistry

The two basic components of zinc oxide–eugenol cements are zinc oxide and eu-genol. Hence, the setting reaction and micro-structure of the cements are essentially the same as those of the impression pastes dis-cussed in Chapter 6. The handling character-istics and physical properties of zinc oxide–eugenol preparations can be altered in sev-eral ways, however. Different particle sizes of zinc oxide and of various additives can alter handling characteristics and working time and increase or decrease strength as required for a particular task. For example, the strength of a Type I cement designed for temporary cementation should be markedly less than that of the Type II cement, which is used for permanent cementation.

Properties

As with other cements, the powder-liquid ratio affects the setting time. The higher the powder-liquid ratio, the faster the set.

Several factors affect the strength of the

cement. In general, the smaller the particle size, the stronger the cement. Substitution of part of the eugenol with orthoethoxybenzoic acid (EBA) results in an appreciable increase in strength, as does the discreet incorporation of polymers.

Zinc oxide–eugenol formulations designed for various uses range in strength from as low as 3 or 4 Mpa (400 or 600 psi) up to 50 to 55 Mpa (7000 to 8000 psi). The properties of some typical zinc oxide–eugenol formulations are listed in Table 22–1.

Manipulation

Zinc oxide–eugenol cements are somewhat less sensitive to manipulative variables than are other cements. Powder-liquid ratios influence the strength properties. Other factors—such as the rate with which powder is added to the liquid and the mixing time—are far less critical than for most other cements.

A cool slab increases working time. This can be helpful when a large amount of powder must be incorporated into a small amount of liquid, as is the case with the intermediate restorative materials. If the slab is cooled below the dew point and water is incorporated into the mix, the set can be accelerated.

Temporary Restorations

Materials used for temporary restorations are expected to last for a short period—a few days to a few weeks at most. They may serve as a treatment while the pulp heals and/or while the permanent restoration is being fabricated.

At one time, *gutta percha*, a thermoplastic natural resin, was popular for this purpose. It did not adapt well, however, to the cavity walls, microleakage ensued, and sensitivity was a common problem. Today, gutta percha is used in conjunction with a zinc oxide–eugenol sealer to obturate root canals. Because of its excellent initial sealing ability and kindness to the pulp, zinc oxide–eugenol is the cement of choice for temporary restorations.

Type I cements are designated for this purpose. Because the restorations will be removed in a short time, the maximum strength as specified by ADA Specification no. 30 for Type I zinc oxide–eugenol cements is 35 MPa.

Zinc oxide–eugenol is particularly useful when a sedative treatment is required to enable the pulp to heal to the point where a permanent restoration can be placed. The relatively low mechanical properties of zinc oxide–eugenol do not permit it to be used where it would be subject to high stress, such as interim coverage of a crown preparation. In those cases, a temporary resin or metal crown is cemented using a zinc oxide–eugenol cement.

Intermediate Restorations

Sometimes the need arises for an *intermediate* restoration, particularly in pediatric dentistry. In cases of rampant caries, for example, the dentist needs to remove all caries quickly to change the oral flora and arrest the caries process. Once the initial clean-up has been accomplished, the dentist can then proceed with placement of the permanent restorations. The interval between removal of the caries and completion of the restorative work may be a matter of several months or longer. During that time, the teeth must be protected by some type of durable restoration.

Materials used in the past for these intermediate restorations include Types II and III zinc silicophosphate cements and Type II zinc phosphate cement. The mechanical properties of both zinc silicophosphate cement and phosphate cement are superior to those of zinc oxide–eugenol. Zinc silicophosphate powder is composed of both silicate and zinc oxide powders. By virtue of its silicate component, the cement contains fluoride, which leaches from the cement, as shown in Figure 21–1 and Table 21–2. It thus has anticariogenic activity. Both cements are irritating to the pulp and require a meticulous cavity preparation.

Because zinc oxide–eugenol cement was a recognized biocompatible material, research centered on the development of this type of material for an intermediate restorative material. Conventional zinc oxide–eugenol cements (described for use as temporary restorations) are deficient in toughness and have inadequate strength and abrasion resistance for use over extended periods.

Several commercial zinc oxide–eugenol products exist—such as those shown in Figure 21–8—in which the longevity of the restoration has been extended for periods of 1 year or longer. In one approach, finely divided polymer filler particles are added. The zinc oxide powder also may be surface-treated with an agent such as propionic acid. The combination of the polymer reinforcement and the surface treatment of the zinc oxide powder increases toughness and abrasion resistance to levels required for an intermediate restorative material. To achieve the properties necessary for this use, a suffi-

ciently high powder-liquid ratio must be used to produce a stiff, putty-like consistency.

Sometimes polycarboxylate cements (discussed in Chapter 22) are used for intermediate restorations. This cement chemically bonds to tooth structure and is gentle on the dental pulp.

CAVITY VARNISHES, LINERS, AND BASES

Before placement of the restoration, the dental pulp may have been irritated or damaged from various sources, such as caries and cavity preparation. The physical and chemical properties of some permanent restorative materials are such that the restoration itself can produce irritation or add to that which already exists.

Irritation induced by restorative materials may stem from a number of sources. Metallic restorations are good thermal conductors: sensitivity caused by thermal shock may occur. Cements that contain phosphoric acid (zinc phosphate, silicate, and zinc silicophosphate) and direct filling resins can produce chemical irritation. Microleakage may be an additional source of irritation. To protect the pulp against these types of insult, cavity varnishes, liners, and insulating bases are used as adjuncts to the restorative materials.

In addition to serving as protective barriers, certain agents have beneficial effects on the vital tooth. Zinc oxide–eugenol compounds, for example, have a palliative effect on the pulp and can aid in reducing sensitivity. Calcium hydroxide accelerates the formation of reparative dentin and is used as a pulp-capping agent. Whenever the slightest possibility of a pulp exposure exists, a layer of calcium hydroxide is applied to the pulpal wall—regardless of the type of restorative material to be used.

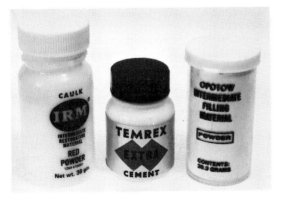

Figure 21–8. Examples of zinc oxide–eugenol cements for intermediate restorations.

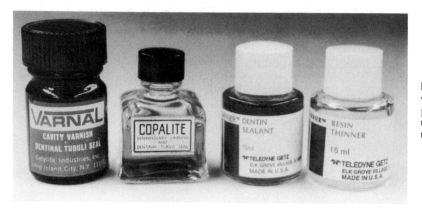

Figure 21-9. Commercial cavity varnishes used to line cavities prior to insertion of restorations and phosphoric acid containing bases.

Cavity Varnishes and Liners

Because varnishes and liners are used for coating the freshly cut tooth structure in the prepared cavity, both technically can be classified as cavity-lining agents. Those materials usually are classified into two groups.

- The typical cavity *varnish* is a natural gum (such as copal or rosin) or a synthetic resin dissolved in an organic solvent (such as acetone, chloroform, or an ether). Typical products are shown in Figure 21-9.
- The second group, called *cavity liners*, are liquid suspensions of calcium hydroxide.

Both varnish and cavity liners are formulated to provide a fluid that is readily painted onto the surfaces of the prepared cavity. The solvent evaporates, leaving a film of the solid components to protect the underlying tooth structure.

Cavity Varnishes

A thin film of varnish on the cavity walls assists in sealing the cavity, reducing leakage around the restoration, particularly in amalgam restorations (Fig. 21-10). The varnish also seals the dentinal tubules and acts as a barrier to reduce the penetration of constituents of the restorative or cementing material. Thus, if a varnish is used under a zinc phosphate cement, it helps to prevent penetration of acid (from the cement) through the dentin into the pulp. Such protection reduces the possibility of postoperative sensitivity.

Cavity varnishes should *not* be used in

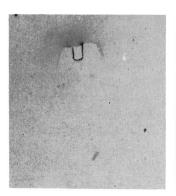
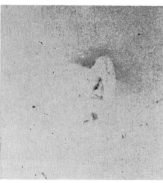

Figure 21-10. Sections through two teeth that were restored with amalgam and then immersed in a radioactive medium. No varnish was used with the amalgam on the left. The black line surrounding the restoration indicates penetration of the margins by the isotope ("marginal leakage"). No leakage occurred in the restoration of the right in which a cavity varnish was applied before inserting the restoration.

some situations, including the following examples:

- Because zinc oxide–eugenol and polycarboxylate cements are nonirritating, cavity varnishes are not required when these cements are used.
- A varnish should not be used for pulp protection under glass ionomer restorations or restorative resins. With glass ionomers, the varnish interferes with bonding to the tooth and the uptake of fluoride from the cement. In the case of resins, varnish interferes with the dentin and enamel bonding agent being used.
- In deep cavities, a base must be used in conjunction with a metallic restoration to protect the pulp from extremes in temperature. A film of varnish placed under a metallic restoration is not an effective thermal insulator. Although varnishes have a low thermal conductivity, the thickness of the film is in the range of only 4 μm—too thin for thermal insulation.

Although a cavity varnish applied to the cavity preparation is not effective in preventing galvanic shock, it helps prevent a secondary problem associated with corrosion—tooth discoloration. Metallic ions released by corrosion from the amalgam restoration often penetrate into enamel and dentin and form colored corrosion products. A cavity varnish aids in reducing penetration of these ions and, thus, discoloration of tooth structure adjacent to the amalgam restoration.

The varnish is applied to the cavity walls in a thin layer by means of a brush, wire loop, or cotton applicator. If the varnish is thick and viscous, it cannot wet the enamel and dentin, thereby eliminating the beneficial effect of the varnish in reducing microleakage. Therefore, the top must be placed back on the varnish bottle immediately after use to prevent evaporation of the solvent. If the varnish becomes viscous, it should be thinned with a suitable solvent or discarded.

Cavity Liners

Cavity liners act as barriers to penetration of irritating substances. They are capable of neutralizing acids contained in the cements and of promoting formation of reparative dentin.

Because calcium hydroxide is dissolved by oral fluids, liners that contain calcium hydroxide do not aid in sealing the cavity and should be kept well away from the margins of the restoration. Hard-setting calcium hydroxide formulations, discussed in the section on bases, have nearly eliminated the use of calcium hydroxide suspensions. When applied to the pulpal wall in a thin layer, hard-setting calcium hydroxide protects the pulp against irritants and promotes reparative dentin. Its handling characteristics are superior to those of calcium hydroxide suspensions.

A thin layer of low-viscosity zinc oxide–eugenol formulation (Type IV) also can be used as a liner, acting as a chemical barrier and having a palliative effect on the pulp. Zinc oxide–eugenol liners usually are not recommended beneath composite resin restorations because they may interfere with the polymerization of the resin.

Glass Ionomer Liners

The newest type of liner is based on the glass ionomer cement. The basic purpose of the glass ionomer liner is different from that of calcium hydroxide liners and cavity varnishes. The primary purpose of a glass ionomer liner is to act as a bonding agent that adheres to both dentin and composite resin and, thus, aids in sealing the cavity and retaining the resin restoration.

A thin layer of glass ionomer lining cement is placed on the dentin surface of the cavity. It is then overlaid with a composite restoration, as diagrammed in Figure 21–11. The glass ionomer cement liner bonds to the dentin and is coated with a dentin bonding

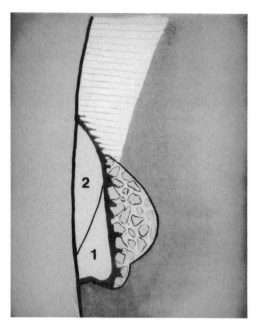

Figure 21-11. Diagram of sandwich technique. The top of the restoration has its cavo-surface in enamel while the bottom is in dentin. The composite resin is placed in increments (1 and 2) over the glass ionomer.

agent to enhance the bond between it and the composite resin. The glass ionomer liner hopefully provides protection from secondary caries. This technique is referred to as the *sandwich technique*. It is particularly useful when margins of the cavity are located in dentin, such as many Class V and II restorations.

Two types of glass ionomer liners are available. Representative products of each can be seen in Figure 21–12. The first is a conventional powder-liquid system, analogous to Type II cements. The basic formulation has been adjusted so that lining cements set a little faster and are more fluid than restorative cements.

The second type is a *light-activated glass ionomer cement*. The light-activated liners also are powder-liquid systems. The powder portion consists of conventional acid-soluble glass particles with a photo-activated accelerator. The liquids are aqueous solutions of

polyacrylic acid or copolymers to which polymerizable methacrylate groups are attached. The two components are mixed, placed on the cavity wall, and then exposed to a resin-curing light. The light activates the accelerator, free radicals are produced, and the pendant methacrylate groups polymerize by way of the addition mechanism.

The mass hardens initially through light-activated addition polymerization of the resin. This is followed by the much slower conventional setting reaction of glass ionomer, which proceeds in the usual manner, as does bonding to tooth structure. With the light-activated ionomer liners, conditioning of the dentin surface with polyacrylic acid is not required. Thicknesses greater than 2 mm do not light-activate adequately.

Both types of glass ionomer cement liners release fluoride in appreciable amounts.

The Cement Base

A layer of cement, called a *base*, is placed under a permanent restoration to encourage recovery of the pulp and to protect it against several types of insult. That insult may come from thermal shock and/or chemical irritation. The base, in essence, serves as a replacement for the dentin that has been damaged by caries and removed during cavity preparation.

Various materials can be used as bases. Zinc phosphate cement (Type II) has been used for this purpose for many years, as have many zinc oxide–eugenol formulations. A commercial zinc oxide–eugenol, shown in Figure 23–13, is an extremely free-flowing formulation designed particularly for this purpose. Polycarboxylate cement is kind to the pulp and is a good thermal insulator, so it is well suited for use as a base.

Two-paste calcium hydroxide formulations that set when mixed together are called *hard-setting calcium hydroxides*. Visible light–activated calcium hydroxide materials

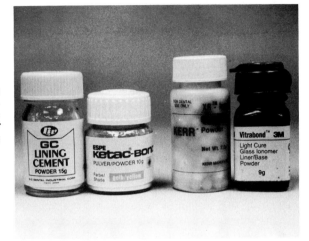

Figure 21-12. Commercial glass ionomer liners. The two at the left are based on conventional powder liquid systems whereas the two at the right are light-activated. (From Phillips RW: *Skinner's Science of Dental Materials,* 9th ed. Philadelphia, WB Saunders Co, 1991.)

also are available. The composition of these materials is quite complicated: they contain several ingredients in addition to the calcium hydroxide. The hard-setting calcium hydroxides can be built up to the thickness required for thermal insulation, usually a minimum of 0.5 μm. Commercial products of this type are shown in Figure 21–13.

Both calcium hydroxide and zinc oxide–eugenol formulations act as barriers against chemical irritation from restorative materials. Even a thin layer of these materials prevents penetration of phosphoric acid from cements. Thus, when thermal insulation is not required, such as with direct filling resins, only a thin layer of a hard-setting calcium hydroxide, analogous to a liner, need be applied to the pulpal wall.

When a zinc phosphate cement base is to be used as a thermal insulating base, a cavity varnish or a thin coat of either zinc oxide–eugenol or hard-setting calcium hydroxide cement should be placed first as a liner on the floor of the cavity to protect the pulp from

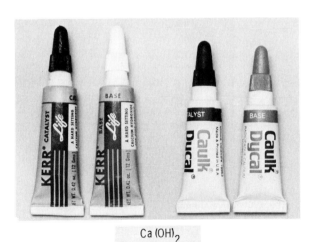
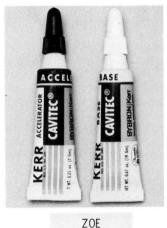

Ca (OH)$_2$ ZOE

Figure 21-13. Commercial cement base products. (From Phillips RW: *Skinner's Science of Dental Materials,* 9th ed. Philadelphia, WB Saunders Co, 1991.)

irritation by the acid cement. This is unnecessary with a polycarboxylate cement base.

The hard-setting calcium hydroxide and zinc oxide–eugenol base materials are sufficiently strong to support condensation of amalgam. Stronger materials, such as zinc phosphate and polycarboxylate cement, should be used as a base for direct gold restorations.

Selected Reading

Croll, T. P., and Phillips, R. W.: Glass ionomer-silver cermet restorations for primary teeth. Quintessence Int. 17:607, 1986.

Duke, E. S., Phillips, R. W., and Blumershine, R.: Effects of various agents in cleaning cut dentine. J. Oral Rehabil. 12:295, 1985.

Goldman, M.: Fracture properties of composite and glass ionomer dental restorative materials. J. Biomed. Mater. Res. 19:771, 1985.

Harper, R. H., Schnell, R. J., Swartz, M. L., and Phillips, R. W.: In vivo measurements of thermal diffusion through restorations of various materials. J. Prosthet. Dent. 43:180, 1980.

Jendresen, M. D., and Phillips, R. W.: A comparative study of four zinc oxide and eugenol formulations as restorative materials. II. J. Prosthet. Dent. 21:300, 1969.

Lind, V., Wennerholm, G., and Nystrom, S.: Contact caries in connection with silver amalgam, copper amalgam and silicate fillings. Acta Odontol. Scand. 22:333, 1964.

Low, T.: The treatment of hypersensitive cervical abrasion cavities using ASPA cement. J. Oral Rehabil. 8:81, 1981.

McKinney, J. E., Antonucci, J. M., and Rupp, N.: Wear and microhardness of a silver-sintered glass ionomer cement. J. Dent. Res. 67:831, 1988.

Mount, G. J.: Restoration with glass-ionomer cement: Requirements for clinical success. Oper. Dent. 6:59, 1981.

Mount, G. J.: The tensile strength of the union between various glass ionomer cements and various composite resins. Austral. Dent. J. 34:136, 1989.

Mount, G. J.: *An Atlas of Glass Ionomer Cements.* London, Martin Dumitz, 1990.

Norman, R. D., Mehra, R. V., Swartz, M. L., and Phillips, R. W.: Effects of restorative materials on plaque composition. J. Dent. Res. 51:1596, 1972.

Norman, R. D., Phillips, R. W. and Swartz, M. L.: Fluoride uptake by enamel from certain dental materials. J. Dent. Res. 39:11, 1960.

Powis, D. R., Follera, T., Merson, S. A., and Wilson, A. D.: Improved adhesion of a glass ionomer cement to dentin and enamel. J. Dent. Res. 61:1416, 1982.

Swartz, M. L., Phillips, R. W. and Clark, H. E.: Long-term fluoride release from glass ionomer cements. J. Dent. Res. 63:158, 1984.

Wilson, A. D.: Adhesion of glass ionomer cements. *In* Allen, K. W. (Ed.): *Aspects of Adhesion.* London, Transcriptor Books, 1975, p. 145.

Wilson, A. D., and Kent, B. E.: A new translucent cement for dentistry. The glass-ionomer cement. Br. Dent. J. 132:133, 1972.

Wilson, A. D., and McLean, J. W.: *Glass Ionomer Cements.* Chicago, Quintessence Publ. Co., 1988.

Reviewing the Chapter

1. List types of cement used for temporary restorations, intermediate restorations, and restoration of anterior teeth.

2. Why is it important to understand the nature and chemistry of silicate in relation to the now popular glass ionomer system?

3. Explain completely the various mechanisms by which a silicate cement provides protection against secondary caries.

4. What are the compositions of a glass ionomer powder and liquid? Describe the setting reaction and structure of the set cement.

5. Is *glass ionomer cement* harder, stronger, and more resistant to solubility than *composite resin?*

6. Describe the manipulation of a Type II glass ionomer cement.

7. What is the mechanism of adhesion of glass ionomer cement to tooth structure?

8. What is the *sandwich technique,* and what are the functions of the glass ionomer liner used in the procedure?

9. Is glass ionomer cement irritating to the pulp? Does it provide protection against secondary caries?

10. Describe the various manipulative steps that must be controlled for clinical success of a glass ionomer cement restoration. What are the common causes for failure?

11. Which material commonly is used for *temporary restorations*? What are its advantages and disadvantages?

12. List the materials used for *intermediate restorations* and the advantages and disadvantages of each.

13. How do the composition and properties of a light-activated glass ionomer differ from those of a conventional glass ionomer cement?

14. What is the difference in composition between a conventional zinc oxide–eugenol cement and one used for an intermediate restoration?

15. Describe the composition of a cavity varnish and a $Ca(OH)_2$ liner. What is the function of such agents?

16. How does one provide thermal protection to the pulp in a deep cavity preparation to be restored with amalgam?

17. What precautions are exercised in the care of a cavity varnish?

18. Discuss the functions of a cement base. What are the various materials used for bases and the characteristics of each?

LUTING CEMENTS

Dental *luting* cements are used to attach numerous types of restorations and appliances to tooth structure. These include inlays, crowns, bridges, laminate veneers, retentive pins, and orthodontic appliances. As indicated in Table 21–1, several cements are used for luting applications. Products representative of the various types are shown in Figure 22–1. Table 22–1 compares typical properties of the different types of luting

cements with American Dental Association (ADA) Specification no. 8 for zinc phosphate cement.

Although variations exist from brand to brand for each kind of cement, manipulative variables can create far greater differences. The importance of correct manipulation cannot be overemphasized; thus, the auxiliary has an important role in the success of the cementation procedure.

TABLE 22–1. Properties of Luting Cements

	Setting Time (min)	Film Thickness (μm)	24-h Compressive Strength		24-h Diametral Tensile Strength		Elastic Modulus		Solubility in Water (% wt)	Pulp Response*
			MPa	psi	MPa	psi	GPa	psi × 10^6		
ADA Spec. 8 Type I	5 Minimum 9 Maximum	25 Maximum	68.7 Minimum	9956	No specification		No specification		0.2 Maximum	No specification
Zinc phosphate	5.5	20	104	15,000	5.5	800	13.5	1.96	0.06	Moderate
ZOE Type I	4–10	25	6–28	800–4000	—	—	—	—	0.04	Mild
ZOE + EBA + alumina Type II	9.5	25	55	8000	4.1	600	5.0	0.73	0.05	Mild
ZOE + polymer Type II	6–10	32	48	7000	4.1	600	2.5	0.36	0.08	Mild
Silicophosphate	3.5–4	25	145	21,000	7.6	1100	—	—	0.4	Moderate
Resin	2–4†	<25	70–172	10,000–25,000	—	—	2.6	0.37	0.0	Moderate
Polycarboxylate	6	21	55	8000	6.2	900	5.1	0.74	0.06	Mild
Glass ionomer	7	24	86	12,500	6.2	900	7.3	1.06	1.25	Mild to moderate

ZOE, Zinc oxide–eugenol; EBA, ortho-ethoxybenzoic acid.
*Based on comparison with silicate cement = severe irritant.
†For chemically activated cements; light-cured and dual-cure cements set immediately on exposure to light.

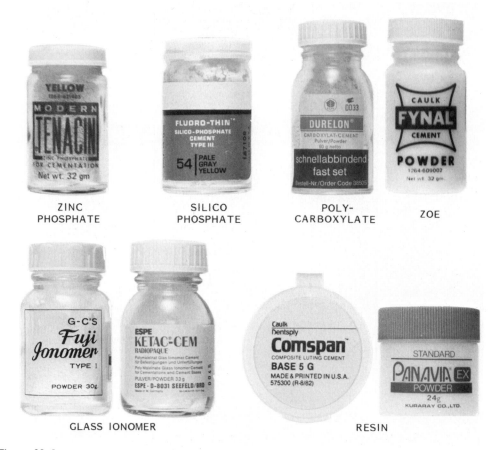

Figure 22–1. Commercial products representative of various kinds of luting cements. (From Phillips RW: *Skinner's Science of Dental Materials,* 9th ed. Philadelphia, WB Saunders Co, 1991.)

ZINC PHOSPHATE CEMENT

Because zinc phosphate is the oldest luting cement, it has the longest clinical "track record" and serves as the benchmark for newer cements. Much of the basic information discussed in the next section also is directly applicable to other types of cements.

Zinc phosphate cement comes as a powder and liquid, which are mixed on a glass slab to the consistency required for the particular application. Figure 22–2 shows a typical mixing slab and spatula, which are used in the following steps:

1. The powder is placed on the slab.
2. *Just* before the mix is made, the liquid is dispensed.
3. After the cement is the proper consistency, it is placed in the oral cavity.
4. A chemical reaction between the powder and the liquid causes the mixture to harden—or *set.*

Composition

The powder is mainly zinc oxide with less than 10 per cent magnesium oxide. The liquid is essentially phosphoric acid and water.

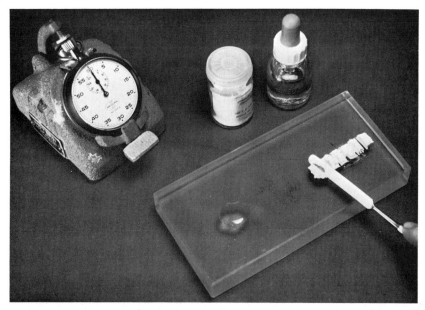

Figure 22–2. Slab and spatula used for mixing zinc phosphate cement. The initial portion of powder is being incorporated into the powder. Note that caps have been placed on the bottles to protect the powder and liquid.

Metallic salts—known as buffering salts—are added to reduce the reaction speed. This provides sufficient working time and helps to secure a smooth, uniform mix.

The composition of the liquid is balanced to that of the powder. The average water content in the liquid is about 33 per cent. The amount is critical because it influences the reaction rate and affects the ultimate properties of the cement. Although the liquid composition for various brands of cement is similar, liquid from one manufacturer should never be used with powder from another manufacturer.

Chemistry of the Setting Reaction

When zinc oxide is mixed with phosphoric acid, a new solid rapidly forms, accompanied by evolution of heat. The liquid first dissolves the surface layer of the powder particles. The resulting reaction then forms zinc orthophosphate.

$$ZnO + H_3PO_4 \rightarrow Zn_3(PO_4)_2 + H_2O$$
$$22–1$$

Zinc oxide + phosphoric acid →
                 zinc phosphate + water

Zinc phosphate continues to form after the mixture is placed in the mouth, continuing the hardening process. The final hardened cement consists of undissolved zinc oxide powder particles suspended in a zinc phosphate matrix. This matrix is the weakest and most soluble component of the set cement.

Setting Time

The setting time of dental cements is measured with a weighted needle—similar to the method used for gypsum products (see Chapter 5). Setting time is defined as the time elapsed from the start of the mix until the needle no longer penetrates the cement surface.

This hardening or setting time must be accurately controlled. The cement should set slowly enough to allow sufficient working time for proper insertion of the restoration in the mouth. But if the setting time is prolonged, the restoration must be held rigidly in the mouth for an inconveniently long time.

Timing and coordination between the dentist and auxiliary are critical in the cementation procedure. Once the cement is the correct consistency, a race begins between the chemical reaction that is thickening the cement and the insertion of the cement into the mouth. Working time is particularly critical when more than one unit is being cemented simultaneously, as with a bridge or orthodontic appliance.

Figure 22–3A shows a correctly seated crown. If the cement hardens too rapidly, the bridge or appliance does not seat completely, as shown in Figure 22–3B. If too much time elapses between mixing and placement, the setting reaction progresses to the point where the cement becomes too thick to squeeze out into a thin film under the casting—the casting then fails to fully seat on the prepared tooth.

With correct manipulation, the setting time for zinc phosphate cement at mouth temperature should be between 5 and 9 minutes. As shown in Table 22–1, this is the ADA Specification for zinc phosphate cement.

The setting time is influenced by the manufacturing process as well as by manipulation. Both composition and particle size of the powder are important. Because the buffering salts and water influence the reaction rate, the composition of the liquid also is critical.

The manufacturing process is continued in the dental office by the person who mixes the powder and liquid to form the cement. The setting time should be sufficiently controlled to provide time for handling the cement. Manipulative factors that influence the setting time include the temperature of the mixing slab and the rate the powder is added to the liquid.

Temperature of the Mixing Slab

Because the rate of any chemical reaction is affected by temperature, the best way to control setting time is to regulate the temper-

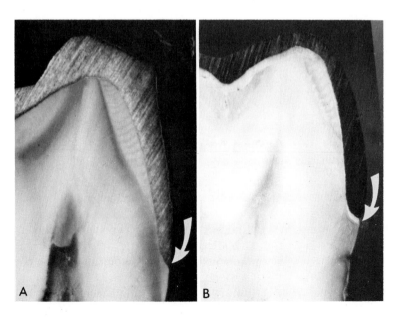

Figure 22–3. Sections through gold crowns cemented with the same mix of zinc phosphate cement. The crown in A was cemented 2.5 minutes after the start of the cement and that in B, at 5 minutes. The casting in B failed to seat, leaving a thick layer of exposed cement at the margin (arrow).

ature of the mixing slab. The chemical reaction proceeds at a slower rate on a cooled mixing slab.

Figure 22–4 shows the effect of slab temperature on the viscosity of cement. The two mixes of zinc phosphate cement were made with the same powder-liquid ratio, but the cement at the top was mixed on a cool slab and the cement at the bottom, on a warm slab. The consistency of the mix in the top photograph is suitable for cementation of cast restorations. The high viscosity of the mix in the bottom photograph makes it unusable for cementation.

For maximum physical properties, a high powder-liquid ratio is desirable. Cooling the mixing slab also permits a maximum amount of powder to be incorporated into the liquid

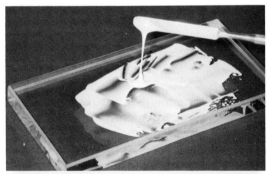

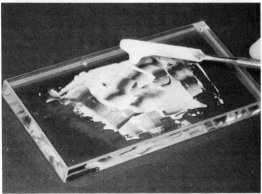

Figure 22–4. Two mixes of cement prepared with identical powder and liquid. The temperature of the slab in the top photograph was 18° C (66° F); the temperature of the slab in the bottom photograph was 29.5° C (85° F).

without unduly increasing the viscosity of the mix.

The slab should not be cooled below the temperature at which moisture condenses from the air—the *dew point.* Moisture condensed on the slab is incorporated into the mixture, affecting setting time and, possibly, impairing the properties.

Rate at Which Powder Is Added to Liquid

The rate at which the powder is added to the liquid is another way to control the setting time. Adding the powder in small amounts, with thorough mixing of each increment, extends the setting time.

Increasing the setting time by using more liquid should be avoided because of the adverse effect on the strength and solubility of the cement.

Water Content of the Liquid

The water content of the liquid is carefully established by the manufacturer and must be maintained. Erratic behavior of the cement often can be traced to incorrect care of the liquid in the dental office. The cap should not be left off the bottle of liquid any longer than necessary, and the liquid component should not be dispensed until just before the mix is made.

Both leaving the cap off the bottle of liquid and leaving the liquid on the mixing slab for any length of time affect water content. The water may evaporate, or the liquid may gain water if the relative humidity in the office is very high. In either case, setting time and properties of the cement are impaired.

Adhesion

Adhesion between the cement and tooth structure is desirable. Many cements—including zinc phosphate, zinc silicophosphate, and zinc oxide–eugenol—do not form an adhesive bond to enamel or dentin. A mechanical interlocking between the cement and the materials being joined is formed instead.

When an inlay is cemented into the prepared tooth, for example, the surfaces of the restoration and the tooth structure are somewhat rough. The cement is forced into those irregularities. After the cement has hardened, these extensions resist shear stresses, thus assisting retention of the inlay. The inlay or crown is held in place primarily by the retention provided in the design of the cavity preparation. This mechanism is shown in Figure 22–5.

The thickness of the film between the casting and the tooth is another factor in retention; the thinner the film, the better the retention. A low viscosity permits the cement to flow into minute surface irregularities and wet the surface. Conversely, a high viscosity prevents the cement from wetting the cavity walls, and the excess cannot flow out from beneath the casting. This results in a thick layer of cement, which prevents the casting from seating completely into the cavity preparation.

The manufacturer controls particle size of the cement powder so that the resulting mixture will extrude into a thin film when the restoration is seated. This particular characteristic of the cement is referred to as the *film thickness*. If the film is thin, the layer of cement between the casting and the prepared cavity does not interfere with the fit of the restoration (see Fig. 22–3).

Manipulative factors that control the thickness of the cement film include the powder-liquid ratio, temperature, and pressure used during cementation of the casting. As listed in Table 22–1, ADA Specification no. 8 states that Type I zinc phosphate cement must have a film thickness no greater than 25 μm. The specification permits a maximum film thickness of 40 μm for Type II cements. (The latter are recommended for uses other than cementation of precision restorations—for example, bases, prefabricated steel crowns, and orthodontic bands.)

Properties other than film thickness also influence the cement bond. The strength of the cement, for example, affects the ease with which the small mechanical interlocks fracture under biting stresses. If they break, mechanical retention from the cement is lost, as shown in the enlargement in Figure 22–5.

Mechanical retention must not be relied on as the primary means of holding the restoration in place. Retention is obtained primarily by the design of the prepared cavity and the accuracy of fit of the casting.

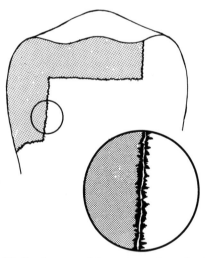

Figure 22–5. Diagram of the suggested mechanism by which a dental cement provides mechanical retention of a gold casting. The cement penetrates into irregularities in the tooth structure and casting. On hardening, this aids in holding restoration in place. The enlargement shows fracture of the tiny cement projections and loss of retention, possibly resulting in dislodgment of the inlay. (From Phillips, R. W., Swartz, M. L., and Norman, R. D.: *Materials for the Practicing Dentist.* St. Louis, C. V. Mosby Co., 1969.)

Strength

The strength of dental cements usually is determined in compression. ADA Specification no. 8 requires a minimum compressive strength of 68.7 MPa (9960 psi) 24 hours after mixing (Table 22–1). Most commercial cements have considerably higher 24-hour compressive strengths—in the range of about 104 MPa (15,000 psi). The cement film is more likely to be subjected to a shear-type stress than a compressive stress when the restoration is placed under masticatory forces. The compressive strength of the cement appears to indicate its mechanical retentive characteristics.

Strength of the cement depends primarily on the powder-liquid ratio. As shown in Figure 22–6, compressive strength increases rapidly as the amount of powder is increased.

The set cement gains strength rapidly, attaining about 75 per cent of its maximum strength during the first hour after mixing. When exposed to water or saliva for long periods, the cement gradually loses strength, probably because of slow disintegration.

Solubility and Disintegration

The solubility and disintegration of a cement in the oral cavity has great clinical sig-

nificance. When the dentist places the inlay or crown into the prepared cavity, excess cement is forced out at the margin between the restoration and the tooth. Regardless of the seating force used, a layer of cement remains between the casting and the tooth. The *cement line* at the casting margin—shown in Figure 22–3—may not be visible to the naked eye. This exposed cement can gradually dissolve, permitting microorganisms and debris to penetrate between the tooth structure and the restoration. The restoration then may become loose, and caries may develop.

From the standpoint of the material, cement solubility probably is the main factor contributing to secondary caries around an inlay or a bridge. Every precaution must be taken to produce a restoration that fits accurately so that the cement can be squeezed out into as thin a thickness as its properties permit. Then the exposed cement layer is minimal. The cement also should be handled in such a manner that the solubility will be as low as possible.

According to ADA Specification no. 8, the maximum solubility of zinc phosphate ce-

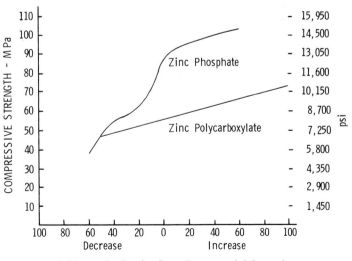

Figure 22–6. Effect of powder-liquid ratio on strength of two cements. Cement specimens were prepared with larger and smaller amounts of powder than the manufacturer's recommendation shown on this figure. (From Phillips RW: *Skinner's Science of Dental Materials*, 9th ed. Philadelphia, WB Saunders Co, 1991.)

ment measured in distilled water is 0.2 per cent. As noted in Table 22–1, most accepted commercial materials have considerably lower solubility. More harmful agents, such as acids, may be present in the mouth, depending on the person's diet, oral flora, and oral hygiene. After a person ingests certain foods, for example, the pH of plaque on the surface of the tooth or restoration may be quite low (acid) for several hours. Disintegration is greatly accelerated in acid solutions (Fig. 22–7). This solubility in acids emphasizes the inherent problems when zinc phosphate cements are exposed to the oral environment. The relative solubility and disintegration rates of the various luting cements in the oral cavity are discussed later in this chapter.

The more powder incorporated into the liquid when making a mix, the greater the number of core particles and the lower the amount of matrix. Because the particles of the original zinc oxide powder are considerably less soluble that the matrix material, the disintegration rate is lower. Thus, the use of a cool slab is essential in providing ample time to incorporate the maximum amount of powder within the limits required to maintain the correct consistency.

Cement is particularly vulnerable to attack by oral fluids during the first 24 hours. To protect the exposed cement during this critical time, the margins of newly cemented restorations and orthodontic bands may be coated with a cavity varnish.

Biological Properties

Because zinc phosphate cements contain phosphoric acid, their pH is quite low at the time they are placed in the mouth. Although the pH rises as the setting reaction progresses, the cement irritates the pulp. In a deep cavity, pulp protective measures are required, as discussed in Chapter 21 with respect to bases and liners. Lower powder-liquid ratios also result in mixes of lower pH—another reason to incorporate as much powder as possible during mixing.

Manipulation

The first part of this chapter has discussed the important manipulative variables that control the rate of the reaction and properties of the cement. The following points summarize the factors to be observed in preparing the mix.

- To reduce the solubility and increase the strength of the cement, the maximum amount of powder possible should be incorporated. A measuring device is not routinely used for proportioning the powder and liquid because the consistency required varies according to the intended purpose. Experience gained in manipulating cement and the handling characteristics desired are the best guides to attaining the correct consistency.
- A cool mixing slab should be used. The surface of the slab should be thoroughly dry.
- The mix should be made by adding small amounts of powder to the liquid (see Fig. 22–2).
- A brisk rotary motion of the spatula (Fig. 22–8) is used to incorporate the powder.
- A considerable portion of the mixing slab should be used.
- A good rule is to spatulate for about 20 seconds before adding the next increment. Mixing usually requires about 1½ minutes.
- The desired consistency is always attained by the addition of more powder and *never* by allowing a thin mix to stiffen.
- If the mix is too stiff, it is discarded and another mix made. More liquid should *never* be added to thin a mix. This rule applies to all cements.

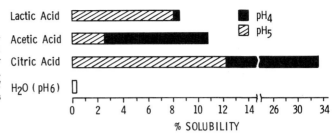

Figure 22–7. Solubility of a zinc phosphate cement when immersed in various media for 1 week. Solutions were changed daily. Solubility is much greater in acids than in distilled water. (From Phillips RW: *Skinner's Science of Dental Materials,* 9th ed. Philadelphia, WB Saunders Co, 1991.)

ZINC SILICOPHOSPHATE CEMENT

Figure 22–1 shows a commercial Type I zinc silicophosphate cement. As noted in Chapter 21, zinc silicophosphate cement systems consist of a phosphoric acid–containing liquid and a powder mixture of zinc oxide and silicate glass. Type I zinc silicophosphate cements form sufficiently thin films to permit cementation of precision castings. Because this cement is somewhat translucent, it is particularly appropriate for porcelain restorations. Fluoride leaches from the cement by virtue of its silicate content, giving it anticariogenic properties (see Fig. 21–1 and Table 21–3.)

As expected, the properties of these cements fall between those of zinc phosphate and silicate cements (see Tables 21–2 and 22–1). Because of the phosphoric acid, they can irritate the pulp, and proper protection

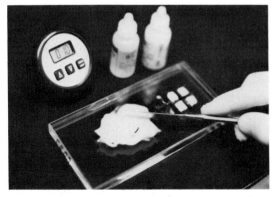

Figure 22–8. In mixing zinc phosphate cement, a rotary motion and a large portion of the slab are used.

is required. This cement has been replaced, to a great extent, by glass ionomer and resin cements.

Like zinc phosphate cements, zinc silicophosphate cements are mixed on a cool, dry slab. The powder usually is incorporated in two or three large increments, with a total mixing time of about 1 minute.

IMPROVED ZINC OXIDE–EUGENOL CEMENT

The biological properties that make zinc oxide–eugenol so useful for temporary restorations and cementation appear to make it attractive as a permanent luting agent. Its low strength, however, precludes its use for permanent cementation.

Zinc oxide–eugenol formulations with improved strengths—48 to 55 MPa (7000 to 8000 psi)—are available through the addition of polymers and inorganic compounds to the powder and ortho-ethoxybenzoic acid (EBA) to the liquid. These cements are referred to as *fortified, reinforced, modified,* or *improved.* Figure 22–1 shows a commercial improved zinc oxide–eugenol cement.

These cements were considered the materials of choice in situations with a potential for postcementation sensitivity. Although ideal from the biological standpoint, the cement presents manipulation problems and has questionable long-term durability in the oral cavity. For these reasons, polycarboxylate cement—which is equally kind to the pulp—has replaced the improved zinc oxide–eugenol cements for this application.

ZINC POLYCARBOXYLATE CEMENTS

Cements of this type are referred to as either *polycarboxylate* or *polyacrylate* cements. This was the first cement system developed that demonstrated a potential for chemical adhesion to tooth structure. Figure 22–1 shows a representative commercial zinc polycarboxylate cement.

Composition and Chemistry of Setting and Adhesion

The composition of the cement powder is similar to that of zinc phosphate cement. Sometimes stannic oxide is substituted for magnesium oxide, and stannous fluoride may be added to modify setting time and improve strength and handling characteristics. In this case, the added fluoride is not released in sufficient amounts for caries protection. The liquid is polyacrylic acid and water.

When zinc oxide powder is mixed with the polyacrylic acid, the zinc reacts with the acid. The cement sets through the formation of a new product, as shown in Figure 22–9. The chemical reaction bonding the cement to the tooth structure appears to be similar to the setting reaction. As shown in Figure 22–9, the calcium ions from the tooth structure substitute for zinc. The bond of the cement to enamel is stronger than that of cement to dentin.

Some polycarboxylate cements are marketed as a powder to be mixed with water. In these products, the cement powder contains freeze-dried polyacrylic acid. When this powder is mixed with water, the acid dissolves and the setting reaction proceeds just like powder–liquid acid systems.

Properties

Although the tensile strengths of polycarboxylate and zinc phosphate cements are similar, the compressive strength of a luting consistency of polycarboxylate cement is lower than that of zinc phosphate cement (see Table 22–1). It is in the range of the stronger improved zinc oxide–eugenol cements—about 55 MPa (8000 psi). Figure 22–6 shows that the strength of these cements is somewhat less affected by small variations in the powder-liquid ratio than the strength of zinc phosphate cement. This is not true, however, of their intraoral solubility.

When mixed at the recommended powder-liquid ratio, polycarboxylate cement is similar to zinc phosphate cement in solubility and disintegration rate in the oral cavity. If the amount of powder in the mix is reduced, the rate of solubility and disintegration dramatically increases. As with other cements, polycarboxylate cement is more soluble in acid than in water.

When the cement is mixed correctly, the mix appears quite viscous. Despite this appearance, the film thickness of the cement should be 25 μm or less.

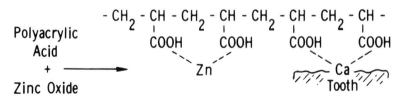

Figure 22–9. Probable setting mechanism and mode of adhesion to tooth structure for a polycarboxylate cement.

The pH of the liquid is quite low—about 1.7. When the liquid is mixed with the powder, the pH rises rapidly as the material sets. Although its acidity at 24 hours is similar to that of zinc phosphate cement, the polycarboxylate cement is much less irritating to the pulp. The pulp reaction is comparable to that produced by zinc oxide–eugenol. The large size of the polyacrylic acid molecule and its tendency to form complexes with tooth structure possibly retard its penetration through the dentin.

Another advantage of polycarboxylate cement is its potential to adhere to tooth structure. Because the bond to noble metals is not greatly superior to that of other types of cements, this characteristic may not be a major factor in increasing the retention of a metallic restoration.

Manipulation

Polycarboxylate cement often is handled incorrectly, and its clinical performance suffers accordingly. Too frequently the auxiliary with experience in mixing zinc phosphate cement uses the same technique with a polycarboxylate cement. Several steps in manipulation are quite different. Important manipulation factors include the following.

- The recommended powder-liquid ratio is about 1.5:1. A proportioner for the powder usually is furnished. At least one product also has a calibrated syringe available for measuring the liquid.
- The cement may be mixed on either a glass slab or a nonabsorbing paper pad. The glass slab is better because it can be cooled to increase the working time, which usually is quite limited.
- The powder is dispensed onto the slab first. The liquid should not be dispensed until just before mixing.
- Exposure of the liquid to the air for only a few minutes results in evaporation of the water, producing an increase in the viscosity of the liquid.

- Polyacrylic acid cement liquids have a limited shelf life. Their viscosity increases with age. A thickened cement liquid should not be used. The viscosity of the resulting mix does not permit seating of the restoration.
- Polycarboxylate liquid should not be stored in a refrigerator. The low temperature causes the liquid to thicken or gel.
- In contrast to mixing zinc phosphate cement, the powder is incorporated with rapid spatulation into the liquid in two or three large increments. The mix should be completed in 30 seconds so that the dentist will have sufficient time to seat the restoration before the viscosity becomes too high.
- A correct mix of polycarboxylate cement is somewhat thick in appearance and has a shiny, glossy surface. It will form a thin strand when picked up by the spatula, as shown in Figure 22–10.
- When the mixing time is prolonged, the cement takes on a dull appearance and becomes tacky, as seen in Figure 22–11. Wetting and bonding to the tooth structure depend on the presence of some liquid polyacrylic acid when the mix comes in contact with

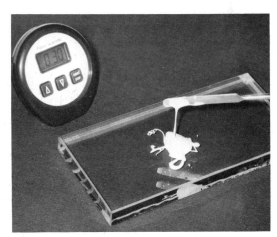

Figure 22–10. Correct mix of a polycarboxylate cement. Completed within 30 seconds, the mix has a glossy surface.

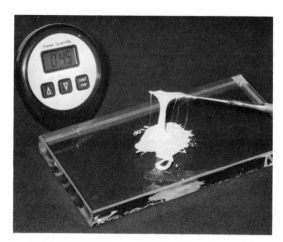

Figure 22–11. If mixing of polycarboxylate cement is prolonged, the cement becomes tacky and dull in appearance.

the tooth. A dull, sticky-appearing cement will not form an adhesive bond.

- The tooth surface must be meticulously clean to achieve a good bond with the cement. One means of cleansing the prepared tooth is with a pumice slurry followed by thorough rinsing and drying.
- Failure of a cemented cast gold restoration often can be traced to loss of retention at the casting-cement interface, possibly caused by a chemically contaminated metal surface left from the acid pickling of the casting. Before cementation, the inside surface of the casting should be cleaned with an air abrasive or carefully abraded with a rotary abrasive tool and then thoroughly rinsed and dried.

GLASS IONOMER CEMENT

The Type I glass ionomer cements—two of which are shown in Figure 22–1—are designed for cementation of restorations and direct-bonded orthodontic brackets.

Composition

The basic compositions and setting reaction of Type I cements are the same as for Type II glass ionomer cements, discussed in Chapter 21. This luting cement is available both as a conventional powder-polyacid liquid system and in the water-settable version. Glass ionomer polyacid liquids have lower viscosity than polycarboxylate liquids. They suffer from similar shelf life limitations. Liquids that have started to thicken (gel) should not be used.

Properties

The compressive strengths of glass ionomer luting cements usually are in the range of zinc phosphate cement, as seen in Table 22–2. The 24-hour solubility in distilled water is higher than that of zinc phosphate and zinc silicophosphate cements. Solubility tests conducted in the oral cavity suggest that both glass ionomer and silicophosphate cements are more resistant to deterioration in oral fluids than either zinc phosphate or polycarboxylate cement.

Glass ionomer cements adhere to tooth structure by a similar mechanism to that just described for polycarboxylate cements (Fig. 22–9). Their bond to enamel is stronger than that to dentin.

Glass ionomer cements are considered relatively kind to the pulp, but the acidity of Type I glass ionomer cement is somewhat greater than that of Type II cement. In deep areas of the cavity, pulp protective measures are advised. More instances of postcementation sensitivity seem to be associated with the water-setting Type I glass ionomer cement than with the polyacid liquid versions. Long-term fluoride release gives Type I glass ionomer cements the potential to inhibit caries.

Manipulation

Most rules for manipulation of polycarboxylate cement apply also to the glass ionomer cements. The prepared tooth structure is carefully cleaned with a pumice-water slurry and dried to attain adhesion of the cement to the tooth. Likewise, the inside surface of the casting must be cleaned.

The recommended powder-liquid ratio varies with different brands but is in the range of 1.25 to 1.5:1. Reduced powder-liquid ratios impair properties; thus, manufacturers' directions relative to proportioning should be followed. The cement can be mixed on a nonabsorbent pad or cooled glass slab. The use of the cool slab to slow the setting reaction is recommended because glass ionomer cement has a relatively short working time. The powder is incorporated with rapid spatulation into the liquid in two or three large increments for a mixing time of 45 seconds.

To obtain adhesion to the tooth, cementation should be done before the cement loses its shiny appearance.

The glass ionomer cement is particularly susceptible to dehydration or to attack by water during setting. To protect the cement from changes in water balance, manufacturers recommend coating all accessible margins of the restoration with a protective material.

RESIN CEMENTS

Resin cements were introduced in the 1950s in the form of lightly filled methylmethacrylate formulations. They were little used because of high polymerization shrinkage, marginal leakage, a tendency for pulpal irritation, and poor handling characteristics. The developments of direct filling composite resins with improved properties, the enamel etch technique, and molecules with a potential to bond to dentin have led to the marketing and acceptance of a large number of resin cements.

Resin cements are used with porcelain and cast ceramic restorations, such as inlays and crowns. The resin cement is the material of choice for cementing composite resin inlays, the attachment of orthodontic brackets, aesthetic ceramic or resin laminate veneers (discussed in Chapter 20), and resin-bonded bridges.

Resin-bonded bridges are considered an intermediate fixed prosthesis for replacing missing teeth. As shown in Figure 22–12, they consist of an artificial tooth *(pontic)* with thin cast metal abutments that fit into shallow preparations in the enamel on the lingual and proximal surfaces of the abutment teeth.

Composition and Chemistry

In composition and chemistry, resin cements are similar to direct filling composite resins (described in Chapter 10), although compositions vary with the product to provide handling characteristics required to perform particular tasks. Because they are used as luting materials, lower viscosities are required than for direct filling composite restorative resin. Hence, most resin cements contain lower filler levels. The resin matrices are BIS-GMA or some other diacrylate resin diluted with low-viscosity monomers. They are filled with inorganic particles in amounts ranging from 30 to 80 per cent by weight, and the filler particles are coated with a silane coupling agent.

Some cements have incorporated the same adhesive mechanisms (such as phosphonates, 4 META, and HEMA) used in dentin bonding agents. These cements are referred to as *adhesive cements.* Other cement systems supply the dentin bonding agent as a separate entity. Bonding to enamel is achieved by the acid etch technique. The cements are polymerized by the same chemical or light activation systems used for restorative resins. Some cements—called *dual-cured* cements—use both mechanisms.

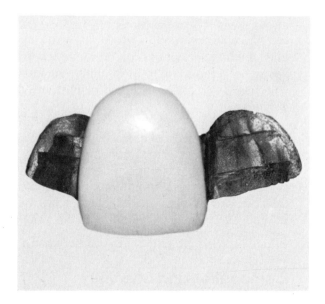

Figure 22-12. Resin-bonded bridge. The cast metal abutments have been etched for retention. (From Phillips RW: *Skinner's Science of Dental Materials,* **9th ed. Philadelphia, WB Saunders Co, 1991.)**

Properties

An outstanding property common to resin cements is their insolubility in oral fluids. As a group, they also tend to be tougher than most cements. As can be seen in Table 22–1, the commercial products vary greatly with respect to most physical properties. These variations undoubtedly are due to differences in formulation. Materials with higher filler contents are stronger and stiffer and have lower polymerization shrinkage and coefficient of expansion than those that contain smaller amounts of filler.

Cements that incorporate dentin adhesives appear to develop reasonably good bond strength. These adhesive cements—like dentin bond agents—have not been in use for sufficient time to document their long-term clinical behavior.

Resin cements are irritating to the pulp, necessitating pulp protection with a calcium hydroxide formulation in deep areas of the cavity preparation. Because resin cements possess no anticariogenic mechanism, adhesion is an important factor in the prevention of leakage leading to recurrent caries.

Techniques and Manipulation

Chemically activated cements are furnished as two-component systems, one containing the peroxide initiator and the other, the amine activator. The two components are mixed on a paper pad by spatulating for 20 to 30 seconds.

The dentist must remove the excess cement from the margins immediately after cementation of the appliance or restoration. If the cement begins to gel before the excess is removed, it may be pulled from beneath margins or edges of the restoration or appliance. It is extremely difficult to remove if it is left until it becomes fully polymerized.

Light-activated cements are single-component systems. Sufficient light must be transmitted through or beneath the appliance or restoration to activate polymerization. This varies with the restoration. Curing time should not be less than 40 seconds. Light of the wavelengths that activate visible light-cured cements transmit through enamel and dentin to a limited extent. Advantage can be taken of this fact to cure beneath some devices—such as metal orthodontic brackets—

by light activation through the surrounding tooth structure.

Dual-cured cements are two-component systems that are mixed for 20 to 30 seconds. Once mixed, the chemically activated polymerization proceeds slowly, allowing time for the cement to be applied to the restoration or appliance and the latter seated in the mouth. Once the restoration or appliance is in position, the cement is light-cured. The visible light-activated polymerization results in immediate hardening of the cement. The chemical activation then continues the polymerization process for up to 24 hours. These materials are particularly useful when thick ceramic restorations limit the amount of activation light that reaches the cement.

Although resin cements bond to etched enamel and can be bonded to dentin through the use of various adhesive agents, they do not adhere to ceramics or metals. The following measures can be taken to achieve a bond to these materials.

- Mechanical interlocking on the tissue surfaces of the metal abutments of resin-bonded bridges may be incorporated into the casting.
- Bridges may be etched to provide a mechanical bond with the cement.
- Metal restorations can be coated with silica and the silica surface then silanated.
- Tissue surfaces of ceramic inlays and laminate veneers may be treated with a silane coupling agent to produce chemical bonding to the resin cement.
- Tissue surfaces of ceramic inlays and laminate veneers may be etched to produce mechanical bonding.
- A wire mesh or undercuts may be added to the backing on metal orthodontic brackets for mechanical retention.
- Ceramic brackets usually are silane-treated and fabricated with mechanical retention or etched.

Summary

Each cement discussed has inherent advantages and disadvantages. In some instances, several cements are appropriate for use in a particular situation. Handling characteristics then may be the major consideration in selecting the luting agent. In other cases, the task to be performed and/or biological factors restrict that choice.

Zinc phosphate has long served as the universal luting cement and is still widely accepted. It has the advantage of good handling characteristics and a proved longevity when used for cementation of well-designed, well-fitting metal restorations. On the other hand, it has the disadvantage of being a pulp irritant lacking in anticariogenic properties. It is opaque and, hence, not appropriate for ceramic restorations.

Both *glass ionomer* and *zinc silicophosphate* cements possess anticariogenic properties and are translucent. Glass ionomer cements have virtually replaced silicophosphate cements because they are kinder to the pulp and bond to tooth structure. These cements are used with cast metal restorations. Their translucence suggests their use in aesthetic ceramic restorations. The glass ionomer cement would be the luting agent of choice for patients with high caries rates.

Both *polycarboxylate* and *improved zinc oxide–eugenol* cements are well tolerated by the pulp. Polycarboxylate cements bond to the tooth and have superior properties and handling characteristics, making them the choice when sensitivity is a problem.

Resin cements are used with composite inlays. They also are good choices with porcelain and cast ceramic restorations. Procedures such as attachment of resin-bonded bridges, ceramic laminate veneers, and orthodontic brackets—all of which involve mechanical bonding to etched enamel—dictate the use of resin cements.

The dental office needs to stock a variety of luting cements.

Selected Reading

Charlton, D. G., Moore, B. K., and Swartz, M. L.: Direct surface pH determinations of setting cements. Oper. Dent., 16:231–238, 1991.

Dennison, J. D., and Powers, J. M.: A review of dental cements used for permanent retention of restorations. Pt. 1: Composition and manipulation. J. Mich. Dent. Assoc. 56:116, 1974.

Dilorenzo, S. C., Duke, E. S., and Norling, B. K.: Influence of laboratory variables on rennin bond strength of an etched chrome-cobalt alloy. J. Prosthet. Dent. 55:27, 1986.

Going, R. E., and Mitchem, J. C.: Cements for permanent luting: A summarizing review. J. Am. Dent. Assoc. 91:107, 1975

Horn, H. *Practical Considerations for Successful Crown and Bridge Therapy: Biological Considerations, Physiologic Considerations, Preventive Factors.* Philadelphia, W. B. Saunders Co., 1976.

Kafalias, M. C., Swartz, M. L., and Phillips, R. W.: Effect of manipulative variables on the properties of a polycarboxylate cement. Aust. Dent. J. 20:73, 1975.

Knibbs, P. J., and Walls, A. W. G.: A laboratory and clinical evaluation of three dental luting cements. J. Oral Rehabil. 16:467, 1989.

Krabbendam, C. A., Ten harkel, H. C., Duijsters, P. P. E., and Davidson, C. L.: Shear bond strength determinations on various kinds of luting cements with tooth structure and cast alloys using a new testing device. J. Dent. 15:77, 1987.

Maijer, R., and Smith, D. C.: A comparison between zinc phosphate and glass ionomer cements in orthodontics. J. Dent. Res. 65:182, 1986 (abstr. no. 781).

Maldonado, A., Swartz, M. L., and Phillips, R. W.: An in vitro study of certain properties of glass ionomer cement. J. Am. Dent. Assoc. 96:785, 1978.

Negm, M. M., Beech, D. R., and Grant, A. A.: An evaluation of mechanical and adhesive properties of polycarboxylate and glass ionomer cements. J. Oral Rehabil. 9:161, 1982.

Norman, R. D., Swartz, M. L., Phillips, R. W., and Sears, C. R.: Properties of cements mixed from liquids with altered water content. J. Prosthet. Dent. 24:410, 1970.

Osborne, J. W., Swartz, M. L., Goodacre, C. J., et al.: A method for assessing the clinical solubility and disintegration of luting agents. J. Prosthet. Dent. 40:413, 1978.

Phillips, R. W., Swartz, M. L., Lund, M. S., et al.: In vivo disintegration of luting agents. J. Am. Dent. Assoc. 114:489, 1987.

Powers, J. M., and Dennison, J. D.: A review of dental cements used for permanent retention of restorations. Pt. 2: Properties and criteria for selection. J. Mich. Dent. Assoc. 56:218, 1974.

Simonsen, R., Thompson, V. P., and Barrack, G.: *Etched Cast Restorations: Clinical and Laboratory Techniques.* Chicago, Quintessence Publishing Co., 1983.

Smith, D. C.: Dental cements. Dent. Clin. North Am. 27(4):763, 1983.

Smith, D. C., and Ruse, N. D.: Acidity of glass ionomer cements during setting and its relation to pulp sensitivity. J. Am. Dent. Assoc. 112:654, 1986.

Smith, D. C., Norman, R. D., and Swartz, M. L.: Dental cements: Current status and future prospects. *In* Reese, J. A., and Valega, T. M. (eds.): *Restorative Dental Materials: An Overview.* London, Quintessence Publishing Co., 1985, pp. 33–74.

Swartz, M. L., Phillips, R. W., and Clark, H. E.: Long-term release from glass ionomer cements. J. Dent. Res. 63:158, 1984.

Swartz, M. L.: Luting cements: A review of current materials. Dental Annual, 1988, p. 232.

Wolff, M. S., Barretto, M. T., Gale, E. N., et al.: The effect of the powder-liquid ratio on in vivo solubility of zinc phosphate and polycarboxylate cements. J. Dent. Res. 64:316, 1985.

Reviewing the Chapter

1. Explain what is meant by a *luting* cement.
2. Give the composition of zinc phosphate and glass ionomer powders and liquids.
3. What is the structure of set zinc phosphate cement?
4. What is the importance of setting time of cements? How is it best controlled?
5. Describe correct mixing and manipulative procedures for each of the following luting cements: zinc phosphate, polycarboxylate, and glass ionomer.
6. What is the significance of the water content of zinc phosphate, polycarboxylate, and glass ionomer cement liquids? What precautions should be taken to preserve water content?
7. Which cements bond to tooth structures? What is the mechanism by which their bonding is achieved?
8. Is it necessary to clean the inside of a pickled gold casting when the cementing agent is glass ionomer or polycarboxylate cement?
9. What effect does the powder-liquid ratio have on the properties of most cements?
10. Discuss relative disintegration rates of zinc phosphate, polycarboxylate, and glass ionomer cements in the oral cavity.

11. Define *film thickness* and give the ADA Specification limit for the film thickness of Type I zinc phosphate cement.
12. What is a *cement line?*
13. Discuss the effect of the various cements on the dental pulp. Which cement usually is recommended for cementation when sensitivity is likely to be a problem?
14. Which luting cements possess anticariogenic properties?
15. Discuss the general composition of resin luting cements. How do the various resin cements differ from one another with respect to properties? What is responsible for these differences?
16. How is polymerization of resin cements accomplished?
17. Which cements are particularly appropriate for cementation of (1) cast ceramic and porcelain restorations, (2) indirect composite inlays, (3) orthodontic brackets and resin-bonded bridges, and (4) cast gold inlays and crowns?
18. What are the principal advantages of resin cement?

CHAPTER 23

DENTAL IMPLANT MATERIALS

TYPES

MATERIALS

Metals

    Stainless Steel

    Cobalt–Chromium–
       Molybdenum-Based
       Alloys

    Titanium and Titanium–
       Aluminum–Vanadium
       Alloy

    Metal with Surface
       Coatings

Ceramics

Polymers and Composites

The replacement of missing tooth structure accounts for a major portion of the clinical dentist's work. The materials discussed to this point are used to fabricate fixed or removable prostheses that are placed into the mouth but do not penetrate the tissue barrier separating the interior of the body from its exterior. A long-term goal of dentistry, however, is the ability to anchor a foreign material into the jaw to replace an entire tooth, either as a single restoration or as a support for a partial or complete denture.

Ancient civilizations used gold and ivory as substitutes for a single tooth or an entire arch. In more modern times, many biomaterials have been used with varying degrees of success. Metals such as platinum, lead, silver, steel, cobalt alloys, and titanium have been used as well as porcelain, carbon, sapphire, alumina calcium phosphates, and even dental acrylic resin.

The use of implants in medicine has become commonplace over the past 35 years. Total hip joint replacements and other prostheses have a history of long-term clinical success and are routine today. The use of implants in dentistry requires the optimization of several important variables to enhance the chances of success, including the following:

- Appropriate material selection and design
- An understanding and evaluation of the biological interaction at the interface between the implant and tissue
- Careful, controlled surgical techniques
- Collaboration between various specialties to optimize patient selection, implant, and prosthodontic geometry
- Follow-up care

With clinical treatment often preceding controlled experimental trials in both animals and humans, many failed implants have contributed to this knowledge. Vitreous carbon is a good example of a material that showed great promise as a dental implant after trials in baboons but failed in controlled human studies. Many unsuccessful implants had been placed clinically before research results had been presented to the dental community.

The dental auxiliary may not be involved in the placement of dental implants but will be otherwise treating patients with implants. As the average age of the dental population increases, so will the demand for dental implants. Both the assistant and the hygienist must have basic familiarity with *dental implantology.*

TYPES

As shown in Figure 23–1, dental implant types fall into the following main categories:

- *Subperiosteal* is a framework that rests on the bony ridge but does not penetrate

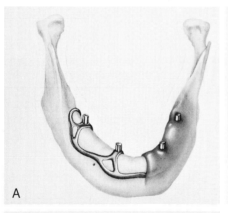

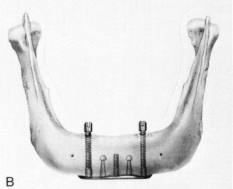

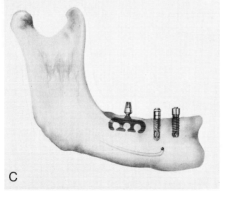

Figure 23–1. Three types of dental implants: *A,* Subperiosteal; *B,* transosteal; and *C,* endosseous. (From Taylor, T. D.: *Dental Implants: Are They for Me?* Chicago, Quintessence Publ. Co., 1990.)

it. The subperiosteal implant has had the longest history of clinical trials, but its long-term success rate is suspect (54 per cent survival rate over 15 years).

- *Transosteal* penetrates completely through the mandible. Considerable success has been reported for the transosteal mandibular staple—success rates of 90 per cent over an 8- to 16-year period—but its use is limited to the mandible.

- *Endosseous* is partially submerged and anchored within the bone. The endosseous implant appears to offer the best solution in terms of fewer clinical limitations and greater success. When careful attention was paid to the surgical technique and follow-up, a specific type of cylindrical screw implant demonstrated a high success rate over a 15-year period. The encouraging results for this implant have paved the way for the introduction of a variety of endosseous implants of varying design and composition. The implants have been shaped as blades, spirals, screws, hollow cylinders, cones, or cylinders with porous surfaces.

Implantation is a lengthy process that involves the following steps.

1. The threaded cylindrical implants are placed into the prepared bony plate and are almost immediately anchored in the cortical bone.

2. Effective stabilization requires the growth of new bone completely surrounding the entire submerged implant—a phenomenon requiring a period of several months during which the implant must remain immobile and unstressed.

3. Once bone has grown into intimate contact with the implant, the device readily transmits forces to the bone, distributing them over a large area with virtually no movement at the interface. This provides stability for the prosthesis supported by the implant.

Implants with porous or irregular surfaces usually are cylindrical. The openings, pores, or irregularities (such as sintered beads) are added to allow bone ingrowth. Although bone ingrowth within the intentional porosities on the implant surface seems to be a logical concept, the results for certain smooth-surfaced, screw-shaped implants suggest that this added retention is not required for long-term success.

The ability of living bone to grow into direct contact and potentially bond with the implant before function has been demonstrated by examination in the electron microscope and has led to the phrase *osseointegration*, which connotes a stable, biocompatible interface void of "fibrous connective tissue." There has been much debate over the nature of this "bony" interface. Irrespective of its actual biology, it appears to provide a successful support mechanism for the implant and is an absolute requirement for success. Its attainment depends on several factors, including the following:

- A material that has a stable surface structure, such as an oxide
- A surgical procedure that ensures a predictable biological response
- Proper design and follow-up for the prosthetic attachments to ensure long-term function

The materials used for these and other, nonendosseous implants are reviewed below.

MATERIALS
Metals

Metals and alloys most commonly are used for dental implants. Surgical-grade stainless steel and cobalt-chromium alloys initially were used because of their acceptable physical properties, relatively good corrosion resistance, and biocompatibility. These materials also had a history of use as

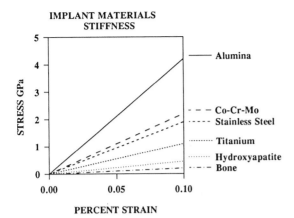

Figure 23–2. Stress–strain curves for various materials used in dental implant devices, as compared with that of bone. (Courtesy of J. Ferracane.)

medical implants, primarily in orthopedic surgery.

Stainless Steel

Surgical stainless steel is an iron-carbon alloy with about 18 per cent chromium for corrosion resistance and 8 per cent nickel. Because surgical stainless steel should not be used in patients allergic to nickel, its use in both medical and dental applications has decreased.

This alloy is the one most subject to crevice and pitting corrosion and stress corrosion cracking. Care must be taken to use and retain the passivated (oxide) surface. Because of the galvanic potential that enhances corrosion, some situations may create a problem. For example, if a bridge of a noble metal alloy touches the abutment heads of a stainless steel implant, an electric circuit is created through the tissues. If the bridge and implant are not in contact, no couple exists, and each device functions independently.

Cobalt–Chromium–Molybdenum-Based Alloys

The composition of the cobalt–chromium–molybdenum-based alloys is approx-

imately 63 per cent cobalt, 30 per cent chromium, and 5 per cent molybdenum with small amounts of carbon, magnesium, aluminum, and nickel. These alloys have a long history of successful implant application, possess outstanding resistance to corrosion, and have a high elastic modulus (Fig. 23–2). They are the least ductile of all the alloy systems, however, and bending must be avoided. This alloy group shows excellent biocompatibility.

Titanium and Titanium–Aluminum–Vanadium Alloy

With its greater corrosion resistance and tissue compatibility, titanium is the most commonly used metal for dental implants. Commercially pure titanium has become one of the materials of choice because of its predictable interaction with the biological environment. It oxidizes *(passivates)* readily on contact with air or tissue fluids. This reactivity is favorable for implant devices and minimizes corrosion. A thin oxide layer forms on a clean surface within a millisecond, making any scratch or nick in the oxide coating essentially self-healing. Also, the low density of titanium (about 4.5 g/cm²) gives it a high strength-weight ratio. In its most common alloyed form, it contains 6 weight per cent aluminum and 4 weight per cent vanadium.

Titanium has a modulus of elasticity about one half that of stainless steel or cobalt–chromium alloys. This is still 5 to 10 times higher than that of bone, as seen in Figure 23–2. Nonetheless, design of the implant is important to distribute stress transfer correctly.

The oxide surface does release titanium ions at a low rate into electrolytes such as blood or saliva. Elevated levels of titanium as well as of other elements present in stainless steel and cobalt–chromium alloys have been found in tissues surrounding implants and in major organs. Although some questions remain to be answered, the long-term clinical applications of these alloys in orthopedic and dental implants suggest that these levels have not been demonstrated to have significant associated sequelae other than the allergic reaction related to nickel.

Metal with Surface Coatings

The design of some implants makes use of a metal substructure that has been coated with a thin layer of a calcium phosphate ceramic or other ceramic materials. The rationale for coating the implant with tricalcium phosphate or hydroxyapatite—both rich in calcium and phosphorus—is to produce a "bioactive" surface to promote bone growth and induce a direct bond between the implant and the hard tissues. A second objective is to provide an interface material whose mechanical properties bridge the gap between bone and the metallic implant, as can be seen in Figure 23–2.

Long-term success of such implants will be dictated by the durability of the coating-metal bond during function as well as the characteristics and uniformity of the coating. Those data are not available.

Ceramics

Because of their outstanding biocompatibility and inert behavior, ceramics are logical materials for dental implants. At least two have been developed, designated as *bioactive* and *bioinert*. As noted earlier, hydroxyapatite has bioactive potential. It has been used mainly as an implant material for alveolar ridge augmentation or for filling bony defects. For these uses, it is produced in a block or granular form that is packed or fitted into the bony site, providing a type of scaffold for new bone growth, much like a bone graft.

The inadequate strength and ductility of this ceramic when bending or tensile forces are developed has limited its use to stress-free applications. As mentioned previously, the use of hydroxyapatite as a coating for

metal substructures addresses the mechanical deficiencies of the material while realizing the benefits of its bioactivity.

Another bioactive material is Bioglass, a dense ceramic made from CaO, Na_2O, P_2O_5, and SiO_2. The suggested bonding mechanism to bone is beyond the scope of this discussion. If its mechanical properties can be improved, Bioglass may become a valuable dental implant material.

One bioinert ceramic that has shown evidence of success in clinical trials is made from aluminum oxide, either as polycrystalline alumina or as single crystal sapphire. Although this ceramic is well tolerated by bone, it does not promote the formation of bone as do the calcium phosphate ceramics and glass. It does, however, possess high strength, stiffness (see Fig. 23–2), and hardness. These implants have either a screw or a blade shape and appear to work optimally when used as abutments for prostheses in partially edentulous mouths.

Polymers and Composites

The application of polymers and composites continues to expand. Polymers have been fabricated in porous and solid forms for tissue attachment and replacement augmentation. They also are used as coatings for force transfer between soft and hard tissues. Some are extremely tough and have been used principally for internal force distribution connectors for osteointegrated implants when the connector is intended to better replicate normal tooth functions. The use of polymeric implants in dentistry is still in the research stage. Polymeric materials have seen extensive use in orthopedic applications that involve articulated joints, such as the hip joint.

The trend for conservative treatment of oral diseases will continue to accelerate. It can be anticipated that dental implants will become a frequent first-option treatment.

Selected Reading

Albrektsson, T., Zarb, G., Worthington, P., and Enksson, A. R.: The long-term efficacy of currently used dental implants: A review and proposed criteria of success. Int. J. Oral Maxillofac. Implants 1:11, 1986.

Hench, J. W., and Hench, L. L.: Tissue response to surface-active materials. In McKinney, R. V., and Lemons, J. E. (eds.): *The Dental Implant*. Littleton, MA, PSG Publishing, 1985, p. 181.

Kay, J. F.: Bioactive surface coatings: Cause for encouragement and caution. Oral Implant 14:43, 1988.

Lemons, J. E., and Phillips, R. W.: Biomaterials for dental implants. In Misch, C. E. (ed.): *Contemporary Implant Dentistry: Diagnosis and Treatment*. St. Louis, C. V. Mosby Co., 1993, pp. 259–278.

Parr, G. R., Gardner, L. K., and Toth, R. W.: Titanium: The mystery metal of implant dentistry. Dental materials aspects. J. Prosthet. Dent. 54:410, 1985.

Williams, D. F. (ed.): *Biocompatibility of Clinical Implant Materials,* Vol. 1. Boca Raton, FL, CRC Press, 1981.

Reviewing the Chapter

1. Name and define the three categories of dental implants.
2. Which type in question 1 has the best success rate over the longest period of clinical use?
3. Which type has the broadest clinical application?
4. Define the term *osseointegration*.
5. Why is the long-term success of a dental implant dependent on osseointegration?
6. What factors are necessary for osseointegration to occur?
7. What metals are used for dental implants? List advantages and disadvantages for each.
8. Which metal appears to be the best choice? Why?
9. What ceramic materials are sometimes applied to the surface of metallic implants? Why?
10. What attractive properties do the ceramic materials offer for use in dental implants?
11. What are two types of ceramic implant materials? Give examples of each type.
12. What potential applications do polymeric materials have as implant materials? What are their limitations?

CHAPTER 24

MISCELLANEOUS MATERIALS

SOLDERING MATERIALS
Requirements for a Dental Solder
Composition
Soldering Procedure
Joining Metal–Ceramic Units
WROUGHT WIRES
Noble Metal Alloy Wires

Base Metal Alloy Wires
Stainless Steel
Cobalt–Chromium–Nickel
    Alloys
Nickel–Titanium Alloys
Titanium Alloys

The previous chapters have discussed the materials most frequently used or encountered by the dental hygienist and assistant. Numerous other materials not usually manipulated by the dental hygienist or assistant also are used in the dental office or laboratory. Some materials are used only in specialized areas of dentistry, such as the stainless steel wires used in orthodontics. An understanding of these materials and procedures is important, however, for the auxiliary to be knowledgeable about their fabrication and their reactions within the oral environment.

SOLDERING MATERIALS

Several components must be joined together in the fabrication of some types of metal dental appliances; for example, individual castings must be joined in assembling a bridge. Likewise, in orthodontics, metals must be joined to the bands that are placed around the teeth. The process of joining these parts is referred to as *soldering*.

Soldering is the joining of metals by fusion with another alloy with a lower melting point than that of any component being joined. After the solder solidifies, the metal parts are joined through the solder. The union of the solder with the metal is the result of primary *(metallic)* bonding. A limited atomic diffusion may occur between the parts and the solder, but the parts being joined should not liquefy or dissolve in the molten solder and their microstructures should not be changed.

Requirements for a Dental Solder

The *fusion temperature* of the solder must be sufficiently lower than that of the parts to be soldered that these parts will not melt or be distorted during soldering. The fusion temperature of the solder should be at least 50° C (90° F) below the fusion temperature of the parts being soldered.

The *flow properties* and *physical adhesion* of the solder to the metal are extremely important. Without such adhesion, there is no soldering action. The solder should flow freely once it is melted. A free-flowing solder spreads easily over clean metal surfaces and penetrates small openings.

The *strength* of the solder should be comparable to that of the parts to be soldered. Hardness and strength of the gold alloy solders decrease as the gold content or *fineness* of the solder increases. For this reason, solders above 650 fine should not be used when considerable stress is involved.

The solder should be *corrosion-resistant.* Solders of greater fineness are superior in this respect to solders with lower gold content. The choice of a solder, as far as *tarnish resistance* is concerned, depends on the type of restoration.

- If the restoration can be removed from the mouth, a solder of lower fineness can be used so that strength need not be sacrificed.
- If the appliance is a temporary one and not in the anterior part of the mouth, or if it is an orthodontic appliance, a solder of lower fineness is indicated. Strength is maintained, and the risk of failure because of any reduction in properties of the metals being soldered is minimized.
- If the restoration is permanent and is not going to be removed and polished frequently, a solder of greater fineness is indicated.

Composition

Composition of gold solders is similar to that of a casting alloy—mainly gold, silver,

and copper. Zinc and tin are added to reduce the fusion temperature and increase fluidity.

Silver solders essentially are alloys of silver, copper, and zinc. They are used in orthodontics because they have melting ranges markedly lower than the gold solders. As noted, their inferior resistance to corrosion usually is not significant in orthodontic appliances.

Soldering Procedure

The soldering procedure has the following basic steps:

1. The bridge is assembled on a master cast and fastened together with *sticky wax.*

2. The assembly is carefully lifted from the master cast and imbedded in a soldering investment with only the joints exposed.

3. The wax is eliminated with boiling water.

4. Cleanliness is the first requisite for a successful solder joint. The parts to be joined must be free of oxides and polishing agents.

5. To keep the surface clean at the soldering temperature, the metal is covered with a *flux* before the solder is applied. Soldering fluxes are ceramic materials that melt and flow over the parts to be soldered at a temperature well below the fusion temperature of the solder. Because they are reducing agents, they dissolve oxides and then keep the parts clean while heat is being applied during the soldering procedure.

6. The solder is applied to the preheated invested assembly and melted.

7. If the solder does not immediately flow smoothly over the area to be soldered, the operation should be discontinued. Further heating volatilizes the base metals in the solder, thereby increasing its fusion temperature, and the parts themselves may melt.

Joining Metal-Ceramic Units

Additional complexity in the terminology and procedure arises when metal-ceramic units are joined by soldering to form a bridge. The soldering may be done either before or after the application of the porcelain to the high-fusing alloy castings. The terms *preceramic* soldering and *postceramic* soldering are used, respectively, to designate these two procedures.

When *presoldering* is used, the fusion temperature of the solder is close to that of the casting alloy, and considerable care is required to prevent melting of the castings. The solder must have a high fusion temperature so that it does not soften and sag during the firing of the porcelain veneer.

A lower fusing solder is used in *postsoldering* because the bridge units now carry the completed porcelain veneer, which has a lower fusion temperature than that of the casting alloy. The heat source can be a flame, an oven, an infrared lamp, or even a laser. To prevent staining and/or roughening of the porcelain veneer, the flux, flame, and investment should not contact the porcelain veneer.

WROUGHT WIRES

Noble Metal Alloy Wires

The use of wrought metal in prosthetic dentistry has steadily declined since the development of precision casting procedures. The principal form in which wrought metal is used is wire. Noble metal alloy wire occasionally is used for the construction of partial denture clasps, but these generally have been replaced by cast clasps. The manipulation of wrought wire is an art. The cast clasp may be more readily contoured to the desired shape by the inexperienced person. Gold alloy wires also were used for the construction of orthodontic appliances; however, base metal wires are now used.

Base Metal Alloy Wires

Four types of base metal alloys are used in constructing the wrought wires, bands,

strips, and other devices used in orthodontic appliances. Each type has a distinctive composition and a particular set of physical properties. All are base metal alloys and owe their corrosion resistance to the process of passivation, as described in Chapter 13.

Stainless Steel

The most commonly used material for orthodontic bands and wires is *austenitic stainless steel.* This corrosion-resistant alloy often is referred to as 18–8 stainless steel because it contains about 18 per cent chromium and 8 per cent nickel. Chromium provides the protection against corrosion.

Stainless steel wires have a relatively high elastic modulus (stiffness), yield strength, and ultimate tensile strength. They cannot be effectively hardened by heat treatment. They can be readily fabricated into appliances by soldering or welding, provided care is taken to avoid excessive heating. The dental assistant who helps to construct orthodontic appliances should be aware that overheating stainless steel wire during soldering can impair its corrosion resistance and degrade its mechanical properties.

Alloys of this general type also are used as crowns for pediatric patients. Generally referred to as *chrome steel,* the preformed crown is used as a restoration on the badly broken down primary tooth where the usual type of restorative material (amalgam) cannot be used. The crown is contoured and adapted for the particular tooth and then cemented in place. This type of preformed crown also may be used as a temporary restoration for the permanent dentition.

Cobalt-Chromium-Nickel Alloys

Cobalt-chromium-nickel–based alloys, drawn into wire, also are used in orthodontics. One particular alloy, Elgiloy, originally was developed for making watch springs and has excellent properties for orthodontic applications.

Their physical properties and soldering and welding are similar to those of stainless steel, but the cobalt-chromium-nickel wires are supplied to the user in different degrees of hardness. The orthodontist also can subject them to a hardening heat treatment after the wire has been bent into shape. This gives the material a potential advantage in terms of ease of fabrication of appliances.

Nickel-Titanium Alloys

In some types of orthodontic treatment, the high elastic moduli of stainless steel and cobalt-chromium-nickel are a disadvantage. Wires with lower stiffness are desired to produce lower forces, longer working distances, and longer times between adjustments.

A particular alloy of nickel and titanium used in orthodontics, called Nitinol, has an elastic modulus about one fourth that of stainless steel. Nitinol wire has the disadvantage that it cannot be soldered or welded and must be joined by mechanical fasteners.

Titanium Alloys

The titanium alloy used in orthodontics is primarily titanium with small amounts of other elements present. It is referred to as beta titanium because of the type of space lattice structure it possesses at room temperature. Beta titanium has about one third the elastic modulus of stainless steel and a significantly higher yield strength than Nitinol.

It also can be welded. Its properties result in a readily formable spring material that will deliver low forces over long deflections.

Titanium alloys owe their excellent corrosion resistance to the passivation of titanium, as noted in Chapter 13.

Selected Reading

Burstone, C. J., and Goldberg, A. J.: Beta titanium: A new orthodontic alloy. Am. J. Orthod. 77:121, 1980.

Goldberg, A. J., and Burstone, C. J.: An evaluation of beta titanium alloys for use in orthodontic appliances. J. Dent. Res. 58:593, 1978.

Rasmussen, E. J., Goodkind, R. J., and Gerberich, W. W.: An investigation of tensile strength of dental solder joints. J. Prosthet. Dent. 41:418, 1979.

Ryge, G.: Dental soldering procedures. Dent. Clin. North Am. November, 1958, pp. 747–757.

Reviewing the Chapter

1. List the requirements of a dental solder. What is the composition of gold and silver solders?
2. Briefly describe the soldering procedure and the precautions that must be exercised.
3. Define what is meant by a soldering *flux* and give the rationale for its use.
4. What are the dental uses for wrought wires? Give the composition of the various types of wires.
5. List the four types of base metal alloys used in constructing orthodontic appliances. Are there certain advantageous characteristics of each?
6. What is Nitinol wire?
7. What are the advantages of beta titanium wire for orthodontic applications?

ABRASION, CUTTING, AND POLISHING MATERIALS

A principal duty of the dental hygienist is the cleaning, abrading, and polishing operation during prophylaxis. This includes not only the teeth but also any restorations and appliances present. The dental assistant also may be involved in similar duties, both intraorally and in the dental laboratory, and even in the margination, finishing, and polishing of restorations in areas where such expanded duties are allowed.

This chapter does not describe in detail the techniques used but outlines principles associated with using the instruments and abrasives intelligently and efficiently. It also seeks to provide a better understanding of the more complex operations performed by the dentist.

CUTTING

The dentist may cut tooth structure with either a hand instrument or a rotating instrument—a dental bur—in a dental handpiece. Several types of dental burs are shown in Figure 25–1. Although the burs have different shapes, all are provided with *blades* or cutting edges. Some blades are spiral, whereas others have slots cut perpendicularly (third from left) to form *serrations*. These serrations increase the cutting efficiency by providing escape channels for debris. Many shapes and sizes are available for various purposes in the preparation and finishing of cavities and restorations.

The blades of most modern dental burs

284

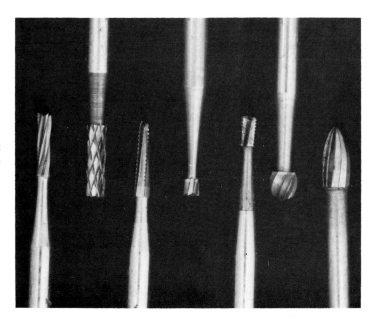

Figure 25-1. Bur types. *Left to right*: Straight fissure (spiral-bladed), straight fissure (double spiral–bladed), tapered dome fine crosscut, inverted cone, pear-shaped fine crosscut, round, and egg-shaped bur.

are made of tungsten carbide and are extremely hard and sharp. The Vickers hardness of tungsten carbide is about 1600, compared with 300 for tooth enamel. This substantial difference in hardness indicates that carbide will cut tooth enamel efficiently with dulling occurring only after considerable use. Some manufacturers may suggest disposal after a single use, however, because heat sterilization may reduce the cutting efficiency and predispose the bur to fracture during use.

As it contacts the tooth, the bur blade penetrates the surface and gradually cuts and shears off some of the tooth structure. The next blade acts in the same manner, and the bur gradually cuts through the tooth structure. Figure 25–2 shows a tooth surface that has been cut by a dental bur. The pattern of tooth removal closely corresponds to the arrangement of the blades of the bur. If the blade is sharp, the surface material is removed with ease and efficiency. The blow of a sharp ax blade against a log cuts away a larger chip of wood, for example, than the same blow with a dull ax blade.

Several factors affect the rate of cutting.

- The faster the blade travels across the tooth surface (i.e., the faster the bur rotates), the faster the cutting. Rotational speeds as high as 400,000 revolutions per minute (rpm) can be obtained with a modern dental handpiece.
- If the cutting rpm is unchanged, the greater the pressure exerted by the bur blade on the tooth, the greater the rate of removal of tooth structure.
- The design of the bur—or the blade—affects the rate of cutting.

In time, any dental bur becomes dull. As it is used, the sharp edge is abraded and rounded until it no longer cuts effectively. If the blade is chipped, it must be replaced. American Dental Association (ADA) Specification no. 23 for dental excavating burs includes requirements for the durability, concentricity, neck strength, and dimensions for various types of burs.

The theory for the use of hand cutting instruments is the same except that the hand instrument is pushed or pulled by hand

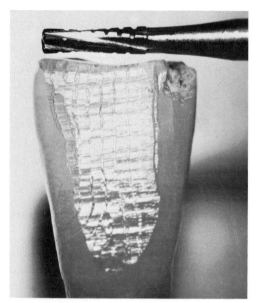

Figure 25-2. Tooth cut by a bur. Note the regular pattern of removal of tooth structure, which corresponds to the regular arrangement of the blades of the cutting tool (bur).

Particle-impregnated polymer abrasives generally are composed of a silicon rubber matrix in which abrasive particles are dispersed. With use, the outermost particles eventually flick off, exposing the matrix. The matrix quickly wears away, making new abrasive particles continuously available.

Abrasive tools manufactured by bonding particles to one another with an adhesive matrix may be given a shape specific to their intended use. Mounted stones, grinding wheels, and even the whetstone used for sharpening hand instruments are examples of this type of abrasive tool. Sandpaper disks and finishing strips are examples of abrasive tools with limited useful lives because comparatively few particles are bonded to a carrier with low durability.

As an abrasive particle acts on a surface, one of three things happens to that particle:

along the surface. The same principles apply as with a rotating instrument. Hand instruments are sterilized for reuse and must be resharpened as they become dull.

ABRASION

Abrasive action also is a cutting action. The difference is that abrasive blades are the sharp edges of randomly located particles, which may be fused to one another, bonded to a carrier with a specific form, or simply remain loose. Abrasive cutting—or grinding—leaves a surface with irregular grooves. The width and depth of the grooves correspond to the size, or grit, of the abrasive particles. A diamond abrasive tool and cut tooth surface are shown in Figure 25–3.

Sandpaper disks, finishing strips, mounted stones, and particle-impregnated polymers are other examples of abrasive tools used in dentistry. Some of these are shown in Figure 25–4.

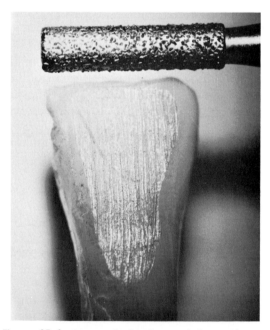

Figure 25-3. Diamond abrasive tool (somewhat enlarged) used in a dental handpiece and a tooth cut by this instrument. Note random pattern of tooth removal, which corresponds to the irregular arrangement of the cutting edges on the tool.

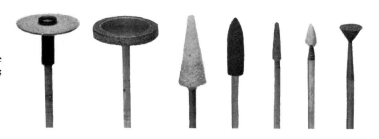

Figure 25–4. Typical dental abrasive tools. Some are used in the oral cavity; others are used in the laboratory.

- The energy required for the particle to cut into the surface may be sufficient to dislodge the particle and remove it from the system.
- The abrasive particle fractures into one or more smaller particles having sharp edges that will produce progressively finer surface scratches, changing the effect to polishing rather than grinding.
- The particle may lose its edge and become rounded as it acts. If this happens, the particle is poorly suited for either grinding or polishing of the particular substrate.

Unbound particle abrasives and polishing agents can be mixed with water, glycerine, or some other liquid medium to produce a paste or *slurry.* The slurry is applied to or rubbed over the surface with a cloth or felt wheel, a brush, or a rubber cup. Because this method of applying an abrasive is particularly well suited to the finishing and polishing of irregularly shaped objects, it is widely used in dentistry, both in the laboratory and in the mouth. Dentures, for example, usually are finished by buffing on a felt wheel with abrasive slurries. The hygienist uses a rubber cup and a slurry of mild abrasive or polishing agent when performing a prophylaxis. Toothpaste is another example of such a system.

Types of Abrasives

Of the many abrading agents used in dentistry, those in the following list are the most common.

EMERY. Emery is a natural oxide of aluminum, sometimes called *corundum.* This widely used abrasive often contains impurities and may vary in its abrasive action.

ALUMINUM OXIDE. This abrasive is a pure form of emery. Sometimes extremely fine particles of aluminum oxide, known as *levigated alumina*, are used for polishing metals.

GARNET. Composed of a number of minerals, garnet is used as an abrasive on dental polishing disks.

PUMICE. Pumice powder, or *flour of pumice*, may be used as an abrasive in dentistry or as a polishing agent during prophylaxis. It is available in various grits or particle sizes. Coarser particles are used as an abrasive in the laboratory. Fine grades are used for dental prophylaxis and as polishing agents for restorations.

ZIRCONIUM SILICATE. This substance is used as a polishing agent during prophylaxis.

DIATOMACEOUS EARTH. This abrasive, sometimes known as *kieselguhr*, is mined. It is used in dentistry not only as an abrasive or a polishing agent but also as a filler in many dental materials, as mentioned in other chapters.

TRIPOLI. Sometimes tripoli is substituted for diatomaceous earth abrasives, although it is not the same substance. It is used for mild abrasive action or polishing.

ROUGE. Rouge is a fine red powder composed of iron oxide (Fe_2O_3). Sometimes it is impregnated on paper disks. It is an excellent polishing agent for gold and noble metal alloys but is dirty to handle.

TIN OXIDE. Tin oxide, or *putty powder,*

is used extensively as a polishing agent for teeth and for metallic restorations in the mouth. Mixed with water, alcohol, or glycerine, it is used in paste form.

SAND. Sand and other forms of quartz may be used as abrasive agents. Sandpaper is a common example in which the sand is impregnated on a paper and used as an abrasive.

CARBIDES. Both *silicon carbide* and *boron carbide* often are used as abrading agents, particularly in the dental stone or bur. Either may be substituted for the diamond chips in the tool shown in Figure 25–3.

DIAMOND. The hardest and most effective abrasive for tooth enamel is composed of diamond chips, as shown in Figure 25–3. The chips are impregnated in a binder to form diamond burs or disks for dental use.

Abrasive Action

As an abrasive particle moves over a surface, it acts as a cutting edge, similar to the dental bur. To be effective, the following three conditions must exist:

- The particle must possess *edge sharpness*—be able to maintain a sharp edge. Materials that are ductile or malleable deform readily and are incapable of holding a sharp edge.
- The hardness of the abrasive must be substantially greater than that of the surface to be abraded. If this condition is not met, the abrasive particle will wear instead of the surface on which it acts.
- The abrasive must not be so brittle that it shatters immediately on striking the substance being abraded. An abrasive particle that maintains its original form during use produces the effect of grinding. One that shatters during use begins its action as an abrasive, but after sequential fracturing, it is more likely to produce polishing effects.

Another feature of abrasive action related to metals is that the metal surface usually is *strain hardened* by the abrasive action and, therefore, becomes harder. The material thus may become more resistant to abrasion during the latter stages of the finishing process. Even soft materials, such as a dental resin, are subjected to surface stresses during either abrasion or polishing.

Other factors that may affect the rate of abrasion are the size of the abrasive particle, the pressure of the abrasive against the surface, and the speed with which the abrasive particle is carried across the surface.

The larger or coarser the abrasive particle, the deeper the scratch and, therefore, the greater the amount of surface material removed. Also, the greater the force with which the abrasive is applied, the deeper the scratch and, therefore, the faster the surface is removed. In this case, caution should be observed that the force is not so great as to pull the abrasive from the binder.

Surfaces subjected to rapid abrasion or polishing heat significantly because of frictional forces between the particles and the effected surface. Heat generated during improper finishing and polishing is capable of producing a warped dental prosthesis, patient discomfort, pulpitis, mercury release from dental amalgam, and other undesirable effects. Increased pressure and cutting rpm also increase heat buildup. Heat generated during abrasion and polishing can be minimized through the use of a water spray, which cools the surface and enhances the efficiency of the abrasion tool by flushing away debris.

POLISHING

The larger the abrasive particle, the deeper the scratch, and conversely, the smaller the abrasive particle, the finer the scratch. If the particle size of the abrasive is sufficiently decreased, the scratches finally become very fine and may disappear entirely with extremely fine abrasives. The surface then acquires a smooth, shiny layer known as a *polish*. This layer is thought to be composed of extremely fine crystals, and its structure is said to be *microcrystalline*.

Although the process is not completely understood, the most recent theory is that polishing agents remove material from the surface, molecule by molecule, and thus produce very smooth surfaces. In the process, fine scratches and irregularities are filled in by the fine particulate being removed. This microcrystalline layer is referred to as the *polish,* or *Beilby, layer.*

The phenomenon of abrasion and polish is shown in Figure 25–5. The photomicrographs show the surface of a typical noble metal alloy casting at three stages in the finishing procedure. A coarse grit of emery produced the deep scratches. The coarse scratches were removed and replaced by smaller scratches when a finer grade of abrasive was used on the surface. Finally, when the surface was buffed with an aluminum oxide polishing agent, the scratches were filled in and a polish layer was formed.

The difference between an abrasive agent and a polishing agent is difficult to define. A simple definition of a polishing agent is that it produces a polish layer on the surface. In practice, the terms are used interchangeably. A given agent having a large particle size may act as an abrasive, whereas the same abrasive having a small particle size polishes the surface. Whether a substance polishes or abrades varies with the properties of the material to which it is applied and the mode and speed of application of the abrasive.

Polishing agents differ in the amount of material they remove from the surface during polishing. Some agents may produce a high surface polish but at the same time remove a considerable amount of material. An agent may have a small particle size but cut rapidly because of the sharpness and hardness of the particles. In such a case, the rate at which material is removed from a surface depends to a considerable degree on the properties of that material.

One agent may be better suited to polishing one substance than another. Levigated alumina, for example, often is used for polishing metal. It produces an excellent polish layer without removing an undue amount of metal. Although levigated alumina imparts a high polish to tooth enamel and dentin, it abrades tooth structure very rapidly in the process. Its use in dentistry should be confined to the polishing of metals.

Aside from aesthetic considerations, a number of reasons exist for desiring highly polished tooth structures and restorations. A smooth surface reduces the potential for the accumulation of food debris. Perhaps equally important, the polished layer on metals aids in preventing tarnish and corrosion. Because the entire surface is protected by a homogeneous polish layer, electrolytic and similar chemical actions are less likely. This point was discussed in Chapter 13.

A Beilby layer may be obtained on enamel surfaces as well as on metal surfaces. A highly polished tooth is more resistant to cariogenic action than a surface that is not polished. A polished tooth surface, for example, is about 15 per cent less soluble in acid than one with a rough surface. Such a consideration stresses the importance of thorough prophylaxis by the hygienist and adequate dental hygiene by the patient.

The polish layer described is inherent and part of the material polished. Such a polish should not be confused with the luster imparted by a wax or lacquer, as in polishing shoes or furniture.

POLISHING TECHNIQUE

All visible scratches should be removed from the surface before polishing is at-

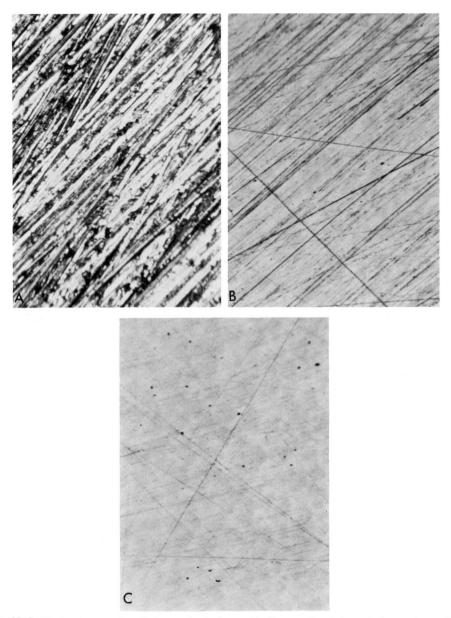

Figure 25-5. Photomicrographs of the surface of a gold alloy casting taken at three stages during polishing. *A*, Scratches produced by the use of coarse abrasive during initial stage of finishing. *B*, Coarse scratches obliterated and replaced by smaller scratches when a finer abrasive is used. *C*, Scratches are virtually eliminated by the action of a polishing agent.

tempted. The gross surface irregularities are first removed by use of a coarse abrasive. As shown in Figure 25–5, a finer-grade abrasive then is used to remove the deep scratches produced by the coarse abrasive. This is followed by the use of finer and finer abrasives until the scratches on the surface are sufficiently small that they can be obliterated by the application of a polishing agent.

In the mouth, one can begin with flour of pumice and then use the following steps.

- The pumice usually is mixed with water or glycerine to a muddy consistency. Water alone may evaporate during the procedure. The use of glycerine prevents such a change in the consistency of the *slurry*.
- A small rubber cup attached to a prophylaxis angle is fitted onto a low-speed dental handpiece motor. Rubber prophylaxis cups are supplied in various shapes, configurations, and flexibilities.
- The rubber cup is dipped into the slurry, which is then carried to the tooth and gently worked over the surface.
- A rotating brush can be manipulated in the same manner, but it is more likely to throw the abrasive off the surface during rotation, resulting in excessive splatter and heat generation.

Under no circumstances should the abrasive or polishing agent be allowed to dry out, or the surface may become scratched and thermal damage may occur.

- If it is necessary to use a finer polishing agent, the areas to be polished as well as the polishing tools should be thoroughly cleansed of all the larger abrasive particles. If one grain of the coarse abrasive remains during the final polishing, the surface will be scratched.
- Commercial polishing pastes contain various other types of polishing agents, such as zirconium silicate for enamel polishing and aluminum oxide, diamond particles, and tin oxide for polishing restorations.

Investigations have been conducted to determine whether tools used for dental polishing can be sterilized. Sound evidence exists that rubber prophylaxis cups cannot be effectively cleansed of embedded debris after a single use, making sterilization efforts impractical. Autoclavable prophylaxis angles are available and, if cleaned and lubricated before steam sterilization, provide effective service. Disposable prophylaxis angles have recently been made available to the profession. Initially, their performance was marginal. Along with improvements relevant to performance and durability, some newer disposable prophy angles offer the operator choices of cup style.

DENTIFRICES

No discussion of the action of abrasives or polishing agents in dentistry would be complete without mentioning the effect of dentifrices on tooth surfaces. Patient education by the auxiliary often involves questions concerning the selection and effect of dentifrices.

The use of a dentifrice and toothbrush by the patient is a most effective means of oral hygiene. Unquestionably, the dentifrice plays an important role in the removal of various types of accumulations from the tooth surface.

Although it is recognized that a dentifrice is not essential for the removal of oral debris and dental plaque by toothbrushing, the use of a dentifrice is essential for the removal of pellicle and stains. A much greater incidence of stained pellicle has been observed within 2 weeks on the teeth of patients who brushed with water only compared with the same people using a dentifrice. On the other hand, there is probably no more controversial subject than that of the effectiveness of dentifrices in cleaning and polishing the teeth.

The primary function of a dentifrice is to assist the patient in keeping the teeth clean and polished. Some dentifrices are more effective than others. The need to use a dentifrice varies appreciably with different people. Inherent differences in the oral flora and in personal habits, such as diet and smoking, influence the rate at which plaque and stained pellicle accumulate on the teeth. Likewise, variations in such factors as the frequency, duration, and thoroughness of toothbrushing modify the ability of any specific dentifrice to maintain tooth cleanliness.

The subject of dentifrices is discussed only from the physical science. A discussion of fluorides and bactericides in dentifrices does not lie within the scope of this text.

Composition

Dentifrices exist today in two forms—pastes and powders. The paste may be opaque or in the form of a translucent gel. Liquid dentifrices have been available, but their inability to prevent the accumulation of stained pellicle resulted in their commercial failure. In terms of usage and commercial sales, more than 98 per cent of the dentifrices used today are pastes. The various components of both types of dentifrices are shown in Table 25–1.

From a functional standpoint, the most important ingredient of a dentifrice is the *abrasive* or *polishing agent*. This material is primarily responsible for the cleaning properties of a dentifrice and is especially necessary for the removal of stained pellicle.

Dentifrice abrasives are insoluble powders that are prepared under carefully controlled conditions to maintain uniform particle size and configuration. Commonly used dentifrice abrasives are calcium pyrophosphate, insoluble sodium metaphosphate, hydrated silica, calcium carbonate, aluminum hydroxide, magnesium oxide, and dibasic calcium phosphate dihydrate. In many instances, a dentifrice is prepared from a blend of two or more types of abrasives, each selected for a specific purpose.

Typical paste-type dentifrices contain 20 to 30 per cent water. This gives the formulation the desired consistency and may serve as a solvent for some of the minor constituents, such as the coloring agent or the fluoride additive.

A *humectant* is included to retard a paste-type dentifrice from drying out if the cap is not replaced on the tube after use and to improve the appearance and consistency of the product. The most commonly used humectants are glycerine, sorbitol, and propylene glycol.

Detergents in dentifrices facilitate the polishing agent and toothbrush in removing various deposits—just as a detergent aids in removing soil from any surface—and enhance the consumer acceptance of the formulation. Examples of commonly used detergents are sodium lauryl sulfate and sodium *N*-lauroyl sarcosinate.

Binders, such as carboxymethylcellulose, are included in paste-type formulations to prevent separation of the liquid and solid components of the dentifrice.

Coloring and *flavoring agents*, added to promote consumer acceptance, are a major consideration for the manufacturer. In addition, the flavor imparts a feeling of freshness and oral cleanliness. Coloring agents typi-

TABLE 25–1. Typical Composition of Dentifrices*

Type of Constituent	Paste-Type Dentifrices (%)	Powder-Type Dentifrices (%)
Abrasive	20–55	90–98
Water	20–25	0
Humectants	20–35	0
Detergents	1–2	1–6
Binders	1–3	0
Color and flavor	1–2	<3
Therapeutic agents	0–1	0–1

*Courtesy of G. Stookey.

cally are certified food dyes, and most of the flavoring agents are mixtures of essential oils and synthetic extracts.

Although an evaluation of the possible therapeutic properties of dentifrices is beyond the scope of this discussion, many formulations contain compounds that may impart additional beneficial characteristics to the dentifrice. In particular, most dentifrices contain *fluoride*—in the form of sodium fluoride, stannous fluoride, or sodium monofluorophosphate—to contribute to the control of dental caries. Some formulations contain *strontium chloride* and other agents that may reduce the sensitivity of exposed dentin or cementum.

The most recent therapeutic agents added to dentifrices are *crystal growth inhibitors*, which retard the mineralization of dental plaque and, therefore, reduce supragingival calculus accretions. This category of additives deserves mention because these agents are primarily soluble pyrophosphates that do not immediately go into solution in human saliva. They have a slight abrasive effect that lasts through the first 100 to 300 brushing strokes. The effect of these products in retarding calculus buildup is, therefore, partly mechanical in nature.

The primary action of soluble pyrophosphates, however, is chemical. In addition to pyrophosphates, other chemotherapeutic agents that inhibit calculus formation are added to dentifrices and prebrush mouth rinses. Their mode of action is of a physiochemical or antimicrobial nature not related to the mechanics of polishing.

From the foregoing overview, the exact composition of dentifrices is quite variable. Only those dentifrices that are developed, tested, and marketed for their therapeutic properties have a constant composition. The other, nontherapeutic dentifrices are in a constant state of formulation modification in an attempt to appeal to other factors that influence product selection by the public.

Abrasion and Polishing of Tooth Structure

The relative abrasive action of several common abrasive and polishing agents on tooth enamel is shown in Table 25–2. Specially designed equipment with water slurries of specific concentrations of abrasives was used to measure abrasiveness in terms of the thickness of enamel removed from teeth during brushing. Interestingly, flour of pumice, which sometimes is used during prophylactic treatment, is highly abrasive and causes as much loss of enamel as does levigated alumina. Daily use of such highly abrasive agents is contraindicated, and abrasives such as pumice are unsuitable for a dentifrice.

Dentin, cementum, and certain restorative materials abrade more quickly than dental enamel, making some polishing techniques inappropriate for less resistant surfaces.

Airborne-particle abrasion (with or without irrigation) has been advocated as an effective means of removing extrinsic stain from dental enamel. Most airborne-particle abrasion systems use sodium bicarbonate and/or calcium carbonate particles mixed

TABLE 25–2. Relative Abrasiveness of Various Compounds on Tooth Enamel*

Abrasive	Abrasion Loss (mm)
Calcium carbonate (extra dense)	0.012
Light chalk (USP)	0.103
Flour of pumice	0.300
Tip alumina	0.300
Dibasic calcium phosphate, dihydrate	0.001
Dibasic calcium phosphate, anhydrous	0.021
Tribasic calcium phosphate	0.001
Calcium pyrophosphate	0.005
Insoluble sodium metaphosphate and dibasic calcium phosphate (equal parts)	0.001

*From Gershon, S., Pokras, H. A., and Rider, T. H.: Dentifrices. Cosmet. Science Technol. 15:296, 1957.

with a compressed air stream surrounded by water spray. They are safe and effective on enamel and metallic surfaces, but their effect on dentin, cementum, restorative composites, and dental resins is that of rapid abrasion and surface destruction.

When used improperly during dental prophylaxis, rubber cups are capable of producing edge gouges on exposed dentin surfaces. Under normal conditions, an experienced dental operator removes an average thickness of 0.24 μm of enamel during the polishing associated with dental prophylaxis. Tooth enamel shows microfine scratches on well-polished surfaces for up to 30 days. Edge gouges produced by improper use of the rubber cup can be sufficiently deep to persist indefinitely.

CERVICAL ABRASION

Although research findings are inconclusive as to the principal offender, facial cervical abrasion of exposed dentin and cementum is partially attributable to frequency and technique of brushing, stiffness of bristles, and dentifrice abrasivity.

A ranking of in vitro abrasivity values for several commercial dentifrices is shown in Table 25–3. The numerical value for the

TABLE 25–3. In Vitro Abrasivity of Various Dentifrices

Dentifrice	Abrasivity
Colgate	44.7
Viadent	52.0
Dentagard	57.5
Zendium	57.9
Pepsodent	61.8
Peak	71.0
Ultra-Brite	81.0
Gleem	86.0
Sensodyne	87.0
Crest	90.0
Aim	93.0
Colgate tartar	94.0
Crest tartar	131.0

*From Cornell, J.: In vitro abrasiveness of dentifrices. *J. Clin. Dent.* 1(Sup A):A9, 1988.

abrasivity is calculated as a percentage of the abrasivity of a standard reference material, Monsanto calcium pyrophosphate.

The ADA considers 250 as the maximum level permitted for a dentifrice. The abrasivity of a dentifrice is a good indicator of the cleansing ability, but abrasivity and polishing effects are not clearly related.

MICROABRASION (ABROSION)

Enamel microabrasion is a relatively new concept that has emerged as a cosmetic procedure useful in the elimination of superficial enamel discolorations and textural aberrations. This process uses 18 per cent hydrochloric acid added to a slurry of abrasive particles (primarily pumice). When this is rubbed slowly onto dental enamel, both abrasion and chemical erosion occur. Because this removal of surface enamel involves two processes, the term *abrosion* has been deemed applicable. This process goes far beyond the normal limits of dental polishing and must involve enamel only. The remaining dental and oral structures are protected by a rubber dam.

Abrosion-treated enamel should be polished immediately with a fluoride-containing prophylaxis paste followed by a 4-minute application of neutral topical fluoride before patient dismissal.

TOOTHBRUSHES

The filaments in toothbrushes are composed almost exclusively of nylon bristles whose tips lie in a flat plane and may be multitufted or end-rounded. The brushes are graded with terms such as hard, medium, and soft. The term hardness is a misnomer in that the reference is to the stiffness of the bristles rather than the material's hardness.

The stiffness of nylon toothbrushes is controlled by the use of different sizes of bristle filaments. The larger the diameter of the filaments, the stiffer the brush. A soft nylon brush, for example, might be composed of

0.20-mm (0.008-in) nylon filaments, whereas the diameter of the filaments of a hard brush would be 0.35 mm (0.014 in). No standardized grading system exists for brushes. A brush graded as hard by one manufacturer might be comparable to another manufacturer's medium or medium-hard brush.

Gingival recession can be a result of incorrect brushing technique as well as incorrect brush selection. Even when used properly, stiff bristles are more likely to cause soft tissue injury than more flexible bristles. Bristle flexibility and toothpaste abrasivity are not major factors in the production of cervical abrasion lesions. Research now supports the frequency and manner of brushing as more likely causes with speculation that excessive occlusal forces and the resulting tooth flexure may contribute significantly to this type of dental lesion.

Selected Reading

Bergstrom J., and Lavstedt, S.: An epidemiologic approach to toothbrushing and dentin abrasion. Community Dent. Oral Epidemiol. 7:57, 1979.

Christensen, R. P., and Bangerter, V. W.: Immediate and long term effects of polishing on enamel and dentin. J. Prosthet. Dent. 57(2):150–160, 1987.

Council on Dental Therapeutics: *Accepted Dental Therapeutics*. 39th ed. Chicago, American Dental Association, 1982, pp. 369–373.

Galloway, S. E., and Pashley, D. H.: Rate of removal of root structure by the use of the prophy-jet device. J. Periodontol. 58(7):464–469, 1987.

Leknes, K. N., and Lie, T.: Influence of polishing procedures on sonic scaling root surface roughness. J. Periodontol. 62(11):659–662, 1991.

Reviewing the Chapter

1. What are the two types of dental burs, in terms of composition?
2. Describe the cutting mechanics of a bur.
3. List the factors that affect the rate of cutting.
4. How does abrasion differ from cutting?
5. Explain the construction of a dental abrasive tool used in a handpiece.
6. How does the cutting of a diamond abrasive stone differ from that of a bur? Are various sizes and shapes of such tools available?
7. How are abrasive or polishing agents used? What is a *slurry*?
8. List the various types of abrasive agents used in dentistry and give the common usage of each.
9. Explain the behavior of an abrasive particle as it is applied to a tooth surface and/or a metal surface.
10. What factors affect the rate of abrasion by such agents?
11. Describe what is meant by a *polish*. Define *Beilby layer*.
12. Discuss the difference between the action and end result of an abrasive agent and a polishing agent.
13. Do polishing agents differ in the amount of material removed from a surface? Explain.
14. Defend the importance of having polished surfaces on all dental structures.
15. Describe the polishing technique as applied to dentistry.
16. What is the primary function of a *dentifrice*?
17. Give the composition of typical paste and powder forms of a dentifrice. Which is most popular?
18. What is the purpose of each component?
19. Discuss the relative abrasive action of common abrasive and polishing agents on tooth enamel. Are any contraindicated for use in a dentifrice?
20. Explain how two dentifrices that contain the same abrasive agents may produce different results in terms of abrasion rate.
21. What would you tell a patient in terms of selection of a commercial dentifrice?
22. Discuss what is meant by a hard or a soft toothbrush.
23. Does the toothbrush have a marked effect on abrasion of tooth structure with a given dentifrice?
24. What is the most common cause for gingival lesions of exposed dentin and cementum?

APPENDIX

Appendix of Conversion Factors

To Convert From	To	Multiply By
Force		
kilograms	pounds	2.2046
kilograms	newtons	9.807
pounds	kilograms	0.4536
pounds	newtons	4.448
newtons	kilograms	0.1020
newtons	pounds	0.2248
Force Per Unit Area		
psi	$MPa(MN/m^2)$	0.006895
psi	kg/cm^2	0.0703
kg/cm^2	$MPa(MN/m^2)$	0.09807
kg/cm^2	psi	14.2233
MN/m^2	psi	145.0
MN/m^2	kg/cm^2	10.1968
Length		
inches	millimeters	25.4
millimeters	inches	0.03937
inches	micrometers (microns)	25,400.00
miocrometers (microns)	inches	0.00003937
Temperature		
Fahrenheit (°F)	Celsius (°C)	5/9 (temp. °F − 32°)
Celsius (°C)	Fahrenheit (°F)	(9/5 temp. °C) + 32°

SI Units
N = newton
MN = meganewton
Pa = pascal
MPa = megapascal

Appendix of the Chemical Elements and Their Symbols

Name	Symbol	Name	Symbol	Name	Symbol	Name	Symbol
Actinum	Ac	Einsteinium	Es	Mendelevium	Md	Ruthenium	Ru
Aluminum	Al	Erbium	Er	Mercury	Hg	Samarium	Sm
Americium	Am	Europium	Eu	Molybdenum	Mo	Scandium	Sc
Antimony	Sb	Fermium	Fm	Neodymium	Nd	Selenium	Se
Argon	Ar	Fluorine	F	Neon	Ne	Silicon	Si
Arsenic	As	Francium	Fr	Neptunium	Np	Silver	Ag
Astatine	At	Gadolinium	Gd	Nickel	Ni	Sodium	Na
Barium	Ba	Gallium	Ga	Niobium	Nb	Strontium	Sr
Berkelium	Bk	Germanium	Ge	Nitrogen	N	Sulfur	S
Beryllium	Be	Gold	Au	Osmium	Os	Tantalum	Ta
Bismuth	Bi	Hafnium	Hf	Oxygen	O	Technetium	Tc
Boron	B	Helium	He	Palladium	Pd	Tellurium	Te
Bromine	Br	Holmium	Ho	Phosphorus	P	Terbium	Tb
Cadmium	Cd	Hydrogen	H	Platinum	Pt	Thallium	Tl
Calcium	Ca	Indium	In	Plutonium	Pu	Thorium	Th
Californium	Cf	Iodine	I	Polonium	Po	Thulium	Tm
Carbon	C	Iridium	Ir	Potassium	K	Tin	Sn
Cerium	Ce	Iron	Fe	Praseodymium	Pr	Titanium	Ti
Cesium	Cs	Krypton	Kr	Promethium	Pm	Tungsten	W
Chlorine	Cl	Lanthanum	La	Protactinium	Pa	Uranium	U
Chromium	Cr	Lead	Pb	Radium	Ra	Vanadium	V
Cobalt	Co	Lithium	Li	Radon	Rn	Xenon	Xe
Copper	Cu	Lutetium	Lu	Rhenium	Re	Ytterbium	Yb
Curium	Cm	Magnesium	Mg	Rhodium	Rh	Yttrium	Y
Dysprosium	Dy	Manganese	Mn	Rubidium	Rb	Zinc	Zn
						Zirconium	Zr

INDEX

Note: Page numbers in *italics* refer to illustrations; page numbers followed by t refer to tables.